NEUROSCIENCE RESEARCH PROGRESS

GLIOMAS

CLASSIFICATION, SYMPTOMS, TREATMENT AND PROGNOSIS

NEUROSCIENCE RESEARCH PROGRESS

Additional books in this series can be found on Nova's website under the Series tab.

Additional e-books in this series can be found on Nova's website under the e-book tab.

NEUROSCIENCE RESEARCH PROGRESS

GLIOMAS

CLASSIFICATION, SYMPTOMS, TREATMENT AND PROGNOSIS

DAVID CORY ADAMSON
EDITOR

New York

Library of Congress Cataloging-in-Publication Data

ISBN: 978-1-63117-868-9

Library of Congress Control Number: 2014938428

Published by Nova Science Publishers, Inc. † New York

Contents

Preface

Gliomas represent some of the most difficult tumors to understand and most challenging to treat. As illustrated in this book, the difficulty in understanding them is apparent in various ways. They have significant diversity in histology, genomic alternations, protein expression, clinical presentation, radiographic appearance, treatment approaches, and ideas of how to cure them. Historically, we have thought of gliomas as representing a group of distinct tumors (e.g., astrocytoma and oligodendroglioma) arising from unique cells of origin and genetic mutations. Our current understanding of the genetic mutations and signaling pathways that drive these tumors has now blurred these distinctions, greatly expanding our knowledge and at the same time, our uncertainty about how to combat these tumors. Added to this complexity is the fact that we are typically talking about tumors that *infiltrate* through an organ that many of us consider the "seat of our souls," where we must exercise the utmost caution in how we deliver treatments with great risks.

In chapter 1, Pineda et al. introduces us to this exciting and complex topic with a broad overview of grading criteria, histological features, common genomic alterations and affected signaling pathways, and current treatments. Most exciting is an extensive discussion on new therapeutic concepts and delivering mechanisms that arise from the complex field of nanotechnology where nanoparticles, nanotubes, and nanocrystals may someday become the Trojan horse.

We often lump together all gliomas in our discussions, but some unique situations warrant a separate discussion. Zhiping Zhou provides a review of the unique set of brainstem gliomas in chapter 2. Zhou discusses the very important and often striking differences in clinical presentation, tumor behavior, molecular characterization, imaging, treatment, and outcome between diffuse intrinsic pontine gliomas and the more focal often exophytic ones. Zhou emphasizes the future role of special drug delivery techniques (e.g., convection enhanced deliver) to this area of the delicate nervous system. In chapter 3, Hwang et al. gives us a tremendous review of gliomas in our pediatric population, where tumors and patients can behave very differently from their adult counterparts.

Before diving into the biology of these tumors driving future therapeutic designs, we briefly discuss surgical and radiotherapeutic aspects of the glioma field. Surgery has always been the cornerstone of therapy, providing the greatest impact on outcome when feasible. Kistka et al. (chapter 4) provide a wonderful review of the current standard of care for surgical management of glioma patients. Even though surgical resection has not dramatically changed the outcome of glioma patients over recent years, the envelope is certainly being pushed as much as possible by utilizing the most sophisticated preoperative imaging and intraoperative tools. This paper focuses on a growing trend to minimize approaches to reduce morbidity, by the use of customized craniotomies, endoscopy, and potential robotics in the near future.

In chapter 5, Gensheimer et al. provides a review of radiation therapy for malignant gliomas, an integral part to the current trimodal standard of care. They described current common imaging characteristics, e.g., MRI and CT, with an excellent description of the limitations that anatomical imaging has with describing the clear biological heterogeneity. They also review more sophisticated functional imaging techniques such as PET, SPECT, and DCE MRI. In this diffuse disease process, they make a strong argument for more efforts at improving locoregional control of tumor progression. More radical radiotherapy forms are discussed, i.e., proton beam vs photon beam vs carbon ion. Past diagnosis and monitoring has depended largely on anatomic imaging modalities, but the future will likely move toward more functional, metabolic, and protein-specific forms of imaging to diagnose, deliver treatments, and monitor response to treatments. In chapter 6, Treglia et al. explains the field of PET tracers being studied in glioma imaging.

Many glioma clinicians would argue that the past decade has witnessed our greatest exploration into the molecular biology that drives gliomagenesis. The sequencing of the human genome at the turn of the century followed now by the development of numerous glioma sequence databases has provided an incomparable amount of information. The latter half of this book is devoted more to this topic. Milinkovic and Tanic explore the role of genomic instability and alterations (chapter 7), Trejo-Solis et al. focuses on molecular pathways driving gliomagenesis (chapter 8), and Patil et al. demonstrate how therapies targeting specific molecules can be analyzed (chapter 9). Milinkovic and Tanic provide a comprehensive review of the genomic alterations common to the malignant glioma glioblastoma, specifically highlighting the differences between primary and secondary glioblastoma and the more recent genomic classification of glioblastoma into Classical, Messenchymal, Proneural, and Neural groups. Hundreds of clinical trials have taught us that simply targeting over-expressed molecules is not enough – we have to develop a smarter strategy. Some experimental strategies target the molecule that affects the most signaling pathways, others combine targeting therapies, while still others focus more targeting a tumor function, e.g., migration or cell death. As an example, Wang et al. in chapter 10 illustrate how one pathway may have key effects in one area of glioma biology, i.e., altered cell death kinetics.

Gliomas pose a unique difficulty in therapy delivery due to their location in brain parenchyma behind a complex blood-brain barrier. Once effective chemotherapies are developed, getting them to the target is another often unsurmountable task. In chapter 11, An et al. review the exciting field of nanoscaled delivery mechanisms being explored for shuttling various genes, proteins, and other tumoricidal agents across the brain's endothelium, through the layers of parenchymal, and to the targeted glioma. This fascinating field requires sophisticated engineering methods and complex knowledge of biological systems on subcellular levels.

The last decade has certainly witnessed significant gains in areas that will contribute to making progress in glioma treatment. In malignant gliomas, we finally have established a trimodal "standard of care" on which all glioma clinicians agree, all glioma patients hopefully receive, and with which we can compare future experimental trials. We have an encyclopedic foundational knowledge of the molecular biology behind these tumors, and now need to figure out where to exploit it. Imaging and drug delivery methods are achieving impressive sophistication. The challenge of the next decade will be to bring focus to our strategies and to channel them through increasingly complex, costly, and lengthy clinical trial designs.

Dr. David Cory Adamson
Associate Professor of Surgery (Neurosurgery)
Duke University Medical Center
Department of Surgery
Division of Neurosurgery
cory.adamson@duke.edu

In: Gliomas: Classification, Symptoms, Treatment and Prognosis ISBN: 978-1-63117-868-9
Editor: David Cory Adamson

Chapter 1

Classification, Histology, Genomic Alterations and New Therapeutic Concepts

Benjamín Pineda[1,•], Norma Y. Hernández-Pedro[1], Roxana Magaña Maldonado[1], Gustavo Vargas Félix[1], Alelí Salazar-Ramiro[1,3], Verónica Pérez de la Cruz[2] and Julio Sotelo[1]

[1] Neuroimmunology and Neuro-Oncology Unit,
Instituto Nacional de Neurología y Neurocirugía,
Mexico City, Mexico
[2] Neurochemistry Unit, Instituto Nacional de Neurología y Neurocirugía, Mexico City, Mexico
[3] Universidad del Valle de México, Mexico

Abstract

Gliomas are primary brain tumors of the central nervous system and they are characterized by great cellular heterogeneity. According to the World Health Organization (WHO) classification of primary brain tumors, gliomas are distinguished by morphological criteria that include morphological similarities of the tumor cells with non-neoplastic glial cells, Thusly, they are classified as astrocytic, oligodendroglial, mixed oligo–astrocytic, or ependymal tumors, and they are graded on a scale of I–IV [astrocytic (grade I–IV); oligodendrogliomas (grade II–III); mixed tumors (grade I–III)] with increasing malignancy.

Recently, the discovery of several genetic alterations and aberrant signaling pathways has made a considerable contribution to our understanding of the genesis and biology of gliomas. To date, four biomarkers have consistently been associated with diagnosis and prognosis in gliomas: the co-deletion of chromosomes 1p/19q, O^6-methylguanine DNA methyltransferase (MGMT) promoter methylation, mutations in

• Phone/Fax: (+52) (55) 56064040. E-mail: benpio76@hotmail.com.

isocitrate dehydrogenase (IDH) IDH1/2 genes and amplification of epidermal growth factor receptor (EGFR). Molecular understanding of gliomas is crucial to improve classification, better predict outcome, select patients in clinical trials, and finally provide specific therapy to individual tumor types.

On the other hand, treatment of gliomas requires a careful selection of one or more interventions, such as surgery, radiotherapy, and chemotherapy. The prognosis for patients with high-grade gliomas is poor, and it has improved little in recent years. The response to chemotherapy is modest and presents with high toxicities. Radiation therapy is moderately effective and it presents limitations due to collateral radiation damage to healthy brain tissue. Other characteristics that limit the therapy of gliomas is the poor drug delivery and inherent chemo- and radio-resistance. Some investigations are focusing on eliminating residual cells with stem-like characteristics that confer resistance and tumor propagation. Other aspects associated with proliferation and the spread of tumors is their microenvironment.

To overcome these limitations in conventional therapy, research in nano- and immune-therapy areas are developing. Nanoparticles are emerging as innovative tools in research and therapies in gliomas due to their capacity of self-assembly, small size, increased stability, biocompatibility, tumor-specific targeting using antibodies or ligands, encapsulation and delivery of antineoplastic drugs, and increasing the contact surface between cells and nanomaterials. The active targeting of nanoparticles through conjugation with cell surface markers could enhance the efficacy of nanoparticles for delivering several agents into the tumoral area while significantly reducing toxicity in living systems.

Recent clinical studies have developed immunotherapies based on the expression of tumoral antigens. This treatment uses peptide vaccines to trigger the immune response against the tumor. Additionally, antibody-toxin complexes known as immunotoxins have been designed. These recombinant proteins consist of a specific antibody or ligand coupled to a toxin protein. The toxins used are byproducts of plants, bacteria and fungi that inactivate eukaryotic protein synthesis.

Developing new therapeutic agents as adjuvants either alone or in combination with chemotherapy to destroy the tumor cells is the major challenge to improve therapy in the near future.

Gliomas Histology and Grading

Histological grading is a mean of predicting the biological behavior of a neoplasm. In the clinical setting, tumor grade is a key factor influencing the choice of therapies, determining the use of adjuvant radiation and specific chemotherapy protocols. According to the World Health Organization (WHO) classification of primary brain tumors, gliomas are distinguished by their morphological criteria that include morphological similarities of the tumor cells with non-neoplastic glial cells. Thusly, they are classified as astrocytic, oligodendroglial, mixed oligo–astrocytic, or ependymal tumors (Louis, Ohgaki et al. 2007).

Grade I is reserved for pilocytic astrocytomas, lesions with low proliferative potential and the possibility of cure following surgical resection alone due to their focality. Diffuse astrocytomas or low-grade astrocytomas (grade II) are poorly defined tumors that infiltrate the parenchyma and obliterate normal gray matter–white matter boundaries. They are generally infiltrative in nature and, despite low-level proliferative activity, often recur. Microscopically there are increased numbers of irregularly distributed astrocytes with mildly atypical nuclei. Diffuse astrocytomas often are classified into one of three subtypes: fibrillary, the most common subtype, protoplasmic, or gemistocytic. Fibrillary astrocytomas are composed of tightly interlacing bundles of small, spindle-shaped cells amid a predominantly fibrillar matrix. Gemistocytic astrocytomas contain plump cells with distinct, round pink cytoplasm arranged on a more delicately interlacing fibrillar matrix, whereas protoplasmic astrocytomas are composed of small, round, regular cells with indistinct cytoplasmic boundaries arranged on a loosely fibrillar stroma.

Some grade II tumors progress to higher grades of malignancy, for example, low-grade diffuse astrocytomas can transform into anaplastic astrocytoma (grade III) and subsequently into glioblastoma (grade IV). Similar transformation occurs in oligodendroglioma and oligoastrocytomas (grade II gliomas) (Louis, Ohgaki et al. 2007).

Microscopically, anaplastic astrocytomas (grade III) are distinguished from grade II tumors by their greater cellularity, increased nuclear pleomorphism, and mitotic activity. In both these and grade IV glioblastomas, tumor cells can be seen infiltrating into surrounding normal brain tissue, often at a great distance from the primary tumor mass. The designation WHO grade IV is assigned to cytologically malignant, mitotically active, necrosis-prone neoplasms typically associated with rapid pre- and postoperative disease evolution and a rapid fatal outcome.

Examples of grade IV gliomas include glioblastoma, and the very rare embryonal and sarcomatous neoplasms. Widespread infiltration of surrounding tissue and a propensity for craniospinal dissemination characterize some grade IV gliomas (DeAngelis 2001; Riemenschneider and Reifenberger 2009).

Glioblastoma (GBM) is the most common malignant primary brain tumor in adults. Approximately 80% of all GBMs develop without any prior history of a glioma and are termed primary GBMs.

The clinical history usually is short, on the order of months, and the patients tend to be older, with a median age of 55 when diagnosed. These tumors tend to be large with lots of edema, central necrosis, and ring enhancement. In 20% of the cases, the patient has an antecedent history of a lower-grade glioma (grade II or III), generally 5 to 10 years previously. These secondary GBMs tend to arise in younger patients, with a median age of 40 years (DeAngelis 2001).

Glioma Genomics

In gliomas, several identified molecular markers are unique to specific histological types or to different grades of malignancy. For example, several specific genes, including TP53, PTEN, CDKN2A, and EGFR, are consistently altered in gliomas (Nigro, Baker et al. 1989; Ueki, Ono et al. 1996; Li, Yen et al. 1997). These alterations tend to occur in a defined order during the progression to a high-grade tumor. The TP53 mutation appears to be a relatively early event during the development of an astrocytoma, whereas the loss or mutation of PTEN and amplification of EGFR are characteristic of higher-grade tumors (Wong, Ruppert et al. 1992; Weber, Sabel et al. 1996; Ohgaki and Kleihues 2007). In oligodendrogliomas, allelic losses of 1p and 19q occur in many WHO grade II tumors, whereas losses of 9p21 are largely confined to WHO grade III tumors (Bigner, Matthews et al. 1999). Some of these markers have diagnostic value, whereas others are useful prognostic factors for patient survival or response to treatment.

Loss of Heterozygosity in 1p and 19q

Although the biological effects of 1p/19q co-deletion remain unclear, this genetic alteration has become an important molecular marker in malignant gliomas. This alteration has recently been found to result from the combined deletion of entire 1p and 19q after unbalanced translocation between chromosomes 1 and 19 [t(1:19)(q10;p10)] (Griffin, Burger et al. 2006; Jenkins, Blair et al. 2006). Loss of heterozygosity (LOH) in 19q13.3 is one of the most common genetic alterations in anaplastic astrocytoma and secondary glioblastoma, but is rare in primary GBM (Nakamura, Yang et al. 2000). Grade II oligodendrogliomas exhibit LOH in 1p and 19q in up to 88% of cases while grade III oligodendrogliomas have the alteration in up to 50 to 70% of cases. LOH of 1p and 19q is common in both grade II and III oligodendrogliomas, and some of these changes probably occur early during tumorigenesis (Rasheed, Wiltshire et al. 1999). In an allelotyping study of oligodendroglial tumors, a high frequency of LOH was found on chromosomes 1, 4, 6, 11, and 19. Also, anaplastic oligodendrogliomas exhibited chromosome 17 LOH. (Zhu, Santarius et al. 1998)

In astrocytic tumors partial 1p and/or 19q deletion is more common. These tumors exhibit 1p/19q loss but only at a 40% frequency, and chromosome 19 abnormalities range from loss of the whole chromosome to a narrow interstitial deletion of 19q13 region. A mutually exclusive pattern of 1p/19q LOH and p53 gene mutations was observed in oligoastrocytomas, suggesting that those with p53 mutations are of astrocytic origin and that tumors with 1p/19q LOH are related to oligodendrogliomas (Maintz, Fiedler et al. 1997; Mizoguchi, Yoshimoto et al. 2012).

Advances in these molecular genetic alterations have contributed considerably to a better understanding, diagnostic classification, and prognostic evaluation. In oligodendrogliomas, the 1p and 19q deletions predict a higher likelihood of response to treatment and define patient subgroups with favorable prognosis. Furthermore, the combined LOH at 1p and 19q has a strong predictive value for chemosensitivity in oligodendrogliomas while the combination of LOH1p and LOH19q define GBM patients with a significantly better survival. Notably, these patients do not exhibit morphological features reminiscent of oligodendroglioma (Ferrer-Luna, Mata et al. 2009).

IDH1

Isocitrate Dehydrogenase 1 (IDH1) gene mutations are found frequently in malignant gliomas and are likely to be involved in the early stage of gliomagenesis, even before TP53 mutations or loss of 1p and 19q (Watanabe, Nobusawa et al. 2009). IDH1 mutations occur in the highly conserved residue R132, which is in the catalytic domain, where it binds to its substrate. Mutations in IDH2 consistently occur at the analogous amino acid R172, which is functionally equivalent to amino acid 132 of IDH1. These mutations have been found in approximately 80% of grades II-III gliomas and secondary GBMs but have been found in less than 10% of primary GBMs (Balss, Meyer et al. 2008; Yan, Parsons et al. 2009). The IDH2 mutations have also been described in gliomas, although at a lower frequency (Hartmann, Meyer et al. 2009; Yan, Parsons et al. 2009). The IDH1 and IDH2 enzymes catalyse oxidative decarboxylation of isocitrate into α-ketoglutarate (aKG), thereby reducing NADP to NADPH (Bolduc, Dyer et al. 1995; Kim, Lee et al. 2007). A heterozygous point mutation in codon 132 impairs the interaction of the enzyme with isocitrate both sterically and electrostatically, and the mutant IDH1 molecules dominantly inhibit the activity of wild-type IDH1 by forming a catalytically inactive heterodimer (Zhao, Lin et al. 2009). The mutations cause reduced formation of aKG and decreased cytoplasmic levels of aKG increase levels of hypoxia-inducible factor subunit HIF-1alpha (Weller, Felsberg et al. 2009; Zhao, Lin et al. 2009), a component of the hypoxia-responsive transcription factor complex that facilitates tumor angiogenesis and growth. Heterozygous IDH mutations confer neomorphic enzyme activity rather than inactivating the enzyme; the mutant enzyme converts aKG to 2-hydroxyglutarate (2-HG). 2HG inhibits 2-oxoglutarate (2OG)-dependent oxygenases that could be associated with tumor progression and lead to an elevated risk of malignant gliomas (Dang, White et al. 2009; Xu, Yang et al. 2011).

Frequent IDH mutations have been shown to be a prognostic marker. Gliomas with IDH mutations are clinically and genetically distinct from gliomas with wild-type IDH genes. Notably, two subtypes of gliomas of WHO grade II or III (astrocytomas and oligodendrogliomas) often carry IDH mutations but no other genetic alterations that are detectable relatively early during the progression of gliomas (Yan, Parsons et al. 2009). A large-scale study revealed IDH1 mutations in 50% to 80% of patients with grade II astrocytoma, oligodendroglioma, or secondary GBM; however, IDH1 mutations were rare in patients with primary GBM (Balss, Meyer et al. 2008; Ichimura, Pearson et al. 2009) Also, the associated with longer overall survival with these mutations are almost exclusively restricted to secondary GBM.

EGFR

The EGFR/PTEN/Akt/mTOR pathway is a key signaling pathway in the development of primary GBM (Kita, Yonekawa et al. 2007). Amplification of the EGFR gene is more frequently in primary GBM (Ekstrand, Sugawa et al. 1992) but it is rarely in secondary GBM (Watanabe, Tachibana et al. 1996). All primary GBM with EGFR amplification show EGFR overexpression and 70 to 90% of those with EGFR overexpression have EGFR amplification (Tohma, Gratas et al. 1998; Biernat, Huang et al. 2004). Approximately half of GBM with EGFR amplification express a mutant form of the receptor (Ekstrand, Longo et al. 1994). The most common mutant is known as EGFRvIII, which is missing exons 2 to 7, resulting in an in-frame deletion of 801 base pairs of the coding sequence of the extracellular domain (Ekstrand, Longo et al. 1994; Nishikawa, Ji et al. 1994). It is associated with constitutive activation of the receptor and failure to attenuate signaling by receptor down-regulation, causes mitogenic effects, and has more powerful transforming activity (Huang, Nagane et al. 1997). The constitutively active EGFRvIII can enhance cell proliferation in part by down-regulation of p27 through activation of the phosphatidylinositol 3-kinase (PI3K)/Akt pathway

(Narita, Nagane et al. 2002). This variant occurs only in GBM with concurrent wild-type EGFR amplification.

The EGFR- and EGFRvIII-mediated pathways are critical for cancer biology and potentially associated with increased proliferation, invasion/metastasis, radio-resistance, and poor survival in patients with GBM (Lo 2010). Stimulation of EGFR also causes an increase of neoplastic angiogenesis and promotes mechanisms of cell migration and invasion of tumors into surrounding nervous tissue. Additionally, frequent mutations of the gene (including EGFRvIII), especially in combination with amplification, lead to hyperactivity of the receptor independently of ligands, and are important factors in malignant biology of gliomas (Bianco, Troiani et al. 2005). EGFRvIII has also been shown to confer resistance to both radiotherapy and chemotherapy (Wikstrand, Hale et al. 1995).

PDGF

Platelet-derived growth factor (PDGF), a major mitogen for connective tissue cells and glia, plays a number of critical roles in normal embryonic development, cellular differentiation, and response to tissue damage, as well as in pathologic processes, such as wound healing, inflammation, and neoplasms (Heldin and Westermark 1990; Reigstad, Varhaug et al. 2005; Goritz, Dias et al. 2011). The PDGF family consists of five members, PDGF-AA,-AB, -BB, -CC, and -DD, which bind to two different tyrosine kinase receptors, PDGF receptor a (PDGFRa) and PDGF receptor b (PDGFRb) (Smith 1976; Heldin and Westermark 1990). There are four PDGF ligands (PDGF-A, PDGF-B, PDGF-C, and PDGF-D) that dimerize and bind to PDGF receptors (PDGFRα and PDGFRβ) (Fredriksson, Li et al. 2004). PDGF-A, PDGF-B, and PDGF-C bind to PDGFRα, while PDGF-B and PDGF-D bind to PDGFRβ. Ligand binding induces autophosphorylation of the PDGFR and propagation of intracellular signals, resulting in changes in cellular behaviors, including proliferation, survival, and migration. Expression of PDGFs and PDGFRs is found even in low-grade gliomas, high-grade gliomas also frequently display high-level expression of PDGF ligands and receptors. Most studies have found that the PDFG-α receptor is overexpressed in 60% to 90% of low- and high grade astrocytomas. By contrast, overexpression of the ligand PDGFA or -B is not very common in low-grade gliomas but is seen in high-grade gliomas, suggesting that this growth factor participates in an autocrine loop in these tumors(Plate, Breier et al. 1992; Hermanson, Funa et al. 1996).

A study tested PDGFRA gain in 166 low-grade diffuse astrocytomas, as well as in 61 oligoastrocytomas and 115 oligodendrogliomas, and correlated these data with other genetic data (IDH1 mutations, TP53 mutations, 1p/19q loss, MET gain) (Kim, Nobusawa et al. 2010; Motomura, Mittelbronn et al. 2012; Pierscianek, Kim et al. 2013). Furthermore, FISH analysis in 6 diffuse astrocytomas with PDGFRA/MET co-gain was carried out to assess whether PDGFRA and MET are co-amplified in single cells or these alterations are observed in different cell populations, since several recent studies in GBM showed amplification of different receptor tyrosine kinase genes (RTKs, PDGFRA, MET, EGFR) in different tumor cells within single tumors(Snuderl, Fazlollahi et al. 2011; Szerlip, Pedraza et al. 2012).

In most of the low-grade diffuse gliomas, the levels of PDGFRA gain detected were relatively low (3–5 copies). However, low-level gain may have significant biologic effects.

For example, PDGFRA gain (~4 copies) was associated with PDGFRA overexpression in non–small cell lung cancer cells, and in a small fraction of squamous cell primary non–small cell lung cancers (McDermott, Ames et al. 2009). Similarly, FISH and quantitative PCR revealed PDGFRA gain (2–6 copies) in 3 of 11 diffuse intrinsic pontine gliomas, and all of those cases showed PDGFRA overexpression (Zarghooni, Bartels et al. 2010). Gain in PDGFRA (3–5 signals per nucleus) detected by chromogenic in situ hybridization was observed in 47% of medulloblastomas and primitive neuroectodermal tumors and was significantly associated with poorer patient outcome (Blom, Roselli et al. 2010).

Some studies have related the overexpression of PDGFRA with unfavorable outcome (Varela, Ranuncolo et al. 2004). In contrast, Ribom et al. showed that PDGFRA overexpression in WHO grade II astrocytomas and oligoastrocytomas was associated with a favorable patient outcome (Ribom, Andrae et al. 2002). Another immunohistochemical study showed an association between PDGFRA expression and a longer survival in patients with WHO grade I-III astrocytomas (Martinho, Longatto-Filho et al. 2009).

PTEN

The tumor suppressor protein, PTEN (phosphatase and tensin homologue deleted on chromosome 10) is a member of the mixed function, serine/threonine/tyrosine phosphatase subfamily of protein phosphatases. Its physiological substrates, however, are primarily 3-phosphorylated inositol phospholipids, which are products of phosphoinositide 3-kinases. PTEN thus antagonizes PI 3-kinase-dependent signaling pathways (Downes, Bennett et al. 2001). The PTEN gene encodes a 403 amino acid protein that is a member of the protein tyrosine phosphatase (PTP) subfamily of protein phosphatases. The role of PTEN is to dephosphorylate PIP3 into PIP2, rendering it incapable of recruiting Akt to the surface of the membrane and thus activating the PI3k/Akt pathway. Loss of PTEN results in accumulation of PIP3. This constitutively activates the PI3k/Akt pathway, inducing tumorigenesis through cell cycle progression, invasion and loss of apoptosis (Downes, Bennett et al. 2001).

PTEN mutations are associated with a wide range of tumors, most frequently endometrial tumors and GBM. PTEN-dependent deregulation of signaling is very frequent in GBM, with mutation occurring in between 5% and 40% of all GBM cases (Srividya, Thota et al. 2011). PTEN mutations occur in tumors from primary and secondary GBM, albeit at a higher frequency in primary GBM (up to 45%)(Kitange, Templeton et al. 2003), while the rate of LOH at 10q, where PTEN is located, is similar between the two at 80% (Behin, Hoang-Xuan et al. 2003)

PTEN mutations have been found in anaplastic astrocytomas, although at a much lower frequency than in GBM. In the largest series studied to date, PTEN mutations were seen in 20 gliomas and homozygous deletions in 7 of 142 GBM tumors, in 1 of 30 pilocytic astrocytomas, and in 2 of 22 oligodendrogliomas. No mutations were detected in 52 astrocytomas, 37 oligoastrocytomas, 15 ependymomas, and 16 ganglio-gliomas (Duerr, Rollbrocker et al. 1998). Bostrom et al. found 9 PTEN gene mutations and 1 deletion among 36 GBMs and none in 34 meningiomas (Bostrom, Cobbers et al. 1998). Other studies reported PTEN mutations in 7 of 25 GBM (Chiariello, Roz et al. 1998), in 5 of 21 high-grade and 1 of 8 low-grade gliomas (Maier, Zhang et al. 1998), in 0 of 15 gemistocytic astrocytomas, and in 2 of 18 anaplastic gemistocytic astrocytomas (Watanabe, Peraud et al. 1998). However, LOH for chromosome 10 loci in high-grade tumors was seen at a much higher frequency in these reports, suggesting the presence of another target tumor-suppressor gene on chromosome 10.

Analyses of PTEN mutations in primary versus progressive tumors showed that PTEN mutations are more common in primary tumors. Ten of 28 primary GBM contained a mutation or deletion of the PTEN gene. By contrast, only 1 of 25 progressive GBM had a PTEN mutation. Moreover, the same PTEN mutation was seen in a tumor progressed from an anaplastic astrocytoma that already had the PTEN mutation (Smith, Tachibana et al. 2001; Ushio, Tada et al. 2003). An analysis found that the 10q loci near PTEN were lost in GBM tumors but were retained in most low-grade tumors; however, the more distal locus around 10q25 was lost in all grades of gliomas (Bostrom, Cobbers et al. 1998).

RB

The pRB is a major protein involved in cell cycle progression from G1 to S phase. CDK4, CDK6 and the hypophosphorylated state pRB bind to the transcription factor E2F, thereby preventing cell cycle progression. Conversely, CDKN2A/CDKN2AINK4A, CDKN2B and CDKN2C, inhibit the different CDKs and are frequently inactivated in GBM. The CDKN2A acts as a cyclin-dependent kinase inhibitor, inhibiting the binding of the CDK4 protein to cyclin D1 and thus preventing phosphorylation of the Rb protein and arresting the cell cycle in the G1 phase (He, Olson et al. 1995; Meyer-Puttlitz, Hayashi et al. 1997). Cyclin D1 overexpression, CDKN2A loss, and pRb inactivation play a key role in glioma tumorigenesis. Alterations in the levels of Rb or p16 expression were seen in 90% of the gliomas studied. The expression of Rb was completely absent or low in 47.5% of GBM and 67.5% of anaplastic astrocytomas. The remainder of the tumors was immunopositive for Rb to varying degrees. Immunoreactivity against p16 was absent in 56% of GBM and 77.5% of anaplastic astrocytomas (Puduvalli, Kyritsis et al. 2000).

RB regulated CDKN2A is located on 9p21, and this chromosomal region is homozygously deleted in at least 30% to 40% of GBM and in approximately 10% of anaplastic astrocytomas, but never in diffuse astrocytomas. Primary GBM often show homozygous deletions of the CDKN2A/p14ARF locus on 9p21 (in 30% to 40% of cases) or amplification of CDK4 and MDM2 on 12q13–15 (in 8% to 13% of cases). Either of these sets of genetic changes will cause disruption of both the p53 and Rb pathways.

P53

The TP53 pathway plays a crucial role in the development of secondary GBM. P53 gene (TP53) mutations are the first detectable genetic alteration in two-thirds of precursor low-grade diffuse astrocytomas; this frequency is similar to that in anaplastic astrocytomas and secondary GBM. P53 mutations also occur in primary GBM, but at a lower frequency (Watanabe, Tachibana et al. 1996; Ohgaki, Dessen et al. 2004). In secondary GBM, 57% of mutations have been reported to be located in the two hotspot codons 248 and 273; however, in primary GBM, mutations were more equally distributed through all exons, with only 17%

transitions at CpG sites, considered to result from deamination of 5-meC, were significantly more frequent in secondary than in primary GBM. Thus, G:C→A:T mutations at CpG sites, particularly in the hotspot codons 248 and 273, seem to be an early event directly associated with malignant transformation in the pathway to secondary GBM. The less specific pattern of TP53 mutations in primary GBM may constitute, at least in part, secondary events due to increasing genomic instability during tumor development (Varela, Ranuncolo et al. 2004).

The p53 pathway frequently is disrupted in all grades of astrocytomas. This can occur by mutation of p53 itself, by overexpression of E3 ubiquitin-protein ligase (MDM2), which degrades p53, or by mutation or deletion of p14ARF, which positively regulates p53 by inhibiting MDM2 expression. It is possible that mutation of p53 in low-grade astrocytomas leads to genomic instability that sets the stage for additional mutations that lead to the formation of higher-grade tumors. TP53 is located on the long arm of chromosome 17 (17p), which frequently is lost in both low-grade and high-grade astrocytomas, suggesting that p53 is the target for this genetic change (Anderson and Allalunis-Turner 2000). Figure 1.

Treatment

Radiation Therapy

Conventional treatment strategy to treat gliomas usually includes standard surgical removal of the tumor, followed by radiotherapy.

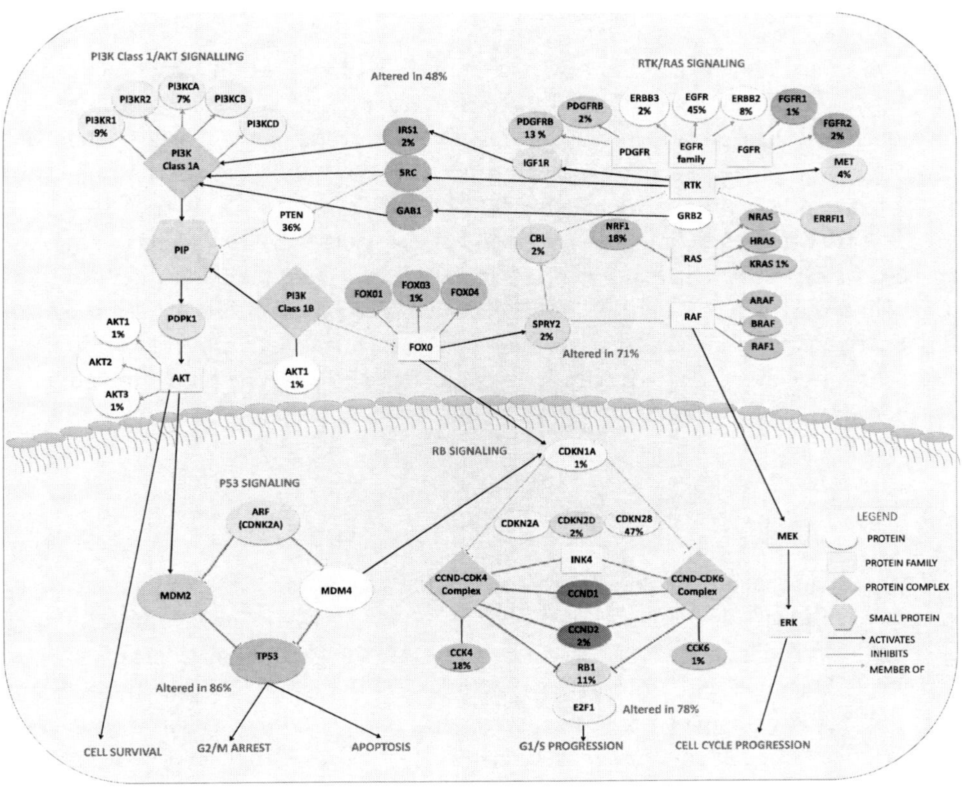

Figure 1. Representation of some pathways altered in gliomas.

Recently, studies show that radiotherapy combined with temozolamide increase the survival rate until 26.5% compared with radiotheraphy alone, being the standard of care (Stupp, Tonn et al. 2010). Numerous retrospective reports have been published on the use of radiation therapy for low-grade gliomas (Leighton, Fisher et al. 2007). These studies are plagued with a myriad of problems, making them inconclusive. In order to contain sufficient patient numbers, most of these reports span decades, sometimes going back as far as the 1940s. The results of these retrospective studies have largely been superseded by the results of three randomized trials, two from the European Organization for Research and Treatment of Cancer (EORTC) and one from the North Central Cancer Treatment Group (NCCG)(Shaw, Arusell et al. 2002). Patients underwent a range of surgical procedures, including biopsy and subtotal or gross total resection. Neither study showed any benefit to the higher dose in terms of overall survival or progression-free survival. If anything, the NCCG study showed a worse survival in patients receiving the higher dose of radiation (64.8 Gy). A statistically significant advantage, however, was observed in the patients who received radiation in terms of progression-free survival (55% versus 35% at 5 years; median time to progression, 5.3 versus 3.4 years). The absence of any difference in survival has supported the position of experts who advocate delaying radiation. Conversely, those favoring upfront radiation in the treatment of low-grade gliomas have cited the improved progression-free survival in the irradiated group, and the fact that at 1 year, seizures were better controlled in the radiation treatment arm. These randomized trials confirmed the importance of certain prognostic factors in low-grade gliomas. In the NCCG trial, three prognostic factors—histologic subtype, patient age, and tumor size—were consistently associated with overall survival in multivariate analysis (Shaw, Arusell et al. 2002). Patients who had greater than 90% of their tumor removed did much better than those who underwent a biopsy. Multivariate analysis of data from the two EORTC trials confirmed that astrocytoma histology, age older than 40 years, and preoperative size greater than 6 cm all were unfavorable prognostic factors but also uncovered a few others, such as tumor crossing midline and the presence of neurologic deficits before surgery (Pignatti, van den Bent et al. 2002).

On the basis of these randomized trials, it is evident that in adults with low-grade gliomas, no difference in survival is achieved whether radiation therapy is given postoperatively or delayed until recurrence. Therefore, a reasonable management strategy would be observation in a patient with a completely resected low-grade glioma. Many investigators, however, still advocate radiation after complete resection in older patients (older than 40 years) or after incomplete resection.

Radiation Therapy for High-Grade Gliomas

The current standard of care in RTOG studies is to define the initial volume as the preoperative lesion with edema as seen on T2- weighted MR images with a 2-cm margin. This volume is treated to 46 Gy, followed by a boost to the gadolinium-enhancing lesion seen on T1-weighted images with a 2.5-cm margin to 60 Gy. By pooling the results of three RTOG studies and using a nonparametric recursive partitioning technique, Curran and associates identified several significant prognostic factors for survival in patients with high-grade gliomas: histologic type, KPS score, age, neurologic function, and duration of symptoms(Curran, Scott et al. 1993).

Radioactive implants also have been used to increase dose locally to the tumor bed. An implantable balloon has been developed for the delivery of brachytherapy (Gliasite). After resection of the tumor, the balloon is placed in the cavity and filled with x-ray contrast medium. The catheter is attached to the balloon and then is brought out through the skull, and an infusion port at the end of the catheter is attached to the skull. A liquid form of 125I (Iotrex), specifically developed for use in the Gliasite, can then be used to fill the balloon 2 to 3 weeks after insertion (Tatter, Shaw et al. 2003). This device provides brachytherapy directly to the resection cavity, with minimal exposure of unaffected brain to the radiation source. The dose for recurrent gliomas is 60 Gy at 1 cm and for metastatic lesions 60 Gy at 0.5 cm. Use of the Iotrex has yielded significant improvements in quality of life and tumor control(Rogers, Rock et al. 2006). This complex mechanism of delivering local radiation therapy has not made it to standard of care regimens, but may be an alternative at centers that can provide it.

Chemotherapy for Gliomas

The role of chemotherapy in the treatment of high-grade astrocytomas has been investigated for more than 30 years. In BTSG 75-01, Green showed that the addition of carmustine (BCNU) or procarbazine to surgery and radiation therapy significantly increased mean survival from 40 weeks to 50 weeks and increased the percentage of patients surviving 18 months to 24%(Green, Byar et al. 1983). In these and most studies of chemotherapy as adjuvant therapy for high-grade astrocytoma, the benefit was greater in patients with anaplastic astrocytoma than in those with GBM. Another well-studied and frequently used chemotherapy regimen is combination therapy with procarbazine, CCNU, and vincristine (i.e., PCV). The PCV regimen clearly is more toxic as a result of myelosuppression and peripheral neuropathy and has been replaced by temozolomide, which has dramatically altered the treatment of high-grade gliomas. Temozolomide is an oral alkylating agent whose levels are not affected by AEDs or other hepatic enzyme inducing drugs. Toxicity with this drug is relatively mild, with good CNS penetration. Patients with a methylated MGMT promoter may have better survival than those without (Baur, Preusser et al. 2010). Even among patients with unmethylated MGMT, a trend toward increased survival is recognized for those receiving temozolomide. These data have made irradiation plus adjuvant temozolomide the standard of care for all patients with GBM regardless of MGMT status (Hegi, Diserens et al. 2005).

Patients with high-grade astrocytomas in whom initial therapy with radiation and temozolomide fails to provide benefit are candidates for participation in phase I/II trials. Such trials include drugs as well as a radiolabeled antibody that is infused directly into the tumor. In patients for whom some interval has elapsed between initial temozolomide therapy and failure, retreatment with low-dose daily temozolomide may be tried. Any benefit from chemotherapy for recurrent disease must be measured against the roughly 4- to 5-month median survival after repeat surgical removal of recurrent high-grade astrocytic tumors. Some patients with recurrent high-grade astrocytomas are offered re-resection with use of either Gliasite (covered earlier under Radiation Therapy for High-Grade Gliomas) or Gliadel (intracavitary biodegradable BCNU wafers), it was approved by the FDA in 2002 to be used during the initial resection (Westphal, Ram et al. 2006). Several institutions have reported a high rate of perioperative craniotomy infection after wafer placement. Irinotecan, a topoisomerase I inhibitor, has been the subject of several studies in patients with recurrent malignant astrocytoma. A respectable 10% to 15% objective imaging response rate has been achieved after thrice-weekly infusions. In two other studies seeking maximal tolerated dose, a marked effect of concomitant enzyme-inducing AEDs was found (Brem, Piantadosi et al. 1995).

Chemotherapy for low-grade astrocytomas usually is reserved for those patients whose unresectable tumors are progressively symptomatic. Radiation therapy traditionally has been used as a first-line treatment for progression. Potential toxicity of any proposed therapy for low-grade gliomas must be balanced against the long natural history. Particularly in younger patients and in those whose tumors have an oligodendroglial component, median survival periods may approach 10 years, with 5-year survival rates of 75% or higher from the time of diagnosis.(Grier and Batchelor 2006) Indeed, some investigators have argued that quality of life considerations, with particular attention to cognitive status, dictate a prolonged "wait and see" policy in patients with suspected low-grade glioma.(Reijneveld, Sitskoorn et al. 2001)Some variants of low-grade glial tumors carry a more ominous prognosis and for the rare situation of multicentric gliomatosis cerebri, chemotherapy may be a reasonable first-line approach (Celli, Nofrone et al. 1994).

Potential considerations in the use of alkylating agents for patients with low-grade astrocytomas should include the risks of hematologic malignancies (5% at 5 years) and sterility. Examination of quality of life outcomes must factor into recommendations for chemotherapy and radiation therapy. The trend over the last 30 years has been for increasing survival times, with a majority of patients receiving only surgery as a first course of treatment (Claus and Black 2006).

Over the past decade, increasing evidence has accumulated to confirm that anaplastic oligodendrogliomas and possibly anaplastic oligoastrocytomas are special types of malignant gliomas that are sensitive to chemotherapy. Although the molecular markers of chemosensitivity, allelic loss of 1p and 19q, have been shown to have prognostic significance in multiple studies, the reason for oligodendroglial chemosensitivity remains unknown. Zlatescu and colleagues have made the clinically interesting observation that allelic loss of 1p and 19q is related to tumor location and extent of tumor spread in the brain (Zlatescu, TehraniYazdi et al. 2001) Anaplastic oligodendrogliomas located in the frontal, parietal, and occipital lobes were significantly more likely to harbor 1p or 19q loss than are histologically identical tumors arising in the temporal lobe, insula, or diencephalon. Frontal tumors tend to have greater bilateral diffuse spread, and investigation of the biologic significance of these growth and invasion differences eventually may have implications for management strategies. In spite of a lack of randomized data with temozolomide in anaplastic oligodendrogliomas, many oncologists are currently using this drug concomitantly with radiation, extrapolating from the experience with GBM (Claus and Black 2006). Most patients with recurrent AOs who received PCV at initial presentation are currently being treated with temozolomide at relapse. Several small trials have shown the safety and efficacy of temozolomide following prior PCV therapy (Yung, Prados et al. 1999; Chinot 2001; van den Bent, Keime-Guibert et al. 2001).

Temozolomide has been used in patients with low-grade oligodendrogliomas or oligoastrocytomas that have recurred. The EORTC conducted one study using temozolomide for patients who had received PCV chemotherapy and irradiation for their initial disease (van den Bent, Chinot et al. 2003) and another study for patients who had received surgery and irradiation without chemotherapy initially. These studies showed 25% to 53% response rates, respectively, to temozolomide. Loss of 1p has been correlated with response to temozolomide for first-line chemotherapy in patients with recurrent oligodendrogliomas (Hoang-Xuan, Capelle et al. 2004; Kouwenhoven, Kros et al. 2006).

The disappointing results with conventional cytotoxic chemotherapy have led to efforts to find more effective and better-tolerated therapies. The challenge of neuro-oncology is to develop new compounds or procedures of gene transfer that specifically target the molecular alterations of glioma tumor cells and restore normal gene expression, cell cycle regulation, and apoptosis (Basso, Ermani et al. 2002). Significant progress is likely to come from some combination of cytotoxic chemotherapy with biologic agents directed at genetic alterations specific to brain tumors, such as growth factor receptors. Receptors are tempting targets because they are extracellular and easily accessible to drugs or antibodies. A number of agents targeted to the EGF receptor and the vIII variant are being tested. These EGFR inhibitors have shown limited utility in the clinic with brain tumors. These inhibitors may be effective only in patients with tumors that have a susceptible target. Receptor tyrosine kinases (RTKs), such as PDGF and insulin-like growth factor (IGF) receptors, regulate cell proliferation and differentiation (Mellinghoff, Wang et al. 2005). Deregulated RTK signaling frequently is found in human astrocytic tumors. Other agents target farnesyl transferase, histone deacetylase, rapamycin (mTOR), protein kinase C, and the ubiquitin-proteosome pathway.

Because gliomas produce specific angiogenic peptides such as VEGF to stimulate new blood vessel formation, angiogenesis inhibitors are a logical drug development target. Hypoxic areas within gliomas may stimulate angiogenesis and promote invasiveness of glial cells. Many of these changes in gene expression are mediated by hypoxia-inducible factor-1 (HIF-1). Many anti-angiogenic agents directed against VEGF, VEGFR, and other targets are in clinical trials. Bevacizumab, a humanized monoclonal antibody against VEGF, showed a 63% radiologic response rate in patients with recurrent high-grade gliomas (Vredenburgh, Desjardins et al. 2007). Although bevacizumab therapy improves progression-free survival as well as overall survival for recurrent GBM patients, essentially all patients ultimately relapse. Continuation of bevacizumab after progression on prior bevacizumab therapy has been associated with improved survival compared to discontinuation of bevacizumab for other oncology patient groups, although have not corroborated for GBM patients (Grothey, Sugrue et al. 2008). The discontinuation of bevacizumab among recurrent GBM patients has been associated with rapid tumor re-growth (Zuniga, Torcuator et al. 2010). Retrospective analyses have demonstrated that additional bevacizumab-based treatment strategies have negligible anti-tumor activity among recurrent GBM patients who have progressed on prior bevacizumab therapy (Iwamoto, Abrey et al. 2009). Similarly poor results have been observed among patients treated with bevacizumab plus irinotecan after progression on bevacizumab monotherapy (Kreisl, Kim et al. 2009). A Phase II study developed to evaluate adults with recurrent GBM who have progressed on prior bevacizumab therapy, were treated with bevacizumab combined to temozolamide or etoposide, demonstrates that combined treatment with bevacizumab, is well-tolerated but is not an effective strategy to overcome bevacizumab resistance in recurrent GBM patients (Reardon, Desjardins et al. 2011).

The transfer of genetic material to tumor cells to make them more susceptible to chemotherapy, or to reverse the alterations that sustain the neoplastic phenotype, has been studied in several centers. Gene therapy strategies include transfecting antioncogenes or drug-activating enzymes to glioma cells. The most extensively studied system is the "suicide gene therapy" with herpes simplex thymidine-kinase (HSV-tk) gene inserted into a replication defective murine retrovirus. Murine fibroblasts are engineered to produce these recombinant retroviruses, which are injected into gliomas, infecting the proliferating tumor cells and making them produce thymidine kinase. The tumor cells then are susceptible to the antiherpes drug ganciclovir, while nondividing brain cells are not infected. Clinical studies using this promising approach have been disappointing because of poor tumor cell transfection efficiency, although some long times to tumor progression have been reported (Ram, Culver et al. 1997; Palu, Cavaggioni et al. 1999; Shand, Weber et al. 1999; Liu, Wang et al. 2007).

Nanomaterial's in Glioblastoma Treatment

Despite considerable advancements in therapy of malignant gliomas in the last years, treatment outcomes are mostly unsatisfactory. A promising way to bypass these impairments and to elicit the specific delivering of drugs to treat tumors within the CNS is the employment of biodegradable polymeric nanoparticles (NPs), which can be loaded with different chemotherapeutic drugs to induce selective toxicity and additionally, modulate cellular and humoral immune responses when looking for a specific immune response against tumoral cells (Banchereau and Palucka 2005). A wide variety of NPs have been designed, each one with particular properties (certain size, shape, and composition) in a scale of strategies such as conjugated to antigens, which are recognized by specific receptors (Klippstein and Pozo 2010); antigens encapsulated within NPs, which offer the ability to protect the antigen from degradation; labeled NPs, which are also recognized by specific receptors and allow an effective tracking of their migration, and the use of NPs as vehicles for specific delivery of chemotherapeutic drugs (Adams and Weiner 2005; Schrama, Reisfeld et al. 2006). Some of the more representative nanoparticles used as carriers and in the treatment of gliomas are described below.

Liposomes

Liposomes are concentric bi-layered vesicles surrounded by a phospholipid membrane. The amphiphilic nature of liposomes, their facility of surface modification, and a good biocompatibility profile make them an appealing solution for increasing the circulating half-life of proteins and peptides. They may contain hydrophilic compounds, which remain encapsulated in the aqueous interior, which may escape encapsulation through diffusion out of the phospholipid membrane. Liposomes can be designed to adhere to cellular membranes to deliver a drug payload or simply transfer drugs through endocytosis (Papahadjopoulos, Portis et al. 1978; Ryman, Jewkes et al. 1978; Lasic, Frederik et al. 1992; Bangham 1995). *In vitro* and *in vivo* experiments have indicated that the activity of a range of drugs or their active metabolites may be enhanced by their encapsulation in liposomes (Chen, Qin et al. 2011; Gong, Wang et al. 2011; Qin, Chen et al. 2011).

Paclitaxel is a chemotherapeutic that inhibits cell division through promotion of the assembly and stabilization of microtubules. Unfortunately, paclitaxel is highly hydrophobic and its absorption across the BBB is also poor. To overcome this limitation, paclitaxel has been conjugated to liposomes (Fellner, Bauer et al. 2002). Recently, Xin et al. determined the potential of Angiopep-conjugated PEG–PCL NPs loaded with paclitaxel as a dual-targeting drug delivery system in the treatment of glioma. Nanoparticles were conjugated to Angiopep (ANG-NP) for enhanced delivery across the BBB as well as for targeting the tumor via lipoprotein receptor-related protein mediated endocytosis.

Curcumin is a polyphenolic compound derived from the Indian spice turmeric. It has been shown to exert antitumor effects in many different cancer cell lines and animal models either by pro-apoptotic, anti-angiogenic, anti-inflammatory, immunomodulatory, and anti-mitogenic effects (Aggarwal, Kumar et al. 2003; Maheshwari, Singh et al. 2006; Hatcher, Planalp et al. 2008). Some potential molecular targets for curcumin include: insulin-like growth factor (IGF), serine threonine protein kinase (Akt), mitogen-activated protein kinase (MAPK), signal transducer, the activator of transcription 3 (STAT3), nuclear factor kappa β (NFκ β), and Notch (Kunnumakkara, Anand et al. 2008; Ravindran, Prasad et al. 2009). These pathways are all thought to be active in malignant brain tumors, raising the possibility that curcumin could be effective in treating these diseases (Atkinson, Nozell et al. 2010; Schmidt, Brunetto et al. 2010).

Celecoxib, a cyclo-oxygenase (COX)-2 inhibitor, has been reported to mediate growth inhibitory effects and to induce apoptosis in various cancer cell lines (Tsujii, Kawano et al. 1998). Celecoxib has been conjugated to Poly DL-lactide-co-glycolide (PLGA) and tested in glioma cells, finding that the celecoxib recovered in the NPs showed similar antitumor activity against U87MG cells and C6 cells in a dose-dependent manner. These results show that PLGA NPs incorporating celecoxib are promising candidates for antitumor drug delivery (Kim, Jeong et al. 2011).

Nanotubes

Self-assembling sheets of atoms arranged in tubes are defined as nanotubes. They may be organic or inorganic in composition and can be produced as single- or multi-walled structures (Li and Zhu 2012). Carbon Nanotubes (CNTs) are formed by rolling sheets of graphite-like carbon with hollow tubes. They are categorized based on the number of carbon layers assembled together: Single-Walled (SW), Double-Walled (DW), and Multi-Walled (MW). The diameters vary according to the number of layers: 0.4–2 nm for SWNTs, 1–3.5 nm for DWNTs, and from 2–100 nm for MWCNTs (Meziani and Sun 2003). The length of these tubes can be extended to tens of micrometers and is dependent on the method of production.

Nanocrystals

Nanocrystals are aggregates of molecules that can be combined into a crystalline form of the drug surrounded by a thin coating of surfactant. They have extensive uses in materials research, chemical engineering, and as quantum dots for biological imaging; there is no carrier material as in polymeric nanoparticles. (Chan and Nie 1998; Dubertret, Skourides et al. 2002; Gao, Cui et al. 2004). Nanocrystalline species may be prepared from a hydrophobic compound and coated with a thin amphiphilic layer. It has been demonstrated that the size and shape of nanocrystals plays an important role in their biological activity (Xiang, Liang et al. 2011).

Some nanocrystals have shown to inhibit the proliferation in different cancer cells lines (Vallhov, Gabrielsson et al. 2007). Silver NPs (Ag-NPs) have recently been the focus of intense research due to their capacity to induce the expression of genes associated with cell cycle progression, DNA damage and apoptosis in human cells at non-cytotoxic doses (Ahamed, Alsalhi et al. 2010). The toxicity of starch-coated Ag-NPs have been studied in normal human lung fibroblast cells (IMR-90) and human GBM cells (U251); uptake of Ag-NPs is predominantly by endocytosis, and partly adhered to membranous surfaces. Once inside, Ag-NPs show a uniform intracellular distribution both cytoplasmic and nuclear. The accumulations of these particles cause DNA damage and reduce cellular ATP content, causing damage in mitochondria and increasing the production of reactive oxygen species (ROS) in a dose-dependent manner in glioma cells.

Also, it has been proposed that Ag-NPs can induce DNA damage leading to cell cycle arreste in G2/M phase and enhanced the apoptotic rate of cancer cells (Carlson, Hussain et al. 2008; AshaRani, Low Kah Mun et al. 2009; Kim, Choi et al. 2009; Asharani, Xinyi et al. 2010).

Dendrimers

Dendrimers are polymer-based macromolecules formed from monomeric or oligomeric units, such that each layer of branching units doubles or triples the number of peripheral groups. These structures are considered as one of the most promising polymer architectures in biomedical applications in recent years (Dhanikula, Argaw et al. 2008; Ren, Kang et al. 2010).(Dhanikula, Argaw et al. 2008; Ren, Kang et al. 2010). Such structures are highly branched, multigenerational NPs consisting of exterior end groups that can be functionalized (Wiener, Brechbiel et al. 1994; Cheng, Thorek et al. 2010; Tan, Wu et al. 2010). Examples include the encapsulation of therapeutic agents inside the dendrimers and attachment of drugs, targeting moieties and functional groups on the surface of them by covalent bounding or physical absorbing, which afforded the possibility to produce the desired multifunctional nanocarriers for drug delivery.

Therapeutic benefit of dendrimers has been evaluated as drug carriers for the treatment of gliomas. These nanomaterials were conjugated to D-glucosamine as the ligand for enhancing their permeability across BBB and tumor targeting. The efficacy of methotrexate (MTX)-loaded dendrimers was established against U87 MG and U343 MG cells. Permeability of rhodamine-labeled dendrimers and MTX-loaded dendrimers across an *in vitro* BBB model and their distribution into vascular human glioma tumor spheroids was also studied. Glucosylated dendrimers were found to be endocytosed in significantly higher amounts than nonglucosylated dendrimers by the cell lines above mentioned. These MTX-loaded dendrimers were also able to kill even MTX-resistant cells highlighting their ability to overcome MTX resistance.

In addition, the amount of MTX-transported across BBB was three to five times more after loading in the dendrimers. Glucosylation further increased the cumulative permeation of dendrimers across BBB and hence increased the amount of MTX available across it. (Yan, Wang et al. 2011).

Altered Immune System in Gliomas

The CNS has been considered an immunologically privileged site owing to its apparent inability to reject intracranial xenografts in older reports (Medawar 1948). The BBB has an important role as it acts as a physical barrier with the lymphatic system. The BBB is mainly composed of astrocytes, microglia, endothelial cells, pericytes; these components contributes to their architecture and stability (Stewart, Magliocco et al. 1987; Rossler, Neuchrist et al. 1992). The capillaries of the BBB consist of a monolayer of endothelial cells coupled by tight junctions and the pericytes provide mechanical stability (Armulik, Abramsson et al. 2005). It is thought that astrocytes provide the specific signals that program endothelial cells to produce and maintain tight junctions (Janzer and Raff 1987). Normally the CNS has a very low level of T-cell infiltration; however, in pathological states the BBB is only a relative barrier to lymphocyte tracking (Goldmann, Kwidzinski et al. 2006).

Since brain tumors reside in an anatomical compartment that lacks a normal lymphatic drainage system, they are separated from normal immunosurveillance (Akopian, Bol'shunov et al. 1978; Sawamura and de Tribolet 1990)]. In spite of the presence of immune cells in GBM, the overall tumor environment is highly immunosuppressive (Bhondeley, Mehra et al. 1988; Black, Chen et al. 1992). Experimentally, brain tumor models that recapitulate GBM-like pathology also show a high degree of immunosuppressive leukocyte infiltration as well as cytokine expression (Tran, Uhl et al. 2007; Mitchell, Cui et al. 2011). The presence of T cells in brain tumors was first describe in both human gliomas and rat brain tumors induced by N-methyl-N-nitrosourea (Stavrou, Anzil et al. 1977). Since then, the effects of brain tumor-derived factors, such as immunosuppressive cytokines, prostaglandins, interleukin 10 (IL-10) and transforming growth factor-beta (TGF-β), which are part of the immunosuppressive tumor environment, have also been described Table 1, (Gomez and Kruse 2006).

Table 1. Agents to promote immunosuppression in the tumor microenvironment

Agents involved in immunosuppression
Interleukin-10 (IL-10)
Transforming growth factor beta (TGF-β)
Cytotoxic T-lymphocyte antigen 4 (CTLA-4)
B- and T- lymphocyte attenuator (BTLA-4)
V-set domain containing T-cell activation inhibitor 1 (B7-H4)
Programmed cell death 1 ligand 1 (PD-L1)
Glucocorticoid-induced TNFR-related protein (GITR)
Indoleamine 2,3 dioxygenase (IDO)
Tryptophan 2,3 dioxygenase (TDO)
Regulatory T cell (Treg)
Myeloid derived suppressor cell (MDSC)
Signal transducer and activator of transcription 3 (STAT 3)
Signal transducer and activator of transcription 5 (STAT 5)

Modified of (Wainwright, Nigam et al. 2012).

Aside from immunosuppressive cytokines, many diverse cells of the immune system that infiltrate brain tumors have been describe, such as T cells (CD4+, CD8+), dendritic cells (DC), macrophages, microglia, B cells, natural killer T (NKT) cells and NK cells (Morimura, Neuchrist et al. 1990; Kiefer, Supler et al. 1994; Curtin, Candolfi et al. 2008). Also, there are T regulatory cells (Tregs) and myeloid-derived suppressor cells (MDSC) which also suppresses T cell function (Prins, Scott et al. 2002; Watters, Schartner et al. 2005; Sonabend, Rolle et al. 2008; Thomas, Kranz et al. 2008).

Glioma cells secrete multiple immunosuppressive factors with diverse effects. The most marked of which is suppressing lymphocyte proliferation. Also, they secrete several factors that are immunomodulatory, such as interleukin-6 (IL-6) and colony stimulating factor-1 (CSF-1). These factors have immune functions such as shifting adaptive immunity to humoral (T H2) responses that may be less effective against solid tumors and/or attracting and stimulating monocytic cells.(Parney, Farr-Jones et al. 2000; Hao, Parney et al. 2002; Bender, Collier et al. 2010). Others, such as vascular endothelial growth factor (VEGF) acts primarily as a pro-angiogenic factor (Norden, Drappatz et al. 2009).

Different molecules recruit different subsets of leukocyte subsets. Accordingly, the chemokine, CCL22, preferentially recruits immunosuppressive Tregs that promote tumorigenesis (Hussain, Kong et al. 2007; Kong, Wei et al. 2009). By contrast, CXCL10 (IP-10) recruits pro-inflammatory IFN-g-expressing CD4+ T cells that promote tumor rejection (Parsa, Waldron et al. 2007). Brain tumor cells produce large amounts of TGF-β that aides in increasing immunosuppressive effector T-cell programs, leading to decreased pro-inflammatory cytokine help and increased GITR by CD4+ effectors, as well as decreased IFN-γ and granzyme B levels by CD8+ T cell effectors (Wainwright, Nigam et al. 2012).

CD4+ T cells have been isolated from human malignant gliomas (Sawamura, Abe et al. 1988). The majority of CD4+ T cells expressing IL-2 receptor alpha (CD25) were not appreciated at the time of the discovery. However, those initial observations were actually describing highly immunosuppressive cellular mediators that we now refer to as regulatory T cells (Tregs; CD4+FoxP3+CD25+) (El Andaloussi, Han et al. 2006; Fecci, Mitchell et al. 2006). Recently, it has been demonstrated that those brain tumor-resident Tregs contribute to the pathogenesis and progression of tumor, as the depletion of these cells increased the survival in experimental mouse brain tumor models (El Andaloussi, Han et al. 2006; Curtin, Candolfi et al. 2008).

CD4+ and CD8+ T cells actively infiltrate brain tumors. CD4+ T cells are enriched for immunosuppressive regulatory T cells (Treg; CD4+FoxP3+), which express high levels of CTLA-4 and GITR. The Tregs that accumulate in brain tumors are primarily thymus derived, or natural Tregs (nTregs). Within the brain tumor microenvironment, nTregs directly and indirectly suppress CD4+ and CD8+ T cells. This occurs through three main mechanisms. First, nTregs directly interact with dendritic cells (DCs) and induce an immunosuppressive phenotype that acts to suppress full CD4+ and CD8+ T-cell activation, thus promoting tumor cell survival. In addition, nTregs produce IL-10 and TGF-b that directly act on effector T cells to downregulate cytotoxic programs that would otherwise promote brain tumor clearance. Finally, nTregs interact via cell surface expression with effector T cells to induce T-cell anergy (Wainwright, Nigam et al. 2012). These immunosuppressive processes promote the persistence and progression of brain tumors (Figure 2).

Moreover, myeloid-derived suppressor cells have profound immunosuppressive implications (Raychaudhuri, Rayman et al. 2011; Kohanbash and Okada 2012).

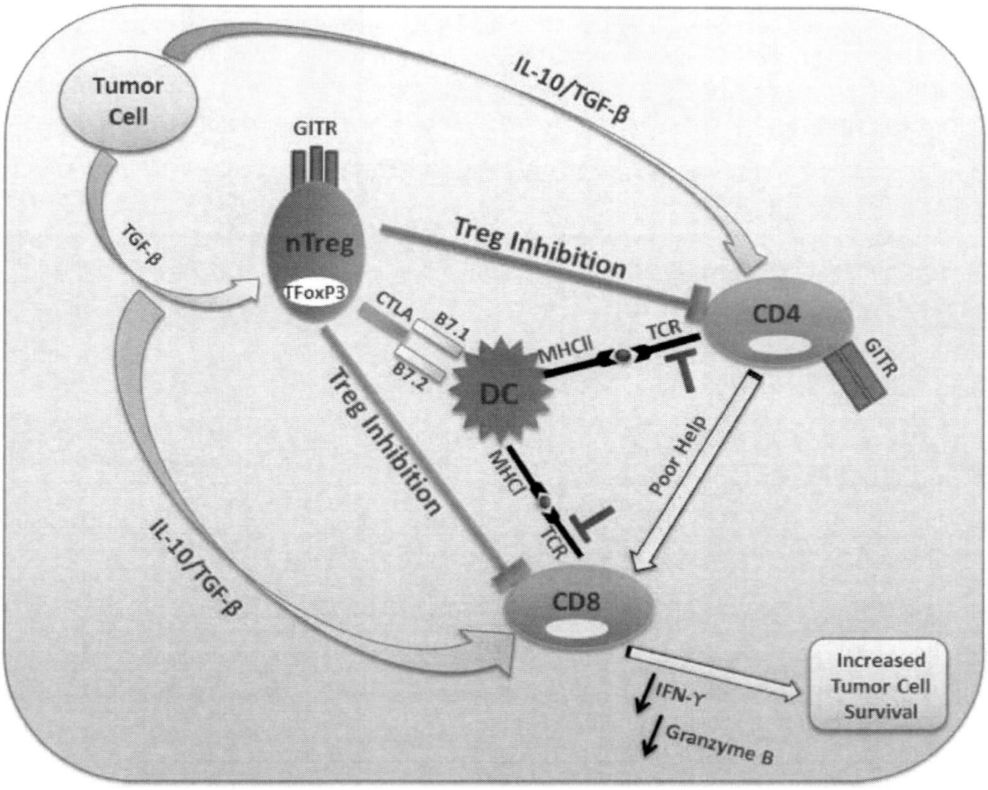

Figure 2. Main interactions between T-cell subtypes and the immunosuppressive signals.

MDSCs were first discovered when it was found that bone marrow hematopoietic progenitor cells in tumor-bearing hosts can suppress T cell blastogenesis (Young, Newby et al. 1987). Due to their immunosuppressive properties, MDSCs were initially believed to consist of granulocytes and monocytes/macrophages (Bronte, Serafini et al. 2001). However, it was shown recently that immunosuppressive MDSCs are inflammatory monocytes and not granulocytes (Gallina, Dolcetti et al. 2006). The MDSC are phenotypically double positive for granulocyte and monocyte markers, His48/CD11bc (rat) or Gr1/CD11b (mouse). MDSCs within tumors also have a potent, immunosuppressive phenotype and produce reactive nitrogen compounds (e.g., peroxynitrites) that have recently been shown to nitrosylate the CD8 and TCR molecules on T cells, thereby inhibiting T cell reactivity. Also, IL-13 produced by NKT cells induces MDSCs to express TGF-β (Umemura, Saio et al. 2008).

Summary

Despite no significant improvement in the survival of glioma patients over the past few decades, the continued study of their biology, histopathology, alterations in genetics, classification and tumor microenvironment has allowed us a better understanding of these deadly brain tumors. This knowledge will eventually allow us to develop better therapeutic strategies based in their unique, often individualistic, molecular characteristics. Personalized medicine will likely become the best way to fight this tumor.

Acknowledgments

This work was supported by National Council of Science and Technology of Mexico (Conacyt) grants CB180851 and FOSSIS 182362.

References

Adams, G. P. and L. M. Weiner (2005). "Monoclonal antibody therapy of cancer." *Nat. Biotechnol.,* 23(9): 1147-1157.

Aggarwal, B. B., A. Kumar, et al. (2003). "Anticancer potential of curcumin: preclinical and clinical studies." *Anticancer Res.,* 23(1A): 363-398.

Ahamed, M., M. S. Alsalhi, et al. (2010). "Silver nanoparticle applications and human health." *Clin. Chim. Acta*, 411(23-24): 1841-1848.

Akopian, V. S., A. V. Bol'shunov, et al. (1978). "[Optical laser interventions on the anterior portion of the eye]." *Vestn. Oftalmol.*, (4): 29-35.

Anderson, C. W. and M. J. Allalunis-Turner (2000). "Human TP53 from the malignant glioma-derived cell lines M059J and M059K has a cancer-associated mutation in exon 8." *Radiat. Res.,* 154(4): 473-476.

Armulik, A., A. Abramsson, et al. (2005). "Endothelial/pericyte interactions." *Circ. Res.,* 97(6): 512-523.

AshaRani, P. V., G. Low Kah Mun, et al. (2009). "Cytotoxicity and genotoxicity of silver nanoparticles in human cells." *ACS Nano*, 3(2): 279-290.

Asharani, P. V., N. Xinyi, et al. (2010). "DNA damage and p53-mediated growth arrest in human cells treated with platinum nanoparticles." *Nanomedicine (Lond),* 5(1): 51-64.

Atkinson, G. P., S. E. Nozell, et al. (2010). "NF-kappaB and STAT3 signaling in glioma: targets for future therapies." *Expert Rev. Neurother.*, 10(4): 575-586.

Balss, J., J. Meyer, et al. (2008). "Analysis of the IDH1 codon 132 mutation in brain tumors." *Acta Neuropathol.*, 116(6): 597-602.

Banchereau, J. and A. K. Palucka (2005). "Dendritic cells as therapeutic vaccines against cancer." *Nat. Rev. Immunol.*, 5(4): 296-306.

Bangham, A. D. (1995). "Surrogate cells or Trojan horses. The discovery of liposomes." *Bioessays,* 17(12): 1081-1088.

Basso, U., M. Ermani, et al. (2002). "Non-cytotoxic therapies for malignant gliomas." *J. Neurooncol.*, 58(1): 57-69.

Baur, M., M. Preusser, et al. (2010). "Frequent MGMT (0(6)-methylguanine-DNA methyltransferase) hypermethylation in long-term survivors of glioblastoma: a single institution experience." *Radiol. Oncol.*, 44(2): 113-120.

Behin, A., K. Hoang-Xuan, et al. (2003). "Primary brain tumours in adults." *Lancet,* 361(9354): 323-331.

Bender, A. M., L. S. Collier, et al. (2010). "Sleeping beauty-mediated somatic mutagenesis implicates CSF1 in the formation of high-grade astrocytomas." *Cancer Res.,* 70(9): 3557-3565.

Bhondeley, M. K., R. D. Mehra, et al. (1988). "Imbalances in T cell subpopulations in human gliomas." *J. Neurosurg*., 68(4): 589-593.

Bianco, R., T. Troiani, et al. (2005). "Intrinsic and acquired resistance to EGFR inhibitors in human cancer therapy." *Endocr. Relat. Cancer*, 12 Suppl. 1: S159-171.

Biernat, W., H. Huang, et al. (2004). "Predominant expression of mutant EGFR (EGFRvIII) is rare in primary glioblastomas." *Brain Pathol.*, 14(2): 131-136.

Bigner, S. H., M. R. Matthews, et al. (1999). "Molecular genetic aspects of oligodendrogliomas including analysis by comparative genomic hybridization." *Am. J. Pathol.*, 155(2): 375-386.

Black, K. L., K. Chen, et al. (1992). "Inflammatory leukocytes associated with increased immunosuppression by glioblastoma." *J. Neurosurg*., 77(1): 120-126.

Blom, T., A. Roselli, et al. (2010). "Amplification and overexpression of KIT, PDGFRA, and VEGFR2 in medulloblastomas and primitive neuroectodermal tumors." *J. Neurooncol.,* 97(2): 217-224.

Bolduc, J. M., D. H. Dyer, et al. (1995). "Mutagenesis and Laue structures of enzyme intermediates: isocitrate dehydrogenase." *Science,* 268(5215): 1312-1318.

Bostrom, J., J. M. Cobbers, et al. (1998). "Mutation of the PTEN (MMAC1) tumor suppressor gene in a subset of glioblastomas but not in meningiomas with loss of chromosome arm 10q." *Cancer Res.,* 58(1): 29-33.

Brem, H., S. Piantadosi, et al. (1995). "Placebo-controlled trial of safety and efficacy of intraoperative controlled delivery by biodegradable polymers of chemotherapy for recurrent gliomas. The Polymer-brain Tumor Treatment Group." *Lancet,* 345(8956): 1008-1012.

Bronte, V., P. Serafini, et al. (2001). "Tumor-induced immune dysfunctions caused by myeloid suppressor cells." *J. Immunother.*, 24(6): 431-446.

Carlson, C., S. M. Hussain, et al. (2008). "Unique cellular interaction of silver nanoparticles: size-dependent generation of reactive oxygen species." *J. Phys. Chem. B.,* 112(43): 13608-13619.

Celli, P., I. Nofrone, et al. (1994). "Cerebral oligodendroglioma: prognostic factors and life history." *Neurosurgery,* 35(6): 1018-1034; discussion 1034-1015.

Claus, E. B. and P. M. Black (2006). "Survival rates and patterns of care for patients diagnosed with supratentorial low-grade gliomas: data from the SEER program, 1973-2001." *Cancer,* 106(6): 1358-1363.

Curran, W. J., Jr., C. B. Scott, et al. (1993). "Recursive partitioning analysis of prognostic factors in three Radiation Therapy Oncology Group malignant glioma trials." *J. Natl. Cancer Inst.,* 85(9): 704-710.

Curtin, J. F., M. Candolfi, et al. (2008). "Treg depletion inhibits efficacy of cancer immunotherapy: implications for clinical trials." *PLoS One,* 3(4): e1983.

Chan, W. C. and S. Nie (1998). "Quantum dot bioconjugates for ultrasensitive nonisotopic detection." *Science,* 281(5385): 2016-2018.

Chen, H., Y. Qin, et al. (2011). "Lactoferrin modified doxorubicin-loaded procationic liposomes for the treatment of gliomas." *Eur. J. Pharm. Sci.*, 44(1-2): 164-173.

Cheng, Z., D. L. Thorek, et al. (2010). "Gadolinium-conjugated dendrimer nanoclusters as a tumor-targeted T1 magnetic resonance imaging contrast agent." *Angew. Chem. Int. Ed. Engl.,* 49(2): 346-350.

Chiariello, E., L. Roz, et al. (1998). "PTEN/MMAC1 mutations in primary glioblastomas and short-term cultures of malignant gliomas." *Oncogene,* 16(4): 541-545.

Chinot, O. (2001). "Chemotherapy for the treatment of oligodendroglial tumors." *Semin. Oncol.*, 28(4 Suppl 13): 13-18.

Dang, L., D. W. White, et al. (2009). "Cancer-associated IDH1 mutations produce 2-hydroxyglutarate." *Nature,* 462(7274): 739-744.

DeAngelis, L. M. (2001). "Brain tumors." *N. Engl. J. Med.*, 344(2): 114-123.

Dhanikula, R. S., A. Argaw, et al. (2008). "Methotrexate loaded polyether-copolyester dendrimers for the treatment of gliomas: enhanced efficacy and intratumoral transport capability." *Mol. Pharm.*, 5(1): 105-116.

Downes, C. P., D. Bennett, et al. (2001). "Antagonism of PI 3-kinase-dependent signalling pathways by the tumour suppressor protein, PTEN." *Biochem. Soc. Trans.*, 29(Pt 6): 846-851.

Dubertret, B., P. Skourides, et al. (2002). "In vivo imaging of quantum dots encapsulated in phospholipid micelles." *Science,* 298(5599): 1759-1762.

Duerr, E. M., B. Rollbrocker, et al. (1998). "PTEN mutations in gliomas and glioneuronal tumors." *Oncogene,* 16(17): 2259-2264.

Ekstrand, A. J., N. Longo, et al. (1994). "Functional characterization of an EGF receptor with a truncated extracellular domain expressed in glioblastomas with EGFR gene amplification." *Oncogene*, 9(8): 2313-2320.

Ekstrand, A. J., N. Sugawa, et al. (1992). "Amplified and rearranged epidermal growth factor receptor genes in human glioblastomas reveal deletions of sequences encoding portions of the N- and/or C-terminal tails." *Proc. Natl. Acad. Sci. U S A,* 89(10): 4309-4313.

El Andaloussi, A., Y. Han, et al. (2006). "Prolongation of survival following depletion of CD4+CD25+ regulatory T cells in mice with experimental brain tumors." *J. Neurosurg.,* 105(3): 430-437.

Fecci, P. E., D. A. Mitchell, et al. (2006). "Increased regulatory T-cell fraction amidst a diminished CD4 compartment explains cellular immune defects in patients with malignant glioma." *Cancer Res.,* 66(6): 3294-3302.

Fellner, S., B. Bauer, et al. (2002). "Transport of paclitaxel (Taxol) across the blood-brain barrier in vitro and in vivo." *J. Clin. Invest.,* 110(9): 1309-1318.

Ferrer-Luna, R., M. Mata, et al. (2009). "Loss of heterozygosity at 1p-19q induces a global change in oligodendroglial tumor gene expression." *J. Neurooncol.*, 95(3): 343-354.

Fredriksson, L., H. Li, et al. (2004). "The PDGF family: four gene products form five dimeric isoforms." *Cytokine. Growth Factor Rev.*, 15(4): 197-204.

Gallina, G., L. Dolcetti, et al. (2006). "Tumors induce a subset of inflammatory monocytes with immunosuppressive activity on CD8+ T cells." *J. Clin. Invest.,* 116(10): 2777-2790.

Gao, X., Y. Cui, et al. (2004). "In vivo cancer targeting and imaging with semiconductor quantum dots." *Nat. Biotechnol.*, 22(8): 969-976.

Goldmann, J., E. Kwidzinski, et al. (2006). "T cells traffic from brain to cervical lymph nodes via the cribroid plate and the nasal mucosa." *J. Leukoc. Biol.*, 80(4): 797-801.

Gomez, G. G. and C. A. Kruse (2006). "Mechanisms of malignant glioma immune resistance and sources of immunosuppression." *Gene Ther. Mol. Biol.*, 10(A): 133-146.

Gong, W., Z. Wang, et al. (2011). "Improving efficiency of adriamycin crossing blood brain barrier by combination of thermosensitive liposomes and hyperthermia." *Biol. Pharm. Bull.*, 34(7): 1058-1064.

Goritz, C., D. O. Dias, et al. (2011). "A pericyte origin of spinal cord scar tissue." *Science,* 333(6039): 238-242.

Green, S. B., D. P. Byar, et al. (1983). "Comparisons of carmustine, procarbazine, and high-dose methylprednisolone as additions to surgery and radiotherapy for the treatment of malignant glioma." *Cancer Treat. Rep.*, 67(2): 121-132.

Grier, J. T. and T. Batchelor (2006). "Low-grade gliomas in adults." *Oncologist*, 11(6): 681-693.

Griffin, C. A., P. Burger, et al. (2006). "Identification of der(1;19)(q10;p10) in five oligodendrogliomas suggests mechanism of concurrent 1p and 19q loss." *J. Neuropathol. Exp. Neurol.*, 65(10): 988-994.

Grothey, A., M. M. Sugrue, et al. (2008). "Bevacizumab beyond first progression is associated with prolonged overall survival in metastatic colorectal cancer: results from a large observational cohort study (BRiTE)." *J. Clin. Oncol.,* 26(33): 5326-5334.

Hao, C., I. F. Parney, et al. (2002). "Cytokine and cytokine receptor mRNA expression in human glioblastomas: evidence of Th1, Th2 and Th3 cytokine dysregulation." *Acta Neuropathol.*, 103(2): 171-178.

Hartmann, C., J. Meyer, et al. (2009). "Type and frequency of IDH1 and IDH2 mutations are related to astrocytic and oligodendroglial differentiation and age: a study of 1,010 diffuse gliomas." *Acta Neuropathol.*, 118(4): 469-474.

Hatcher, H., R. Planalp, et al. (2008). "Curcumin: from ancient medicine to current clinical trials." *Cell Mol. Life Sci.,* 65(11): 1631-1652.

He, J., J. J. Olson, et al. (1995). "Lack of p16INK4 or retinoblastoma protein (pRb), or amplification-associated overexpression of cdk4 is observed in distinct subsets of malignant glial tumors and cell lines." *Cancer Res.,* 55(21): 4833-4836.

Hegi, M. E., A. C. Diserens, et al. (2005). "MGMT gene silencing and benefit from temozolomide in glioblastoma." *N. Engl. J. Med.,* 352(10): 997-1003.

Heldin, C. H. and B. Westermark (1990). "Platelet-derived growth factor: mechanism of action and possible in vivo function." *Cell Regul.,* 1(8): 555-566.

Hermanson, M., K. Funa, et al. (1996). "Association of loss of heterozygosity on chromosome 17p with high platelet-derived growth factor alpha receptor expression in human malignant gliomas." *Cancer Res.,* 56(1): 164-171.

Hoang-Xuan, K., L. Capelle, et al. (2004). "Temozolomide as initial treatment for adults with low-grade oligodendrogliomas or oligoastrocytomas and correlation with chromosome 1p deletions." *J. Clin. Oncol.*, 22(15): 3133-3138.

Huang, H. S., M. Nagane, et al. (1997). "The enhanced tumorigenic activity of a mutant epidermal growth factor receptor common in human cancers is mediated by threshold levels of constitutive tyrosine phosphorylation and unattenuated signaling." *J. Biol. Chem.*, 272(5): 2927-2935.

Hussain, S. F., L. Y. Kong, et al. (2007). "A novel small molecule inhibitor of signal transducers and activators of transcription 3 reverses immune tolerance in malignant glioma patients." *Cancer Res.,* 67(20): 9630-9636.

Ichimura, K., D. M. Pearson, et al. (2009). "IDH1 mutations are present in the majority of common adult gliomas but rare in primary glioblastomas." *Neuro. Oncol.*, 11(4): 341-347.

Iwamoto, F. M., L. E. Abrey, et al. (2009). "Patterns of relapse and prognosis after bevacizumab failure in recurrent glioblastoma." *Neurology,* 73(15): 1200-1206.

Janzer, R. C. and M. C. Raff (1987). "Astrocytes induce blood-brain barrier properties in endothelial cells." *Nature*, 325(6101): 253-257.

Jenkins, R. B., H. Blair, et al. (2006). "A t(1;19)(q10;p10) mediates the combined deletions of 1p and 19q and predicts a better prognosis of patients with oligodendroglioma." *Cancer Res.*, 66(20): 9852-9861.

Kiefer, R., M. L. Supler, et al. (1994). "In situ detection of transforming growth factor-beta mRNA in experimental rat glioma and reactive glial cells." *Neurosci. Lett.,* 166(2): 161-164.

Kim, S., J. E. Choi, et al. (2009). "Oxidative stress-dependent toxicity of silver nanoparticles in human hepatoma cells." *Toxicol. In Vitro*, 23(6): 1076-1084.

Kim, S. Y., S. M. Lee, et al. (2007). "Regulation of singlet oxygen-induced apoptosis by cytosolic NADP+-dependent isocitrate dehydrogenase." *Mol. Cell Biochem.*, 302(1-2): 27-34.

Kim, T. H., Y. I. Jeong, et al. (2011). "Preparation of polylactide-co-glycolide nanoparticles incorporating celecoxib and their antitumor activity against brain tumor cells." *Int. J. Nanomedicine*, 6: 2621-2631.

Kim, Y. H., S. Nobusawa, et al. (2010). "Molecular classification of low-grade diffuse gliomas." *Am. J. Pathol.*, 177(6): 2708-2714.

Kita, D., Y. Yonekawa, et al. (2007). "PIK3CA alterations in primary (de novo) and secondary glioblastomas." *Acta Neuropathol.*, 113(3): 295-302.

Kitange, G. J., K. L. Templeton, et al. (2003). "Recent advances in the molecular genetics of primary gliomas." *Curr. Opin. Oncol.*, 15(3): 197-203.

Klippstein, R. and D. Pozo (2010). "Nanotechnology-based manipulation of dendritic cells for enhanced immunotherapy strategies." *Nanomedicine,* 6(4): 523-529.

Kohanbash, G. and H. Okada (2012). "Myeloid-derived suppressor cells (MDSCs) in gliomas and glioma-development." *Immunol. Invest.*, 41(6-7): 658-679.

Kong, L. Y., J. Wei, et al. (2009). "A novel phosphorylated STAT3 inhibitor enhances T cell cytotoxicity against melanoma through inhibition of regulatory T cells." *Cancer Immunol. Immunother.*, 58(7): 1023-1032.

Kouwenhoven, M. C., J. M. Kros, et al. (2006). "1p/19q loss within oligodendroglioma is predictive for response to first line temozolomide but not to salvage treatment." *Eur. J. Cancer,* 42(15): 2499-2503.

Kreisl, T. N., L. Kim, et al. (2009). "Phase II trial of single-agent bevacizumab followed by bevacizumab plus irinotecan at tumor progression in recurrent glioblastoma." *J. Clin. Oncol.*, 27(5): 740-745.

Kunnumakkara, A. B., P. Anand, et al. (2008). "Curcumin inhibits proliferation, invasion, angiogenesis and metastasis of different cancers through interaction with multiple cell signaling proteins." *Cancer Lett.*, 269(2): 199-225.

Lasic, D. D., P. M. Frederik, et al. (1992). "Gelation of liposome interior. A novel method for drug encapsulation." *FEBS Lett.,* 312(2-3): 255-258.

Leighton, C., B. Fisher, et al. (2007). "The dose-volume interaction in adult supratentorial low-grade glioma: higher radiation dose is beneficial among patients with partial resection." *J. Neurooncol.*, 82(2): 165-170.

Li, J., C. Yen, et al. (1997). "PTEN, a putative protein tyrosine phosphatase gene mutated in human brain, breast, and prostate cancer." *Science,* 275(5308): 1943-1947.

Li, J. J. and K. D. Zhu (2012). "Spin-based Optomechanics with Carbon Nanotubes." *Sci. Rep.,* 2: 903.

Liu, Y., Q. Wang, et al. (2007). "TGF-beta2 inhibition augments the effect of tumor vaccine and improves the survival of animals with pre-established brain tumors." *J. Neurooncol.,* 81(2): 149-162.

Lo, H. W. (2010). "EGFR-targeted therapy in malignant glioma: novel aspects and mechanisms of drug resistance." *Curr. Mol. Pharmacol.*, 3(1): 37-52.

Louis, D. N., H. Ohgaki, et al. (2007). "The 2007 WHO classification of tumours of the central nervous system." *Acta Neuropathol.*, 114(2): 97-109.

Maheshwari, R. K., A. K. Singh, et al. (2006). "Multiple biological activities of curcumin: a short review." *Life Sci.,* 78(18): 2081-2087.

Maier, D., Z. Zhang, et al. (1998). "Somatic deletion mapping on chromosome 10 and sequence analysis of PTEN/MMAC1 point to the 10q25-26 region as the primary target in low-grade and high-grade gliomas." *Oncogene*, 16(25): 3331-3335.

Maintz, D., K. Fiedler, et al. (1997). "Molecular genetic evidence for subtypes of oligoastrocytomas." *J. Neuropathol. Exp. Neurol.,* 56(10): 1098-1104.

Martinho, O., A. Longatto-Filho, et al. (2009). "Expression, mutation and copy number analysis of platelet-derived growth factor receptor A (PDGFRA) and its ligand PDGFA in gliomas." *Br. J. Cancer*, 101(6): 973-982.

McDermott, U., R. Y. Ames, et al. (2009). "Ligand-dependent platelet-derived growth factor receptor (PDGFR)-alpha activation sensitizes rare lung cancer and sarcoma cells to PDGFR kinase inhibitors." *Cancer Res.,* 69(9): 3937-3946.

Medawar, P. B. (1948). "Immunity to homologous grafted skin; the fate of skin homografts transplanted to the brain, to subcutaneous tissue, and to the anterior chamber of the eye." *Br. J. Exp. Pathol.,* 29(1): 58-69.

Mellinghoff, I. K., M. Y. Wang, et al. (2005). "Molecular determinants of the response of glioblastomas to EGFR kinase inhibitors." *N. Engl. J. Med.*, 353(19): 2012-2024.

Meyer-Puttlitz, B., Y. Hayashi, et al. (1997). "Molecular genetic analysis of giant cell glioblastomas." *Am. J. Pathol.*, 151(3): 853-857.

Meziani, M. J. and Y. P. Sun (2003). "Protein-conjugated nanoparticles from rapid expansion of supercritical fluid solution into aqueous solution." *J. Am. Chem. Soc.*, 125(26): 8015-8018.

Mitchell, D. A., X. Cui, et al. (2011). "Monoclonal antibody blockade of IL-2 receptor alpha during lymphopenia selectively depletes regulatory T cells in mice and humans." *Blood,* 118(11): 3003-3012.

Mizoguchi, M., K. Yoshimoto, et al. (2012). "Molecular characteristics of glioblastoma with 1p/19q co-deletion." *Brain Tumor Pathol.*, 29(3): 148-153.

Morimura, T., C. Neuchrist, et al. (1990). "Monocyte subpopulations in human gliomas: expression of Fc and complement receptors and correlation with tumor proliferation." *Acta Neuropathol.*, 80(3): 287-294.

Motomura, K., M. Mittelbronn, et al. (2012). "DMBT1 homozygous deletion in diffuse astrocytomas is associated with unfavorable clinical outcome." *J. Neuropathol. Exp. Neurol.*, 71(8): 702-707.

Nakamura, M., F. Yang, et al. (2000). "Loss of heterozygosity on chromosome 19 in secondary glioblastomas." *J. Neuropathol. Exp. Neurol.*, 59(6): 539-543.

Narita, Y., M. Nagane, et al. (2002). "Mutant epidermal growth factor receptor signaling down-regulates p27 through activation of the phosphatidylinositol 3-kinase/Akt pathway in glioblastomas." *Cancer Res.,* 62(22): 6764-6769.

Nigro, J. M., S. J. Baker, et al. (1989). "Mutations in the p53 gene occur in diverse human tumour types." *Nature,* 342(6250): 705-708.

Nishikawa, R., X. D. Ji, et al. (1994). "A mutant epidermal growth factor receptor common in human glioma confers enhanced tumorigenicity." *Proc. Natl. Acad. Sci. U S A,* 91(16): 7727-7731.

Norden, A. D., J. Drappatz, et al. (2009). "Antiangiogenic therapies for high-grade glioma." *Nat. Rev. Neurol.*, 5(11): 610-620.

Ohgaki, H., P. Dessen, et al. (2004). "Genetic pathways to glioblastoma: a population-based study." *Cancer Res.,* 64(19): 6892-6899.

Ohgaki, H. and P. Kleihues (2007). "Genetic pathways to primary and secondary glioblastoma." *Am. J. Pathol.*, 170(5): 1445-1453.

Palu, G., A. Cavaggioni, et al. (1999). "Gene therapy of glioblastoma multiforme via combined expression of suicide and cytokine genes: a pilot study in humans." *Gene Ther.,* 6(3): 330-337.

Papahadjopoulos, D., A. Portis, et al. (1978). "Calcium-induced lipid phase transitions and membrane fusion." *Ann. N Y Acad. Sci.,* 308: 50-66.

Parney, I. F., M. A. Farr-Jones, et al. (2000). "Human glioma immunobiology in vitro: implications for immunogene therapy." *Neurosurgery*, 46(5): 1169-1177; discussion 1177-1168.

Parsa, A. T., J. S. Waldron, et al. (2007). "Loss of tumor suppressor PTEN function increases B7-H1 expression and immunoresistance in glioma." *Nat. Med.*, 13(1): 84-88.

Pierscianek, D., Y. H. Kim, et al. (2013). "MET gain in diffuse astrocytomas is associated with poorer outcome." *Brain Pathol.*, 23(1): 13-18.

Pignatti, F., M. van den Bent, et al. (2002). "Prognostic factors for survival in adult patients with cerebral low-grade glioma." *J. Clin. Oncol.*, 20(8): 2076-2084.

Plate, K. H., G. Breier, et al. (1992). "Platelet-derived growth factor receptor-beta is induced during tumor development and upregulated during tumor progression in endothelial cells in human gliomas." *Lab. Invest.,* 67(4): 529-534.

Prins, R. M., G. P. Scott, et al. (2002). "Irradiated tumor cell vaccine for treatment of an established glioma. II. Expansion of myeloid suppressor cells that promote tumor progression." *Cancer Immunol. Immunother.*, 51(4): 190-199.

Puduvalli, V. K., A. P. Kyritsis, et al. (2000). "Patterns of expression of Rb and p16 in astrocytic gliomas, and correlation with survival." *Int. J. Oncol.*, 17(5): 963-969.

Qin, Y., H. Chen, et al. (2011). "Liposome formulated with TAT-modified cholesterol for improving brain delivery and therapeutic efficacy on brain glioma in animals." *Int. J. Pharm.*, 420(2): 304-312.

Ram, Z., K. W. Culver, et al. (1997). "Therapy of malignant brain tumors by intratumoral implantation of retroviral vector-producing cells." *Nat. Med.*, 3(12): 1354-1361.

Rasheed, B. K., R. N. Wiltshire, et al. (1999). "Molecular pathogenesis of malignant gliomas." *Curr. Opin. Oncol.*, 11(3): 162-167.

Ravindran, J., S. Prasad, et al. (2009). "Curcumin and cancer cells: how many ways can curry kill tumor cells selectively?" *AAPS J.*, 11(3): 495-510.

Raychaudhuri, B., P. Rayman, et al. (2011). "Myeloid-derived suppressor cell accumulation and function in patients with newly diagnosed glioblastoma." *Neuro. Oncol.*, 13(6): 591-599.

Reardon, D. A., A. Desjardins, et al. (2011). "Phase II study of metronomic chemotherapy with bevacizumab for recurrent glioblastoma after progression on bevacizumab therapy." *J. Neurooncol.*, 103(2): 371-379.

Reigstad, L. J., J. E. Varhaug, et al. (2005). "Structural and functional specificities of PDGF-C and PDGF-D, the novel members of the platelet-derived growth factors family." *FEBS J.*, 272(22): 5723-5741.

Reijneveld, J. C., M. M. Sitskoorn, et al. (2001). "Cognitive status and quality of life in patients with suspected versus proven low-grade gliomas." *Neurology*, 56(5): 618-623.

Ren, Y., C. S. Kang, et al. (2010). "Co-delivery of as-miR-21 and 5-FU by poly(amidoamine) dendrimer attenuates human glioma cell growth in vitro." *J. Biomater. Sci. Polym. Ed.*, 21(3): 303-314.

Ribom, D., J. Andrae, et al. (2002). "Prognostic value of platelet derived growth factor alpha receptor expression in grade 2 astrocytomas and oligoastrocytomas." *J. Neurol. Neurosurg. Psychiatry*, 72(6): 782-787.

Riemenschneider, M. J. and G. Reifenberger (2009). "Astrocytic tumors." *Recent Results Cancer Res.*, 171: 3-24.

Rogers, L. R., J. P. Rock, et al. (2006). "Results of a phase II trial of the GliaSite radiation therapy system for the treatment of newly diagnosed, resected single brain metastases." *J. Neurosurg.*, 105(3): 375-384.

Rossler, K., C. Neuchrist, et al. (1992). "Expression of leucocyte adhesion molecules at the human blood-brain barrier (BBB)." *J. Neurosci. Res.*, 31(2): 365-374.

Ryman, B. E., R. F. Jewkes, et al. (1978). "Potential applications of liposomes to therapy." *Ann. N Y Acad. Sci.*, 308: 281-307.

Sawamura, Y., H. Abe, et al. (1988). "Isolation and in vitro growth of glioma-infiltrating lymphocytes, and an analysis of their surface phenotypes." *J. Neurosurg.*, 69(5): 745-750.

Sawamura, Y. and N. de Tribolet (1990). "Immunobiology of brain tumors." *Adv. Tech. Stand. Neurosurg.*, 17: 3-64.

Schmidt, A. L., A. L. Brunetto, et al. (2010). "Recent therapeutic advances for treating medulloblastoma: focus on new molecular targets." *CNS Neurol. Disord. Drug Targets,* 9(3): 335-348.

Schrama, D., R. A. Reisfeld, et al. (2006). "Antibody targeted drugs as cancer therapeutics." *Nat. Rev. Drug Discov.,* 5(2): 147-159.

Shand, N., F. Weber, et al. (1999). "A phase 1-2 clinical trial of gene therapy for recurrent glioblastoma multiforme by tumor transduction with the herpes simplex thymidine kinase gene followed by ganciclovir. GLI328 European-Canadian Study Group." *Hum. Gene Ther.*, 10(14): 2325-2335.

Shaw, E., R. Arusell, et al. (2002). "Prospective randomized trial of low- versus high-dose radiation therapy in adults with supratentorial low-grade glioma: initial report of a North

Central Cancer Treatment Group/Radiation Therapy Oncology Group/Eastern Cooperative Oncology Group study." *J. Clin. Oncol.*, 20(9): 2267-2276.

Smith, J. S., I. Tachibana, et al. (2001). "PTEN mutation, EGFR amplification, and outcome in patients with anaplastic astrocytoma and glioblastoma multiforme." *J. Natl. Cancer Inst.*, 93(16): 1246-1256.

Smith, T. C. (1976). "Toleration and bioavailability of gemfibrozil in healthy men." *Proc. R. Soc. Med.*, 69 Suppl. 2: 24-27.

Snuderl, M., L. Fazlollahi, et al. (2011). "Mosaic amplification of multiple receptor tyrosine kinase genes in glioblastoma." *Cancer Cell*, 20(6): 810-817.

Sonabend, A. M., C. E. Rolle, et al. (2008). "The role of regulatory T cells in malignant glioma." *Anticancer Res.*, 28(2B): 1143-1150.

Srividya, M. R., B. Thota, et al. (2011). "Homozygous 10q23/PTEN deletion and its impact on outcome in glioblastoma: a prospective translational study on a uniformly treated cohort of adult patients." *Neuropathology,* 31(4): 376-383.

Stavrou, D., A. P. Anzil, et al. (1977). "Immunofluorescence study of lymphocytic infiltration in gliomas. Identification of T-lymphocytes." *J. Neurol. Sci.*, 33(1-2): 275-282.

Stewart, P. A., M. Magliocco, et al. (1987). "A quantitative analysis of blood-brain barrier ultrastructure in the aging human." *Microvasc. Res.*, 33(2): 270-282.

Stupp, R., J. C. Tonn, et al. (2010). "High-grade malignant glioma: ESMO Clinical Practice Guidelines for diagnosis, treatment and follow-up." *Ann. Oncol.*, 21 Suppl. 5: v190-193.

Szerlip, N. J., A. Pedraza, et al. (2012). "Intratumoral heterogeneity of receptor tyrosine kinases EGFR and PDGFRA amplification in glioblastoma defines subpopulations with distinct growth factor response." *Proc. Natl. Acad. Sci. U S A*, 109(8): 3041-3046.

Tan, M., X. Wu, et al. (2010). "Peptide-targeted Nanoglobular Gd-DOTA monoamide conjugates for magnetic resonance cancer molecular imaging." *Biomacromolecules,* 11(3): 754-761.

Tatter, S. B., E. G. Shaw, et al. (2003). "An inflatable balloon catheter and liquid 125I radiation source (GliaSite Radiation Therapy System) for treatment of recurrent malignant glioma: multicenter safety and feasibility trial." *J. Neurosurg.*, 99(2): 297-303.

Thomas, D. L., D. M. Kranz, et al. (2008). "Experimental manipulations of afferent immune responses influence efferent immune responses to brain tumors." *Cancer Immunol. Immunother.*, 57(9): 1323-1333.

Tohma, Y., C. Gratas, et al. (1998). "PTEN (MMAC1) mutations are frequent in primary glioblastomas (de novo) but not in secondary glioblastomas." *J. Neuropathol. Exp. Neurol.*, 57(7): 684-689.

Tran, T. T., M. Uhl, et al. (2007). "Inhibiting TGF-beta signaling restores immune surveillance in the SMA-560 glioma model." *Neuro. Oncol.*, 9(3): 259-270.

Ueki, K., Y. Ono, et al. (1996). "CDKN2/p16 or RB alterations occur in the majority of glioblastomas and are inversely correlated." *Cancer Res.,* 56(1): 150-153.

Umemura, N., M. Saio, et al. (2008). "Tumor-infiltrating myeloid-derived suppressor cells are pleiotropic-inflamed monocytes/macrophages that bear M1- and M2-type characteristics." *J. Leukoc. Biol.*, 83(5): 1136-1144.

Ushio, Y., K. Tada, et al. (2003). "Correlation of molecular genetic analysis of p53, MDM2, p16, PTEN, and EGFR and survival of patients with anaplastic astrocytoma and glioblastoma." *Front. Biosci.*, 8: e281-288.

Vallhov, H., S. Gabrielsson, et al. (2007). "Mesoporous silica particles induce size dependent effects on human dendritic cells." *Nano Lett.,* 7(12): 3576-3582.

van den Bent, M. J., O. Chinot, et al. (2003). "Second-line chemotherapy with temozolomide in recurrent oligodendroglioma after PCV (procarbazine, lomustine and vincristine) chemotherapy: EORTC Brain Tumor Group phase II study 26972." *Ann. Oncol.*, 14(4): 599-602.

van den Bent, M. J., F. Keime-Guibert, et al. (2001). "Temozolomide chemotherapy in recurrent oligodendroglioma." *Neurology,* 57(2): 340-342.

Varela, M., S. M. Ranuncolo, et al. (2004). "EGF-R and PDGF-R, but not bcl-2, overexpression predict overall survival in patients with low-grade astrocytomas." *J. Surg. Oncol.*, 86(1): 34-40.

Vredenburgh, J. J., A. Desjardins, et al. (2007). "Phase II trial of bevacizumab and irinotecan in recurrent malignant glioma." *Clin. Cancer Res.,* 13(4): 1253-1259.

Wainwright, D. A., P. Nigam, et al. (2012). "Recent developments on immunotherapy for brain cancer." *Expert Opin. Emerg. Drugs,* 17(2): 181-202.

Watanabe, K., A. Peraud, et al. (1998). "p53 and PTEN gene mutations in gemistocytic astrocytomas." *Acta Neuropathol.*, 95(6): 559-564.

Watanabe, K., O. Tachibana, et al. (1996). "Overexpression of the EGF receptor and p53 mutations are mutually exclusive in the evolution of primary and secondary glioblastomas." *Brain Pathol.*, 6(3): 217-223; discussion 223-214.

Watanabe, T., S. Nobusawa, et al. (2009). "IDH1 mutations are early events in the development of astrocytomas and oligodendrogliomas." *Am. J. Pathol.*, 174(4): 1149-1153.

Watters, J. J., J. M. Schartner, et al. (2005). "Microglia function in brain tumors." *J. Neurosci. Res.,* 81(3): 447-455.

Weber, R. G., M. Sabel, et al. (1996). "Characterization of genomic alterations associated with glioma progression by comparative genomic hybridization." *Oncogene,* 13(5): 983-994.

Weller, M., J. Felsberg, et al. (2009). "Molecular predictors of progression-free and overall survival in patients with newly diagnosed glioblastoma: a prospective translational study of the German Glioma Network." *J. Clin. Oncol.*, 27(34): 5743-5750.

Westphal, M., Z. Ram, et al. (2006). "Gliadel wafer in initial surgery for malignant glioma: long-term follow-up of a multicenter controlled trial." *Acta Neurochir.,* (Wien) 148(3): 269-275; discussion 275.

Wiener, E. C., M. W. Brechbiel, et al. (1994). "Dendrimer-based metal chelates: a new class of magnetic resonance imaging contrast agents." *Magn. Reson. Med.*, 31(1): 1-8.

Wikstrand, C. J., L. P. Hale, et al. (1995). "Monoclonal antibodies against EGFRvIII are tumor specific and react with breast and lung carcinomas and malignant gliomas." *Cancer Res.,* 55(14): 3140-3148.

Wong, A. J., J. M. Ruppert, et al. (1992). "Structural alterations of the epidermal growth factor receptor gene in human gliomas." *Proc. Natl. Acad. Sci. U S A*, 89(7): 2965-2969.

Xiang, Y., L. Liang, et al. (2011). "Chloride channel-mediated brain glioma targeting of chlorotoxin-modified doxorubicine-loaded liposomes." *J. Control. Release*, 152(3): 402-410.

Xu, W., H. Yang, et al. (2011). "Oncometabolite 2-hydroxyglutarate is a competitive inhibitor of alpha-ketoglutarate-dependent dioxygenases." *Cancer Cell*, 19(1): 17-30.

Yan, H., D. W. Parsons, et al. (2009). "IDH1 and IDH2 mutations in gliomas." *N. Engl. J. Med.,* 360(8): 765-773.

Yan, H., J. Wang, et al. (2011). "Imaging brain tumor by dendrimer-based optical/paramagnetic nanoprobe across the blood-brain barrier." *Chem. Commun. (Camb),* 47(28): 8130-8132.

Young, M. R., M. Newby, et al. (1987). "Hematopoiesis and suppressor bone marrow cells in mice bearing large metastatic Lewis lung carcinoma tumors." *Cancer Res.,* 47 (1): 100-105.

Yung, W. K., M. D. Prados, et al. (1999). "Multicenter phase II trial of temozolomide in patients with anaplastic astrocytoma or anaplastic oligoastrocytoma at first relapse. Temodal Brain Tumor Group." *J. Clin. Oncol.,* 17(9): 2762-2771.

Zarghooni, M., U. Bartels, et al. (2010). "Whole-genome profiling of pediatric diffuse intrinsic pontine gliomas highlights platelet-derived growth factor receptor alpha and poly (ADP-ribose) polymerase as potential therapeutic targets." *J. Clin. Oncol.*, 28(8): 1337-1344.

Zhao, S., Y. Lin, et al. (2009). "Glioma-derived mutations in IDH1 dominantly inhibit IDH1 catalytic activity and induce HIF-1alpha." *Science*, 324(5924): 261-265.

Zhu, J. J., T. Santarius, et al. (1998). "Screening for loss of heterozygosity and microsatellite instability in oligodendrogliomas." *Genes Chromosomes Cancer*, 21(3): 207-216.

Zlatescu, M. C., A. TehraniYazdi, et al. (2001). "Tumor location and growth pattern correlate with genetic signature in oligodendroglial neoplasms." *Cancer Res.,* 61(18): 6713-6715.

Zuniga, R. M., R. Torcuator, et al. (2010). "Rebound tumour progression after the cessation of bevacizumab therapy in patients with recurrent high-grade glioma." *J. Neurooncol.,* 99 (2): 237-242.

In: Gliomas: Classification, Symptoms, Treatment and Prognosis ISBN: 978-1-63117-868-9
Editor: David Cory Adamson

Chapter 2

Brainstem Gliomas

Zhiping Zhou*
Department of Neurological Surgery
Weill Medical College of Cornell University
New York, NY, US

Abstract

Brainstem gliomas are a heterogeneous group of tumors occurring in the brainstem. They occur more often in children than in adults. Based on the location, focality and growth patterns, they are classified into four groups: focal gliomas (tectal and other locations), dorsal exophytic gliomas, cervicomedullary gliomas and diffuse intrinsic pontine gliomas (DIPG). DIPG accounts for approximately 80% of all brainstem gliomas.

Brainstem gliomas are typically astrocytomas. Focal, dorsal exophytic and cervicomedullary gliomas are usually pilocytic astrocytoma (WHO grade I) and fibrillary astrocytoma (WHO grade II). Other low-grade gliomas with indolent growth are also seen. DIPGs are typically anaplastic astrocytoma (WHO grade III) and glioblastoma multiforme (WHO grade IV).

There are significant advances in the last a few years concerning the molecular genetics of brainstem gliomas. DIPGs are genetically complex and distinct from both adult and pediatric supratentorial high-grade gliomas (HGG). The most notable commonly mutated genes in DIPGs include platelet-derived growth factors (PDGF) and their receptors (PDGFR), and recurrent adenine-to-thymine transversions in the H3F3A gene encoding a lysine-to-methionine missense at position 27 (K27M) of histone H3.3. The most notable mutations in nondiffuse brainstem gliomas occur in the BRAF gene.

The clinical behavior and presentation of brainstem gliomas are highly variable, depending on the anatomic location and pattern of growth of the tumor, age of the patient and certain other factors. Initial presentation is usually a combination of cranial neuropathies, long tract signs, signs and symptoms of increased intracranial pressure, and ataxia. Diagnosis of brainstem gliomas is based on clinical presentation and imaging studies, and needs to address the location and nature of the lesion. MRI is the preferred imaging modality.

* Zhiping Zhou, MD, PhD, Email: zhz2004@med.cornell.edu.

Brainstem glioma patients are treated by a multidisciplinary team including neurosurgeons, non-surgical specialists and other therapists. Treatment includes management of pain, bulbar symptoms and motor impairment, relief of hydrocephalus and general support. Some nondiffuse brainstem gliomas are amenable to surgical resection while DIPGs are unresectable. The outcomes of brainstem gliomas depend on the location and pathological grade of the tumors. Focal, dorsal exophytic and cervicomedullary gliomas typically have fairly good prognoses. In contrast, the median survival of DIPG patients is only about one year despite numerous investigational therapies.

Introduction

Brainstem gliomas are a heterogeneous group of tumors occurring in the brainstem and cervicomedullary junction. They occur more often in children than in adults. Brainstem tumors, according to data prior to early 1980s, represent 10-20% of all central nervous system neoplasms in the pediatric population (Panitch and Berg, 1970; Farwell et al., 1977; Albright et al., 1983). Approximately 90% of brainstem tumors are gliomas in origin (Pierre-Kahn et al., 1993).

Diffuse intrinsic pontine glioma (DIPG) is the most common type representing approximately 80% of brainstem gliomas (Freeman and Farmer, 1998; Hargrave et al., 2006). They have a dismal prognosis with a median survival of only a year. Their natural history is often compared to but worse than that of supratentorial glioblastoma seen primarily in the adult population. Nondiffuse brainstem gliomas, including focal, dorsal exophytic and cervicomedullary gliomas, are encountered less often and have a better prognosis. However, if untreated, they could also lead to progressive brainstem dysfunction and ultimately death.

Epidemiology

True incidence studies of brainstem gliomas are lacking. According to the Central Brain Tumor Registry of the United States, there were 400-450 cases of brainstem gliomas in children under the age of 19 years old per year between 2006 and 2010 in the U.S., representing 10.4% of primary central nervous system tumors (Ostrom et al., 2013). This number is higher than those previously estimated for the period between 1970s and 1990s (Smith et al., 1998). The increase is thought primarily to be a result of increased detection by the use of magnetic resonance imaging (MRI) and better data reporting as opposed to a true increase in the incidence of these tumors.

The most common age at diagnosis for DIPG is 5-9 years old with a median of 6.5 years, but cases have been seen in all age groups from infants to adults (Kaplan et al., 1996; Freeman and Farmer, 1998). Nondiffuse brainstem gliomas have roughly the same age distribution.

Neurofibromatosis type 1 (NF1) patients have higher incidence of brainstem gliomas. These tumors, whether diffuse or nondiffuse, appear to have a more benign course compared with tumors from patients without NF1 (Ullrich et al., 2007).

There does not appear to be a sex predilection in any of the brainstem tumor subgroups (Kaplan et al., 1996; Freeman and Farmer, 1998). Because of the low incidence and lack of diagnosis in less developed countries, there is not sufficient data to determine if there is a geographic propensity. No specific risk factors, either environmental or infectious, have been described to be related to the incidence of brainstem gliomas.

Classification

Brainstem gliomas are classified based on their location, focality and growth patterns. Classification systems were created using the current form of imaging available. Brainstem gliomas can be broadly categorized as diffuse intrinsic pontine glioma (DIPG) and nondiffuse brainstem gliomas. Nondiffuse brainstem gliomas can be further classified into three groups: focal gliomas (tectal and other locations), dorsal exophytic gliomas and cervicomedullary gliomas.

DIPG accounts for approximately 80% of brainstem gliomas in children (Freeman and Farmer, 1998; Hargrave et al., 2006). Surgical resection is not possible due to the location and infiltrative nature of the tumor. The standard of care for DIPG is radiation therapy. They have a median survival of about 10-12 months (Hargrave et al., 2006).

Focal gliomas account for about 5% of brainstem gliomas in children. They may be located anywhere within the brainstem but are rarely in the ventral pons. Most focal gliomas occur in the midbrain, especially the tectum of the midbrain. Focal gliomas in other areas of the brainstem, such as the medulla, are less often seen. As a result, most discussions about focal gliomas focus on tectal gliomas. Focal gliomas have well defined margins. They usually have an indolent course, and depending on location, may be amenable to surgical resection. The majority of tectal glioma patients have non-communicating hydrocephalus at initial presentation due to compression of the cerebral aqueduct. Focal gliomas have a good prognosis (Robertson et al., 1995).

Dorsal exophytic gliomas account for 10-15% of brainstem gliomas in children. They present insidiously with a long history of nonspecific headache and vomiting. They are often amenable to surgical resection. These tumors have a good outcome after surgical resection (Pollack et al., 1993).

Cervicomedullary gliomas account for 5-10% of brainstem gliomas in children. They arise from the lower medulla or the upper cervical spinal cord. They may be amenable to surgical resection if primarily exophytic and mostly near the surface. These may have extensions into the cerebellar peduncles and cerebellum. Long-term tumor control can be achieved in most patients with surgical resection alone (Weiner et al., 1997; Young Poussaint et al., 1999).

Pathology and Pathophysiology

Brainstem gliomas are typically astrocytomas. Focal, dorsal exophytic and cervicomedullary gliomas are usually pilocytic astrocytomas (WHO grade I) and fibrillary astrocytomas (WHO grade II). Other more rare low-grade gliomas with indolent growth patterns such as ganglioglioma are also seen. DIPGs are typically anaplastic astrocytomas (WHO grade III) or glioblastoma multiforme (WHO grade IV). Growth of low-grade gliomas typically respect fiber tracts and pial borders. In contrast, high-grade gliomas grow and expand without respecting anatomic boundaries of these surrounding tissues.

70-90% of DIPGs are anaplastic astrocytoma (WHO grade III) and glioblastoma multiforme (WHO grade IV) if biopsied before radiation therapy is given (Cartmill and Punt, 1999; Wolff et al., 2008; Wolff et al., 2010). The remainders are mainly fibrillary astrocytoma (WHO grade II). At a later stage, invasion of adjacent levels of the brainstem and cerebellar peduncles is common. At autopsy, the vast majority of DIPGs are high-grade and more than 50% have disseminated within the neuraxis (Sethi et al., 2011).

Most focal gliomas are low-grade (Hoffman et al., 1980; Robertson et al., 1995). Low-grade gliomas seen in this subgroup include pilocytic astrocytoma, fibrillary astrocytoma and ganglioglioma. Most tectal gliomas cause hydrocephalus at an early stage due to compression on the cerebral aqueduct.

Dorsal exophytic gliomas arise from subependymal glial tissue. Over 90% of these tumors are pilocytic astrocytomas (Khatib et al., 1994) that grow along the path of least resistance. As a result, most of the tumor extends into the fourth ventricle rather than infiltrating the brainstem ventrally. Tumors that extend laterally and/or ventrally into the brainstem are usually more aggressive and of higher grade on pathological examination.

Cervicomedullary gliomas arise from either the lower medulla or upper cervical spinal cord. Most of them are low-grade astrocytomas, but gangliogliomas and ependymomas are also seen (Epstein and Farmer, 1993; Weiner et al., 1997). Tumors with epicenters in the upper cervical cord grow dorsally into the cisterna magna. Those with epicenters in the lower medulla grow centrifugally as focal nodules.

Molecular Genetics

Partially because of the low incidence of brainstem gliomas, their molecular genetics is less studied compared with some more common primary central nervous system tumors. However, there are some significant advances in the last a few years concerning the molecular genetics of both DIPG and focal brainstem gliomas.

DIPGs are genetically complex and distinct from both adult and pediatric supratentorial high-grade gliomas (HGG). Recent evidence points to platelet-derived growth factor (PDGF) and its receptors (PDGFR) as among the major driving forces of tumorigenesis in the majority of cases (Becher et al., 2010; Paugh et al., 2010; Zarghooni et al., 2010; Paugh et al., 2011; Puget et al., 2012). Another growth factor receptor, epidermal growth factor receptor (EGFR), shows strong immunohistochemistry staining in about 27% of cases (Zarghooni et al., 2010), and amplification of the gene at a rate of 7-9% (Zarghooni et al., 2010; Paugh et al., 2011). Unlike the case in pediatric supratentorial HGG, *CDKN2A* deletion is non-existent (Barrow et al., 2011; Paugh et al., 2011) or only occurs at a low rate (3%) (Puget et al., 2012) in DIPG. Amplification of *CDK4* and *CDK6* in DIPG occurs at a rate of 7% and 11.6%, respectively (Paugh et al., 2011). Approximately 50% of DIPG have *TP53* mutations (Zhang et al., 1993; Badhe et al., 2004) and three groups report loss of a region of 17p containing the *TP53* gene in 31%, 57% and 64% of cases, respectively (Louis et al., 1993; Zarghooni et al.,

2010; Barrow et al., 2011). In approximately 50% of DIPG patients, allelic loss of a region of 10q where the *PTEN* gene is located is observed (Louis et al., 1993; Cheng et al., 1999; Cheng and Wu, 1999).

Histone H3, which forms part of the nucleosome core, plays an essential role in the epigenetic regulation of DNA replication and gene transcription. Recent studies of histone mutations indicate DIPGs are also epigenetically distinct from pediatric supratentorial HGG. Recurrent adenine-to-thymine transversions in the *H3F3A* gene, encoding a lysine-to-methionine missense at position 27 (K27M) of histone H3.3, is seen in 60-75% of DIPGs (Khuong-Quang et al., 2012; Wu et al., 2012), significantly higher than that in pediatric supratentorial glioblastoma multiforme (GBM) (14-19%) (Schwartzentruber et al., 2012; Wu et al., 2012). The *H3F3A* mutation is not present in the matching germline DNA samples (Wu et al., 2012), suggesting its somatic nature. The K27M mutation is found in 66-77% of pretreatment DIPG samples (Khuong-Quang et al., 2012; Wu et al., 2012), indicating that it is not the result of a selection or mutation process secondary to therapies.

In contrast to the H3.3K27M mutation profiles, a guanine-to-adenine transition in *H3F3A*, resulting in a glycine-to-arginine missense at position 34 (G34R) of H3.3, is identified in 10-14% of pediatric supratentorial GBMs (Schwartzentruber et al., 2012; Wu et al., 2012) but not in any of the 90 DIPG samples analyzed by two groups (Khuong-Quang et al., 2012; Wu et al., 2012).

The presence of mutations in the *HIST1H3B* gene, which encodes histone H3.1, is less conclusive. One study found that the adenine-to-thymine transversion that encodes the K27M missense was present in 18% (9/50) of DIPGs (Wu et al., 2012), whereas another group did not detect the mutation in any of their DIPG samples (0/27) (Khuong-Quang et al., 2012).

There have been fewer molecular genetic studies of nondiffuse brainstem gliomas. Similar to what was seen in the cerebellum and cerebral hemispheres, recently it was reported that *BRAF* gene mutation are often observed in pediatric pilocytic astrocytomas located in the brainstem. These mutations include *BRAF-KIAA1549* fusion (Forshew et al., 2009; Yu et al., 2009; Hawkins et al., 2011; Horbinski et al., 2012), V600E point mutation (Schindler et al., 2011) and some less frequent mutations. *BRAF-KIAA1549* fusion occurs at a rate of 47-63% in brainstem pilocytic astrocytomas (Yu et al., 2009; Hawkins et al., 2011).

Clinical Presentation

The clinical behavior and presentation of brainstem gliomas are highly variable, depending on the anatomic location and pattern of growth of the tumor, age of the patient and certain other factors. Symptom evolution reflects aggressiveness of the tumor. Low-grade tumors typically present with an insidious course over several months of gradual symptom progression. By comparison, a shorter and more abrupt onset of symptoms is indicative of higher-grade tumors.

Nondiffuse gliomas are often low-grade lesions with expectedly slow growth. Symptoms are insidious in onset and may not be readily appreciated. Careful history taking, including comparison to photographs, may be necessary to evaluate subtle changes associated with cranial nerve dysfunction in these slow-growing tumors. DIPGs, in comparison, typically present with a short prodrome of symptoms (usually 1-2 months or shorter) (Kaplan et al., 1996).

In brainstem gliomas, the pattern of symptoms reflects the extent of the tumor. Diffusely growing tumors are associated with multiple and bilateral cranial neuropathies, long tract signs and ataxia. Hydrocephalus in these tumors is uncommon at initial presentation. Nondiffuse gliomas often present with isolated cranial neuropathies, signs and symptoms of increased intracranial pressure, and ataxia. Rarely, hemiparesis may be part of the clinical presentation.

Brainstem glioma patients can have a combination of the following at presentation. Cranial neuropathies are common in most tumors of the brainstem. Simultaneous involvement of multiple cranial nerves is more frequently encountered with diffuse lesions. Focal lesions, in contrast, are often associated with more limited cranial nerve involvement. Midbrain involvement is often associated with oculomotor deficits, and lesions of the lower brainstem are frequently found to have lower cranial nerve involvement resulting in changes in voice, dysphagia and/or aspiration pneumonias.

Long tract signs, including motor dysfunction and hyperreflexia, are most often associated with diffusely growing tumors or focal tumors of the cervicomedullary junction. Long tract signs are often conspicuously absent with dorsal exophytic gliomas (Pollack et al., 1993).

In brainstem glioma patients, ataxia can be a result of loss of proprioceptive sensation, CN VIII involvement and/or invasion of cerebellar peduncles by the tumor. Ataxia is frequently seen in DIPG patients.

Obstructive hydrocephalus is usually the first sign seen in focal tectal gliomas as a result of the tumor compressing the cerebral aqueduct. Hydrocephalus and its associated signs and symptoms are also often seen in dorsal exophytic gliomas which grow dorsally into the fourth ventricle resulting in the obstruction of normal cerebrospinal fluid (CSF) flow.

Failure to thrive is commonly encountered in infants with tumors of the cervicomedullary junction due to lower cranial nerve dysfunction resulting in swallowing difficulties.

Diffuse Intrinsic Pontine Gliomas

DIPG patients usually have an acute onset and present with a history of rapid deterioration of 1-2 months or even shorter. Physical examination reveals classic brainstem signs: cranial nerve deficits, long tract signs and ataxia, or combinations of the three. At least two of the triad need to be present along with MRI evidence to establish the diagnosis of DIPG.

Bilateral and multiple cranial nerve involvement is frequent in DIPG. Abducens (CN VI) palsy is the most frequent cranial neuropathy at presentation (Freeman and Farmer, 1998). Facial palsy is also frequently seen at initial presentation. Involvement of CN VIII causes deafness and contributes to ataxia. Lower cranial nerve involvement causes aspiration, and difficulty in speech, swallowing and maintaining normal head positions.

These children often present with severe limb weakness and hyperreflexia, resulting in their difficulty to walk and sometimes even to sit. Long tract involvement also causes loss of tactile, nociceptive and proprioceptive sensations, causing numbness and contributing to ataxia.

In DIPG patients, both CN VIII involvement and loss of proprioceptive sensation contribute to ataxia. Invasion of cerebellar peduncles is also common in DIPG, which is another factor contributing to ataxia.

DIPG patients may also have other symptoms including headache, nausea and vomiting etc. indicating increased intracranial pressure from edema or hydrocephalus. Approximately 10% of DIPG patients have hydrocephalus at initial presentation (Freeman and Farmer, 1998).

Focal Gliomas

Focal gliomas can occur anywhere in the brainstem, but rarely in the vental pons. Their clinical presentations depend on the location.

Focal tectal gliomas have an insidious clinical course and often compress on the cerebral aqueduct to cause a non-communicating hydrocephalus (Robertson et al., 1995; Bowers et al., 2000). As a result the initial presentation is usually those signs reflecting increased intracranial pressure: headache, vomiting, diplopia and papilledema.

Focal gliomas in the midbrain tegmentum and the medulla are usually larger than tectal gliomas and present with cranial nerve dysfunction, long tract signs and ataxia (Robertson et al., 1995; Ueoka et al., 2009).

Dorsal Exophytic Gliomas

Dorsal exophytic gliomas grow into the fourth ventricle and typically present with signs and symptoms of increased intracranial pressure including headache, nausea and/or vomiting, lethargy, downward gaze preference, changes in vision and cranial nerve palsies (including abducens palsy). Infants with these tumors may present primarily with failure to thrive. Long tract signs are rare with these tumors (Pollack et al., 1993).

Cervicomedullary Gliomas

Cervicomedullary gliomas usually have an indolent course because the majority of these tumors are slow growing low-grade lesions. Two presenting syndromes have been described based on the epicenter of these tumors (Epstein and Wisoff, 1987). Medullary syndrome often presents as a failure to thrive secondary to nausea, vomiting or dysphagia. Also seen with this syndrome are sleep apnea, dysarthria and recurrent upper respiratory tract infections. Cervical cord syndrome presents with progressive myelopathy with spasticity and weakness. Hydrocephalus is unusual in cervicomedullary gliomas.

Imaging Studies

Diagnosis of brainstem gliomas is based on clinical presentations and imaging studies. MRI is the imaging method of choice because of its high resolution and ability to differentiate the nature of lesions (tumor vs. inflammation etc.), which is especially important in the diagnosis of DIPG.

MRI enables identification of important anatomic features and localization of tumors with multi-planar views. It allows a precise evaluation of the growth pattern and accurate preoperative diagnosis in most cases. Both T1- and T2-weighted axial and sagittal sequences should be obtained for the basic studies.

Other useful sequences include fluid attenuated inversion recovery (FLAIR), diffusion tensor imaging (DTI), gradient echo (GRE) and susceptibility weighted imaging (SWI). DTI tractography may be useful in evaluating the relationship between the tumor and white matter tracts (Helton et al., 2008), which can be a part of the preoperative planning for nondiffuse brainstem gliomas.

Diffuse Intrinsic Pontine Gliomas

DIPGs are diagnosed with clinical presentation and magnetic resonance imaging. Since the publication of the Children's Cancer Group (CCG) report in 1993 (Albright et al., 1993), when a brainstem tumor presents with typical symptoms and radiological appearance, it is usually considered that these findings are diagnostic and a biopsy is rarely performed. If, however, the clinical or radiological presentation is not typical, where brainstem encephalitis or an inflammatory process of the pons cannot be ruled out, a stereotactic biopsy would be needed before initiating radiation therapy and/or chemotherapy.

DIPGs infiltrate widely (Figure 1). MRI scans show infiltrative expansion of the pons that is typically hypointense on T1-weighted, hyperintense on T2-weighted and FLAIR images, and has no significant dorsal exophytic component. Involvement of adjacent levels of the brainstem and/or cerebellar peduncles is common. Envelopment of the basilar artery is commonly present in DIPG showing the tumor growing ventrally outside of the boundary of the brainstem. Contrast enhancement with gadolinium is variable, with no enhancement being common (Mauffrey, 2006).

Enhancement, if present, is usually patchy, without known prognostic significance. Neuraxis dissemination of DIPG can be seen on MRI in more than 50% of patients during progression (Sethi et al., 2011). In some cases the tumor may show atypical features including prominent enhancement and/or hypointense T2-weighted/FLAIR signals.

Magnetic resonance spectroscopy (MRS) is helpful in the differential diagnosis when the tumor shows atypical features. Increased Cho/NAA (choline/N-acetyl aspartate) and Cho/Cr (choline/creatine) ratios in DIPG are useful in differentiating it from brainstem encephalitis, demyelination and other inflammatory processes when clinical and MRI presentations are atypical (Thakur et al., 2006; Porto et al., 2007).

However, the differentiating power of MRS is limited in NF1-associated DIPG (Porto et al., 2007).

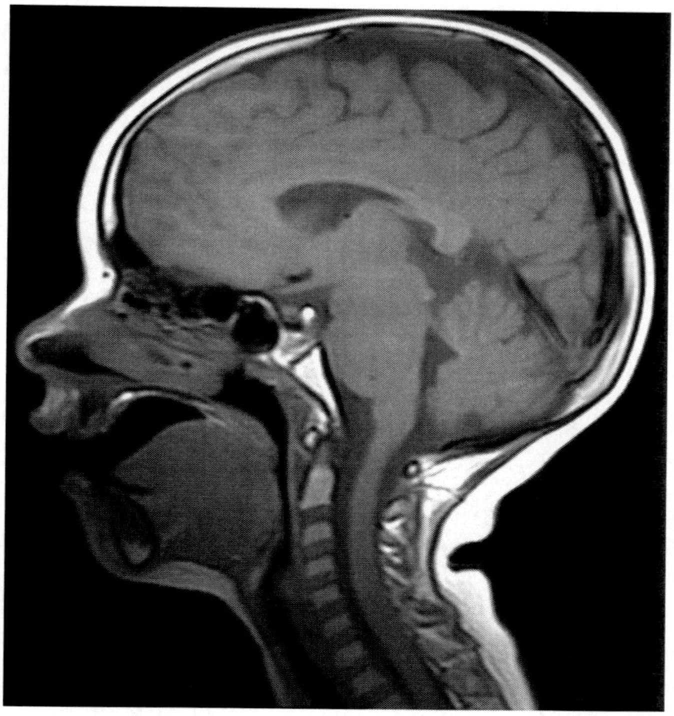

A

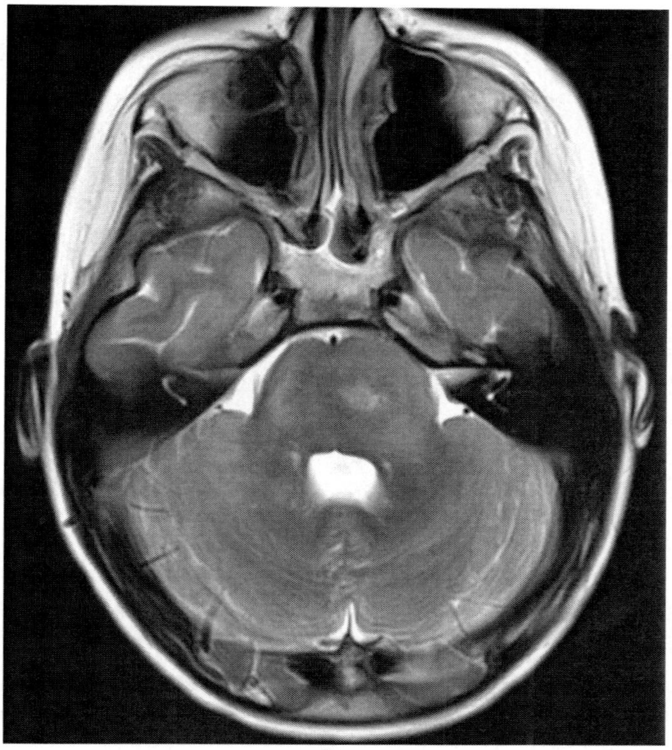

B

Figure 1. (Continued)

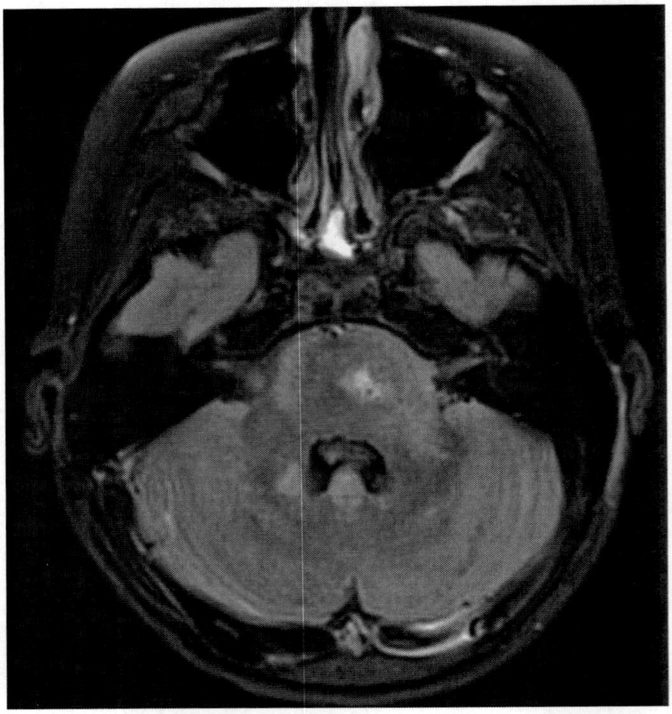

C

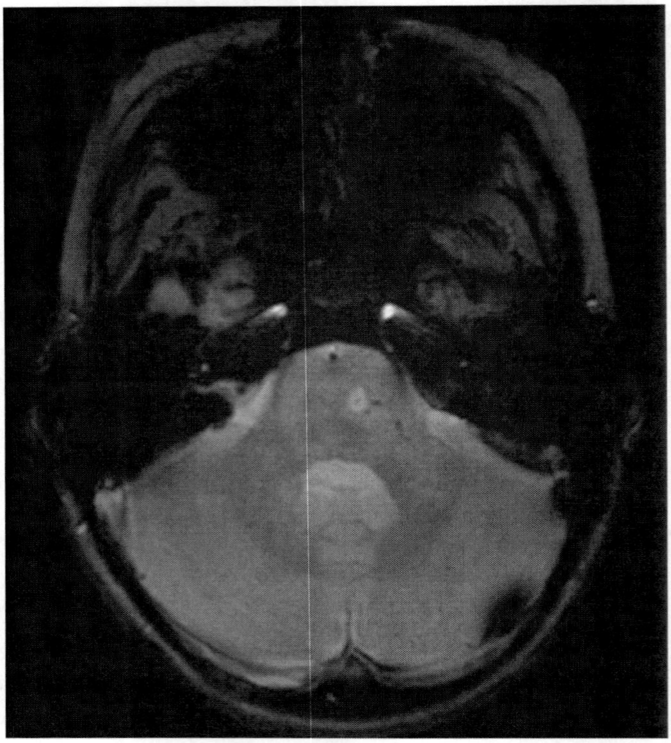

D

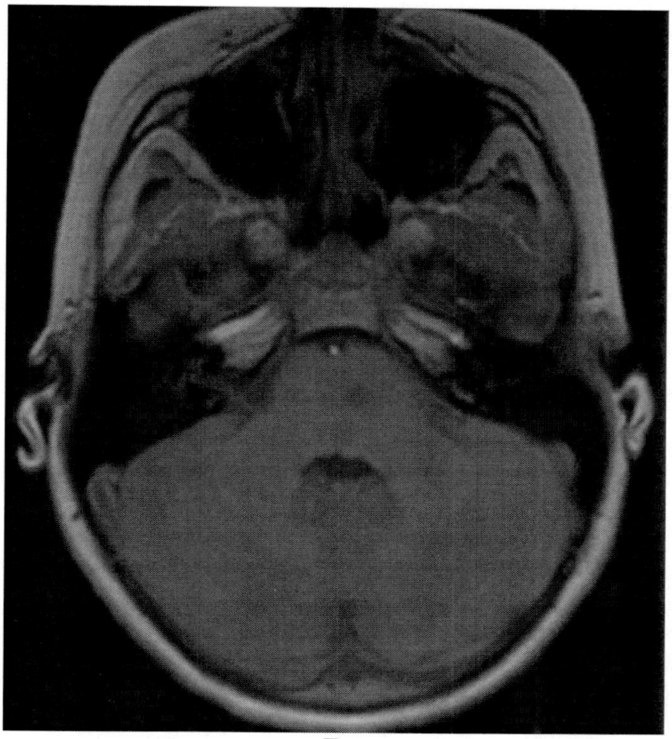

E

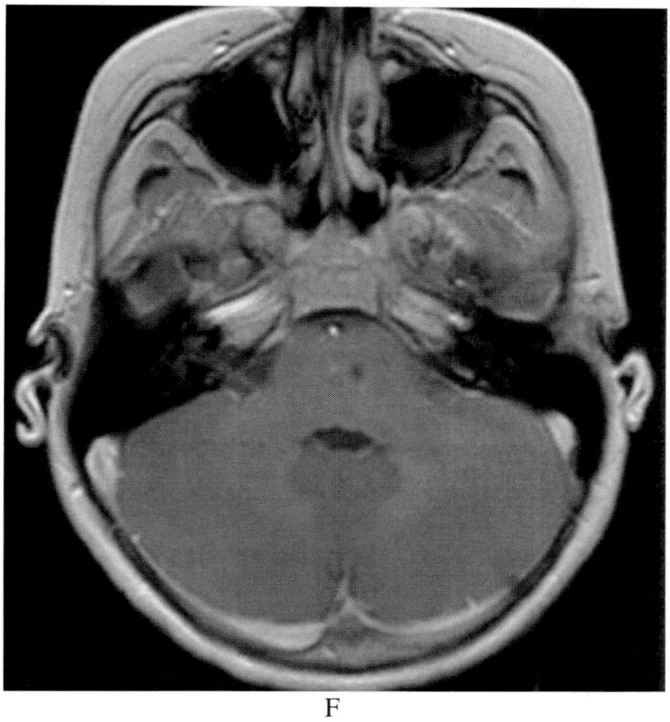

F

Figure 1. (Continued)

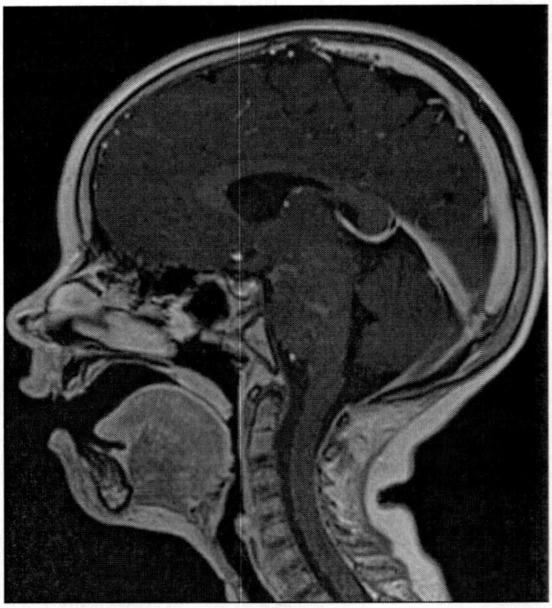

G

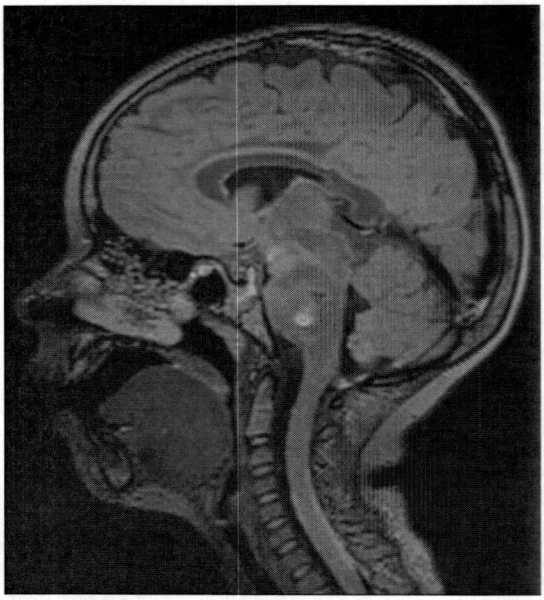

H

Figure 1. Imaging Presentation of a DIPG. These representative images were acquired from the same patient in one study. Note the heterogeneity of the tumor and the small cysts presumably from necrosis of the tumor core. **A.** T1-weighted image sagittal view shows the ventral expansion of the pons. **B.** T2-weighted image, axial view. Note the diffuse border between the tumor and the surrounding brain tissue, making it essentially impossible to pinpoint its location. **C.** FLAIR image, axial view. Note the diffuse border. **D.** T2*-weighted image, axial view. **E.** T1-weighted FLAIR image, axial view, pre-contrast. **F.** T1-weighted FLAIR image, axial view, post-contrast. Note the enhancement around the cyst. **G.** 3D T1-weighted image, sagittal view, post-contrast. Note the patchy enhancement inside the tumor. **H.** 3D FLAIR image, sagittal view, post-contrast. Note the ring enhancement.

Focal Gliomas

Before the availability of computed tomography (CT) and MRI for the diagnosis of intracranial lesions, focal tectal gliomas could only be found in autopsy evaluations. In the 1950s, when CSF diversion procedures were not as universally successful as of today, Kernohan and Sayre stated that tectal gliomas were "in all probability the smallest tumors in the human body that lead to the death of the patient (Kernohan and Sayre, 1952)."

Focal gliomas are focal lesions on MRI. Focal tectal gliomas are usually isointense on MRI and show up as a thickened tectal plate. Tectal gliomas rarely enhance with gadolinium (Robertson et al., 1995; Bowers et al., 2000). Central calcification may be noted rarely (Daglioglu et al., 2003). Hydrocephalus is seen in the vast majority of tectal gliomas, causing symptoms for which the patients are seeking medical attention.

Focal gliomas in other areas of the brainstem are usually hypointense on T1-weighted and hyperintense on T2-weighted images. The margins are well defined in focal tegmentum and medullary gliomas, and most are more or less round or spherical. They are frequently cystic with an intense rim enhancement after intravenous contrast agent administration. Most midbrain focal gliomas show upward extension to the thalamus and downward extension to the pons.

Dorsal Exophytic Gliomas

Dorsal exophytic gliomas typically erupt through the pia/ependyma early in their growth, so imaging will show the bulk of tumor outside of the brainstem. Imaging of patients suspected of dorsal exophytic gliomas should include MRI studies with and without intravenous gadolinium of the brain to differentiate this type of tumor from tumors in the fourth ventricle such as primitive neuroectodermal tumors (PNETs). On MRI, dorsal exophytic gliomas appear as a dorsal exophytic expansion into the fourth ventricle or below the cerebellum. They usually demonstrate sharply demarcated hypointense signals on T1-weighted and hyperintense on T2-weighted images. Bright homogeneous contrast enhancement and hydrocephalus are common MRI findings (Khatib et al., 1994).

Cervicomedullary Gliomas

Imaging of patients suspected cervicomedullary gliomas should include MRI studies with and without intravenous gadolinium of the brain and cervical spine to determine the extent of tumor growth and involvement.

Cervicomedullary gliomas arise from either the lower medulla or upper cervical spinal cord. The growth pattern of the tumor will give some hints as to their epicenters and what structures are being placed at risk by tumor growth. Tumors with epicenters in the upper cervical cord will have their rostral growth blocked by the decussating fibers of the sensory and motor pathways. Instead, the tumor curves dorsally to grow into the cisterna magna at the cervicomedullary junction. Tumors with epicenters in the lower medulla grow centrifugally as focal nodules pushing the surrounding fibers to their side (Epstein and Farmer, 1993).

Cervicomedullary gliomas appear as solid masses within the above-described areas. They are hypointense on T1-weighted and hyperintense on T2-weighted images. They typically enhance homogeneously upon gadolinium injection.

Diagnosis and Differential Diagnosis

Diagnosis of brainstem gliomas is based on clinical presentations and imaging studies and needs to address the location and nature of the lesion.

It is expected that the patient's clinical course, examination and imaging studies be in agreement. With nondiffuse brainstem gliomas this congruence often prompts surgical intervention (resection and/or relief of hydrocephalus), particularly for those located at the cervicomedullary junction or dorsal exophytic in growth.

Incongruent presentation and clinical studies suggests the need for biopsy prior to definitive treatment. In cases with disagreement between the imaging findings and clinical course (i.e., rapidly progressive course with imaging consistent with a focal or low-grade lesion), frozen sections should be obtained at the time of surgery prior to progressing to an aggressive resection. These instances may be representative of a more malignant tumor in which case the potential for iatrogenic injury during resection outweighs the potential benefit of an extensive resection.

Differential diagnosis includes other tumors in the brainstem and adjacent regions and other lesion types. Other tumors include lymphoma, metastatic tumors, germinoma and non-germinomatous germ cell tumors, PNET, hemangioblastoma, lipoma, and acoustic neuroma. Some of these tumors typically arise from nearby regions and may encroach into the brainstem, e.g., primary intracranial germ cell tumors usually occur in the pineal region and can invade the brainstem. The majority of non-germinomatous germ cell tumors can be differentiated by testing for secreted markers in the blood and CSF such as α-fetoprotein (AFP) and β-human chorionic growth hormone (β-hCG). PNET occurring in the brainstem, even though relatively rare, can appear similar to DIPG or nondiffuse brainstem gliomas. Because of the difference in treatment options from those for brainstem gliomas, it should be carefully differentiated when suspected. Lesions of other types include infectious, autoimmune, inflammatory, vascular and metabolic lesions.

The role of biopsy in the diagnosis of DIPG remains intensely debated (Leach et al., 2008; Wilkinson and Harris, 2008). Before the wide adoption of MRI in the diagnosis of brainstem gliomas, biopsy was performed to confirm diagnosis and provide information on prognosis. However, biopsy has been only performed infrequently since the mid-1990s. Of note is that since the Children's Cancer Group (CCG) report in 1993 (Albright et al., 1993), MRI has superseded biopsy as the main method of diagnosing DIPG. As better methods to characterize tumors become available and more molecularly targeted therapies have become available or are under development in recent years, there is increasing interest to perform biopsy more frequently in clinically diagnosed DIPGs. Brainstem biopsy may be safe with low morbidity and mortality rates when performed properly (Pincus et al., 2006; Pirotte et al., 2007; Roujeau et al., 2007). Surveys show that parents of children with DIPG are generally amenable to biopsy, even if the results may not benefit the patient (Bartels et al., 2011). Various focus groups have been holding discussions on criteria for recommending biopsy.

Some investigational protocols of DIPG have included biopsy and molecular characterization as mandatory components in stratifying subjects for experimental therapy.

Treatment

Treatment of brainstem gliomas includes management of pain, bulbar symptoms and motor impairment, relief of hydrocephalus and general support. Brainstem glioma patients should be cared for by a multidisciplinary team including neurosurgeons, non-surgical specialists and other therapists.

Surgical intervention is indicated for certain nondiffuse brainstem gliomas. Tectal gliomas are usually indolent and present with hydrocephalus. Hydrocephalus is relieved by endoscopic third ventriculostomy (ETV) or ventricular shunt placement. Early resection of tectal gliomas is controversial. Dorsal exophytic gliomas are the most amenable to surgical resection in brainstem gliomas. The goal is to remove the exophytic component, and when safe, followed by debulking of the intrinsic component. Surgical resection is typically recommended early for cervicomedullary gliomas. Subtotal resection can be safely performed in most cases.

Adjuvant therapy for brainstem gliomas depends on the tumor location, pathological diagnosis and extent of previous surgical resection. Radiation therapy is the standard of care for DIPG, but it is not recommended as an early treatment for nondiffuse brainstem gliomas if pathology shows a low-grade glioma. It is usually used in patients with high-grade pathology, upon clinical and imaging evidence of progression, or late in the disease course (Freeman and Farmer, 1998; Ueoka et al., 2009). Stereotactic radiosurgery is also used in nondiffuse brainstem gliomas. Chemotherapy has limited use in the management of brainstem gliomas. It is mainly used for high-grade pathology or at the late stage of the disease.

Diffuse Intrinsic Pontine Glioma

Surgical resection of DIPG is not safe because of its location and infiltrative nature. Biopsy is not indicated for patients with typical clinical presentation and MRI findings. Hydrocephalus, if present, should be treated with either an ETV or a shunt. Histological confirmation might be needed if imaging or clinical history is not typical for a DIPG, or if an investigational protocol requests it.

The standard of care for DIPG is external beam radiation therapy, typically delivered at 1.8Gy/fraction for 30-33 fractions in North America. Significant clinical improvement occurs in 85% of patients receiving radiation therapy, but the improvement is usually transient, lasting only 3-4 months, before progressive decline in clinical status returns (Hargrave et al., 2006). For children younger than 3 years of age with DIPG, radiation therapy is usually avoided, and chemotherapy is used instead.

Various chemotherapeutic regimens have been studied either alone or in combination with radiation therapy, including: carboplatin (Allen et al., 1999; Doz et al., 2002); carboplatin plus etoposide (Walter et al., 1998); carboplatin, etoposide plus vincristine (Jennings et al., 2002); cisplatin plus cyclophosphamide (Kretschmar et al., 1993); cisplatin, etoposide, cyclophosphamide plus vincristine (Jennings et al., 2002); CCNU, vincristine plus prednisone (Jenkin et al., 1987); vincristine plus etoposide (Korones et al., 2008); trophosphamide plus etoposide (Wolff et al., 2002); etoposide, vincristine plus cyclosporine A (Greenberg et al., 2005); tamoxifen (Broniscer et al., 2000); topotecan (Blaney et al., 1996; Sanghavi et al., 2003; Bernier-Chastagner et al., 2005); temozolomide (Broniscer et al., 2005; Jalali et al., 2010; Cohen et al., 2011); and pegylated interferon α-2b (Warren et al., 2012). However, up to date, no chemotherapeutic agent, either alone or in combination, or in conjunction with radiation therapy, has altered the natural history of DIPG. Similarly, studies utilizing high-dose, marrow-ablative chemotherapies with autologous bone marrow or peripheral hematopoietic stem cell rescue have been ineffective in extending survival (Dunkel et al., 1998; Jakacki et al., 1999; Bouffet et al., 2000). Many patients are enrolled in clinical trials of new agents or previously used agents in previously untested combinations.

Focal Gliomas

Most tectal gliomas in children have indolent growth patterns with few symptoms except those caused by hydrocephalus. Early resection of focal tectal gliomas is controversial and infrequently done. Often, these tumors are managed by relief of hydrocephalus, followed by clinical observation and periodic MRI scans (Walker et al., 1999; Sandri et al., 2006). Treatment of the hydrocephalus typically includes ETV to restore CSF flow. Shunting is an alternative or can be considered for patients who fail ETV. Surgical resection may be considered on rare occasions.

Focal gliomas in other areas of the brainstem, including tegmentum and medulla, are usually indicated for surgical resection. Tissue diagnosis before radical resection is indicated for lesions with atypical clinical and imaging findings. For those patients initially put on observation, when tumor progression is observed, biopsy or sometimes radical resection is indicated. Transventricular endoscopic biopsy may be performed with or without CSF diversion when the tumor is adjacent to a ventricle's walls (Ahn and Goumnerova, 2010). Stereotactic biopsies may be considered for lesions that cannot be approached with endoscopy where accurate histological diagnosis is warranted but more aggressive surgical resection is deemed unsafe. Surgical resection of focal, well-circumscribed lesions provides not only a tissue diagnosis but also a prolonged event-free survival in many cases.

Conventional radiation therapy has demonstrated limited efficacy in patients with focal gliomas. Tumors with high-grade features should be treated with radiation therapy after recovery from surgery or when surgery is not indicated, while low-grade tumors may be observed and treated only if there is subsequent tumor progression (Freeman and Farmer, 1998; Ueoka et al., 2009). Implantation of iodine-129 (^{129}I) or iodine-125 (^{125}I) seeds has been used in some patients with acceptable tumor control. ^{125}I is an alternative to resection, external beam radiation therapy and chemotherapy in children with progressively symptomatic low-grade gliomas in deep and eloquent areas where high postoperative morbidity would be expected with open surgery (Korinthenberg et al., 2011). Stereotactic radiosurgery has been used as an alternative means for managing focal brainstem gliomas (Yen et al., 2007). Its use has been reported in patients with progressive tumor growth or worsening neurological deficits.

The role of chemotherapy has not been well evaluated for focal brainstem gliomas. In general, for tumors that total or subtotal resection has been performed on and subsequently progress, chemotherapy may be considered with or without radiation therapy. In children younger than 3 years old, chemotherapy may be used alone in attempts to delay the need for radiation therapy.

Dorsal Exophytic Gliomas

Dorsal exophytic gliomas are the group most amenable to surgical resection among brainstem gliomas, and total or near total resection alone usually results in a good prognosis (Pollack et al., 1993; Khatib et al., 1994). Long-term event-free survival is expected when these tumors are simply shaven down to the level of the floor of the fourth ventricle. Debulking of the intrinsic component should only be attempted when considered safe, and should not be pursued aggressively. Tumor specimens should be sent early for frozen sections. A high-grade lesion is an indication to halt the surgery, as there is no proven long-term benefit to debulking aggressive lesions. Resection of the tumor takes place primarily within the fourth ventricle on the extra-axial part. In instances where there is a large intramedullary component to the tumor or if it is felt that damage to the functional tissues of the brainstem would be unavoidable, subtotal, instead of gross total, resection should be attempted. Some have advocated that resection carried to the level of the floor of the fourth ventricle confers a sufficient balance between disease control and preservation of neurological function by minimizing the risk of injuring functional brainstem tissues. In patients with findings consistent with an obstructive hydrocephalus who have not previously undergone a CSF diversion procedure (e.g., ETV or shunting), placement of an external ventricular drain may be considered.

Radiation therapy is used for inoperable tumors or recurrent disease not amenable to re-resection (Freeman and Farmer, 1998; Ueoka et al., 2009). Treatment primarily consists of conventional external beam radiation therapy with 30-33 daily fractions of 1.8Gy/fraction (Schild et al., 1998; Skowronska-Gardas, 2003; Hoffman and Yock, 2009). The use of stereotactic radiation therapy and radiosurgery has also been examined in small cohorts. Chemotherapy has no proven efficacy in the treatment of dorsal exophytic gliomas (Allen and Siffert, 1996).

Cervicomedullary Gliomas

Cervicomedullary gliomas are treated in a fashion similar to that of an intramedullary spinal cord glioma or a focal glioma of the medulla depending on the location of the epicenter. When attempting surgical resection, specimens should be sent early for frozen sections. Identification of a high-grade lesion is an indication to halt the surgery, as there is no proven long-term benefit to debulking aggressive lesions. Surgical resection should begin with internal debulking from the center to periphery.

As the majority of these tumors are low grade, surgery is typically the initial treatment modality. Radiation therapy should be reserved for advanced or recurrent diseases not amenable to surgical resection (Freeman and Farmer, 1998; Ueoka et al., 2009). Treatment primarily consists of conventional fractionated external beam radiation given at 1.8Gy/fraction for 30-33 fractions (Schild et al., 1998; Skowronska-Gardas, 2003; Hoffman and Yock, 2009). The use of stereotactic radiation therapy and radiosurgery has also been examined in small cohorts. Although a number of trials have examined the efficacy of chemotherapy in the treatment of DIPG, no role has been defined for its use in the treatment of cervicomedullary tumors (Allen and Siffert, 1996).

Outcomes

The outcome of brainstem gliomas depends on the location and pathological grade of the tumor. Focal, dorsal exophytic and cervicomedullary gliomas typically have a fairly good prognosis. In contrast, the median survival of DIPG patients is only about one year despite numerous investigational therapies. In both DIPG and nondiffuse brainstem gliomas, patients with neurofibromatosis, older age, and longer duration of symptoms before diagnosis are thought to have a more favorable outcome (Ullrich et al., 2007).

Diffuse Intrinsic Pontine Gliomas

External beam radiation therapy transiently improves the neurological condition in 85% of DIPG patients, but the disease usually progresses within 3-4 months. No treatment has been shown to be effective at the time of progression. Clinical deterioration is usually fast once progression is detected. Median survival is 10-12 months. Only 10% of patients survive beyond two years after diagnosis (Hargrave et al., 2006). Children under the age of 3 years, young adults over 18 and those with NF1 may have a better prognosis.

Focal Gliomas

Lesions typical of tectal gliomas on imaging studies usually need treatment for hydrocephalus only and rarely progress over many years. Hydrocephalus can be well managed in tectal gliomas. ETV for tectal gliomas has a success rate exceeding 70% and as high as 90%. Focal gliomas in other areas of the brainstem, especially if the pathology is pilocytic astrosytoma, can be cured by gross total resection but long-term follow-up is necessary. One study noted a 4-year progression-free survival rate of 94% and an overall 4-year survival rate of 100% in 17 patients with focal midbrain gliomas, which included tectal gliomas (Robertson et al., 1995). Stereotactic radiosurgery may be an effective primary treatment or adjunct to open surgery for focal brainstem gliomas. After gamma knife radiosurgery, most patients improved or stabilized but some worsened (Yen et al., 2007).

Dorsal Exophytic Gliomas

Dorsal exophytic gliomas are generally amenable to surgical resection. Gross total or subtotal resection can be achieved in most cases. They have a good outcome after surgical resection. Among 18 patients who underwent surgery, 17 survived and only four showed evidence of radiological progression after a median follow-up of 113 months (Pollack et al., 1993). Subsequent progression may require re-resection or radiation therapy.

Cervicomedullary Gliomas

Tumor control can be achieved by surgical resection in most patients with cervicomedullary gliomas. 5-year progression-free survival rate is 60% and overall 5-year survival rate about 90% after surgical resection alone (Weiner et al., 1997).

Recent Advances and Future Directions

Because of the dismal prognosis of DIPG and the lack of therapeutic efficacy of current chemotherapies, innovative approaches are urgently needed for the disease. One promising drug delivery method that may improve the outcome of DIPG patients is convection-enhanced delivery (CED). Another recent advance is the molecular characterization of DIPG, which may provide guidance for developing new therapies.

Convection-Enhanced Delivery

The blood-brain barrier (BBB) presents a significant obstacle to achieving therapeutic concentrations of systemically delivered agents in brain tumors. CED is a method of local delivery that bypasses the BBB (Bobo et al., 1994). CED is typically accomplished by inserting a small-bore cannula directly into a tumor followed by drug infusion through the cannula. Experimental studies have led to the recognition that CED can be characterized by several common features:

- Local drug concentration can exceed that achieved with systemic administration by several thousand times.
- Systemic exposure by efflux into the vasculature is minimal.
- Tissue penetration by CED is well beyond that achieved by other local delivery methods that rely on diffusion rather than bulk flow such as drug-impregnated polymers.
- Distribution is preferentially along white matter tracts, a pattern reminiscent of glioma cell invasion.
- CED can be used to deliver macromolecules such as monoclonal antibodies or recombinant toxins, which is not possible by systemic administration in the brain parenchyma or tumor.

It is hypothesized that CED is ideally suited for the treatment of DIPG based on several features particular to this disease such as the tumor's relative compact growth pattern, its tendency to migrate along white matter fibers, the rarity of large cysts and the lack of cavitary changes from radiation therapy.

The safety of CED in the brainstem has been well established in rodents and non-human primates (Laske et al., 1997; Lonser et al., 2002; Sandberg et al., 2002; Nguyen et al., 2003; Croteau et al., 2005; Lonser et al., 2007; Krauze et al., 2008). The tolerability of several therapeutic agents delivered using CED into the brainstem has also been investigated and most of them proven to be safe at high concentrations (Souweidane et al., 2004a; Souweidane et al., 2004b; Murad et al., 2006; Murad et al., 2007; Szerlip et al., 2007; Luther et al., 2008; Luther et al., 2010). This approach has been safely used on a limited clinical basis.

Although it is clear that certain limitations exist in the application of CED for the treatment of DIPG, currently existing preclinical data are sufficient to guide the design of clinical studies. Decisions in the design of these studies include the selection of an appropriate agent or agents, surgical techniques, parameters of infusion, timing of treatment and methods of assessing distribution, local concentration, safety and therapeutic efficacy. These questions, however, should not be perceived as a barrier to clinical implementation, but rather as goals for early phase clinical studies. Based on current preclinical data, CED may serve as the basis for a new approach in the treatment of DIPG.

Molecular Characterization of Diffuse Intrinsic Pontine Gliomas

A promising advance that may aid the development of therapies for DIPG is the recent molecular characterization of this tumor. As discussed in the Molecular Genetics section, four groups independently discovered that PDGF and the PDGFR are amplified or over-expressed in the majority of these tumors (Becher et al., 2010; Paugh et al., 2010; Zarghooni et al., 2010; Paugh et al., 2011; Puget et al., 2012). Less common are mutations in another growth factor receptor, EGFR (Zarghooni et al., 2010; Paugh et al., 2011). Other common mutations include *H3F3A* (Khuong-Quang et al., 2012; Wu et al., 2012), *TP53* (Zhang et al., 1993; Badhe et al., 2004) and its chromosomal region (Louis et al., 1993; Zarghooni et al., 2010; Barrow et al., 2011), and allelic loss of a region of 10q where the *PTEN* gene is located (Louis et al., 1993; Cheng et al., 1999; Cheng and Wu, 1999). Like in adult malignant gliomas, the interleukin-13 receptor subtype IL-13Rα2 is highly expressed in DIPG (Joshi et al., 2008; Okada et al., 2008).

Some of these genetic aberrations have been used as the basis for DIPG animal models that could be powerful tools for studying the disease, e.g., Becher et al. designed a mouse model of DIPG based on PDGF overexpression (Becher et al., 2010). Ways to therapeutically target these genetic aberrations include, but are not limited to, inhibiting enzymatic activities, passive immunotherapy such as therapeutic antibodies, active immunotherapy such as therapeutic vaccines *etc*. Some of these are already under study. There are therapeutic monoclonal antibodies targeting PDGFR, namely IMC-3G3 (ImClone Systems, Bridgewater, New Jersey) and MEDI-575 (MedImmune LLC., Gaithersburg, Maryland), that need to be tested for efficacy in treating DIPG, preferably delivered through CED into the tumor since they are macromolecules unable to cross the BBB. There are numerous small molecule tyrosine kinase inhibitors with strong inhibitory effects on PDGFR and/or EGFR kinases, and inhibitors of downstream signaling molecules such as AKT and mTOR, that are undergoing clinical trials for the treatment of DIPG. There are also targeted recombinant toxins, e.g.,

IL13-PE38QQR, utilizing IL-13 as the targeting moiety to target tumor cells overexpressing IL-13 receptors. An IL-13Rα2 epitope is also used as an ingredient in a therapeutic vaccine for childhood gliomas (Pollack et al., 2013). Even though biopsy of DIPG is far from being routine, when these targeted therapies come to clinical use, it would be ideal for the tumor to be pre-screened for specific targets of those agents.

Conclusion

Brainstem gliomas are a heterogeneous group of neoplasms with considerably diverse natural histories and prognoses. They are classified into four groups based on their location, focality and growth patterns. Diffuse intrinsic pontine gliomas (DIPG) account for approximately 80% of brainstem gliomas. The overwhelming majority of them are high grade. They are not resectable and the standard of care involves external beam radiation therapy. They have a dismal prognosis. The vast majority of focal, dorsal exophytic and cervicomedullary gliomas is low grade, often amenable to surgical resection and has a more favorable outcome.

Developing an effective therapy for DIPG remains frustrating as neither new schedules of radiation therapy nor chemotherapeutic regimens being studied have improved survival of these patients. As better molecular characterization methods become available, there are increasing calls to perform biopsy and tissue diagnosis in clinically diagnosed DIPGs. Recent molecular characterization of DIPG identified some genetic aberrations that could be effective therapeutic targets, including PDGF and PDGF receptors. There are both large and small molecule agents targeting these genetic aberrations that are either available or under development. However, most of these agents are unable to cross the blood-brain barrier (BBB) to reach the tumor. Convection-enhanced delivery (CED) is a drug delivery method to bypass the BBB. It has proven capability to deliver high local drug concentrations and the safety of its use in the brainstem has been established in small and large animals and a small number of patients. CED, combined with conventional chemotherapeutic drugs and novel targeted agents, has the potential to produce an effective treatment for DIPG.

References

Ahn ES, Goumnerova L (2010) Endoscopic biopsy of brain tumors in children: diagnostic success and utility in guiding treatment strategies. *J. Neurosurg. Pediatr.* 5:255-262.

Albright AL, Price RA, Guthkelch AN (1983) Brain stem gliomas of children. A clinicopathological study. *Cancer* 52:2313-2319.

Albright AL, Packer RJ, Zimmerman R, Rorke LB, Boyett J, Hammond GD (1993) Magnetic resonance scans should replace biopsies for the diagnosis of diffuse brain stem gliomas: a report from the Children's Cancer Group. *Neurosurgery* 33:1026-1029; discussion 1029-1030.

Allen J, Siffert J, Donahue B, Nirenberg A, Jakacki R, Robertson P, DaRosso R, Thoron L, Rosovsky M, Pinto R (1999) A phase I/II study of carboplatin combined with hyperfractionated radiotherapy for brainstem gliomas. *Cancer* 86:1064-1069.

Allen JC, Siffert J (1996) Contemporary chemotherapy issues for children with brainstem gliomas. *Pediatr. Neurosurg*. 24:98-102.

Badhe PB, Chauhan PP, Mehta NK (2004) Brainstem gliomas--a clinicopathological study of 45 cases with p53 immunohistochemistry. *Indian J. Cancer* 41:170-174.

Barrow J, Adamowicz-Brice M, Cartmill M, MacArthur D, Lowe J, Robson K, Brundler MA, Walker DA, Coyle B, Grundy R (2011) Homozygous loss of ADAM3A revealed by genome-wide analysis of pediatric high-grade glioma and diffuse intrinsic pontine gliomas. *Neuro Oncol.* 13:212-222.

Bartels U, Hawkins C, Vezina G, Kun L, Souweidane M, Bouffet E (2011) Proceedings of the diffuse intrinsic pontine glioma (DIPG) Toronto Think Tank: advancing basic and translational research and cooperation in DIPG. *J. Neurooncol.* 105:119-125.

Becher OJ, Hambardzumyan D, Walker TR, Helmy K, Nazarian J, Albrecht S, Hiner RL, Gall S, Huse JT, Jabado N, MacDonald TJ, Holland EC (2010) Preclinical evaluation of radiation and perifosine in a genetically and histologically accurate model of brainstem glioma. *Cancer Res*. 70:2548-2557.

Bernier-Chastagner V, Grill J, Doz F, Bracard S, Gentet JC, Marie-Cardine A, Luporsi E, Margueritte G, Lejars O, Laithier V, Mechinaud F, Millot F, Kalifa C, Chastagner P (2005) Topotecan as a radiosensitizer in the treatment of children with malignant diffuse brainstem gliomas: results of a French Society of Paediatric Oncology Phase II Study. *Cancer* 104:2792-2797.

Blaney SM, Phillips PC, Packer RJ, Heideman RL, Berg SL, Adamson PC, Allen JC, Sallan SE, Jakacki RI, Lange BJ, Reaman GH, Horowitz ME, Poplack DG, Balis FM (1996) Phase II evaluation of topotecan for pediatric central nervous system tumors. *Cancer* 78:527-531.

Bobo RH, Laske DW, Akbasak A, Morrison PF, Dedrick RL, Oldfield EH (1994) Convection-enhanced delivery of macromolecules in the brain. *Proc. Natl. Acad. Sci. USA* 91:2076-2080.

Bouffet E, Raquin M, Doz F, Gentet JC, Rodary C, Demeocq F, Chastagner P, Lutz P, Hartmann O, Kalifa C (2000) Radiotherapy followed by high dose busulfan and thiotepa: a prospective assessment of high dose chemotherapy in children with diffuse pontine gliomas. *Cancer* 88:685-692.

Bowers DC, Georgiades C, Aronson LJ, Carson BS, Weingart JD, Wharam MD, Melhem ER, Burger PC, Cohen KJ (2000) Tectal gliomas: natural history of an indolent lesion in pediatric patients. *Pediatr. Neurosurg*. 32:24-29.

Broniscer A, Leite CC, Lanchote VL, Machado TM, Cristofani LM (2000) Radiation therapy and high-dose tamoxifen in the treatment of patients with diffuse brainstem gliomas: results of a Brazilian cooperative study. Brainstem Glioma Cooperative Group. *J. Clin. Oncol.* 18:1246-1253.

Broniscer A, Iacono L, Chintagumpala M, Fouladi M, Wallace D, Bowers DC, Stewart C, Krasin MJ, Gajjar A (2005) Role of temozolomide after radiotherapy for newly diagnosed diffuse brainstem glioma in children: results of a multiinstitutional study (SJHG-98). *Cancer* 103:133-139.

Cartmill M, Punt J (1999) Diffuse brain stem glioma. A review of stereotactic biopsies. *Childs Nerv. Syst*. 15:235-237; discussion 238.

Cheng Y, Wu H (1999) [Recent advances on molecular biology of diffuse astrocytoma]. Zhonghua Bing Li Xue Za Zhi 28:165-168.

Cheng Y, Ng HK, Zhang SF, Ding M, Pang JC, Zheng J, Poon WS (1999) Genetic alterations in pediatric high-grade astrocytomas. *Hum. Pathol.* 30:1284-1290.

Cohen KJ, Heideman RL, Zhou T, Holmes EJ, Lavey RS, Bouffet E, Pollack IF (2011) Temozolomide in the treatment of children with newly diagnosed diffuse intrinsic pontine gliomas: a report from the Children's Oncology Group. *Neuro Oncol.* 13:410-416.

Croteau D, Walbridge S, Morrison PF, Butman JA, Vortmeyer AO, Johnson D, Oldfield EH, Lonser RR (2005) Real-time in vivo imaging of the convective distribution of a low-molecular-weight tracer. *J. Neurosurg.* 102:90-97.

Daglioglu E, Cataltepe O, Akalan N (2003) Tectal gliomas in children: the implications for natural history and management strategy. *Pediatr. Neurosurg.* 38:223-231.

Doz F, Neuenschwander S, Bouffet E, Gentet JC, Schneider P, Kalifa C, Mechinaud F, Chastagner P, De Lumley L, Sariban E, Plantaz D, Mosseri V, Bours D, Alapetite C, Zucker JM (2002) Carboplatin before and during radiation therapy for the treatment of malignant brain stem tumours: a study by the Societe Francaise d'Oncologie Pediatrique. *Eur. J. Cancer* 38:815-819.

Dunkel IJ, Garvin JH, Jr., Goldman S, Ettinger LJ, Kaplan AM, Cairo M, Li H, Boyett JM, Finlay JL (1998) High dose chemotherapy with autologous bone marrow rescue for children with diffuse pontine brain stem tumors. Children's Cancer Group. *J. Neurooncol.* 37:67-73.

Epstein F, Wisoff J (1987) Intra-axial tumors of the cervicomedullary junction. *J. Neurosurg.* 67:483-487.

Epstein FJ, Farmer JP (1993) Brain-stem glioma growth patterns. J Neurosurg 78:408-412.

Farwell JR, Dohrmann GJ, Flannery JT (1977) Central nervous system tumors in children. *Cancer* 40:3123-3132.

Forshew T, Tatevossian RG, Lawson AR, Ma J, Neale G, Ogunkolade BW, Jones TA, Aarum J, Dalton J, Bailey S, Chaplin T, Carter RL, Gajjar A, Broniscer A, Young BD, Ellison DW, Sheer D (2009) Activation of the ERK/MAPK pathway: a signature genetic defect in posterior fossa pilocytic astrocytomas. *The Journal of pathology* 218:172-181.

Freeman CR, Farmer JP (1998) Pediatric brain stem gliomas: a review. *Int. J. Radiat. Oncol. Biol. Phys.* 40:265-271.

Greenberg ML, Fisher PG, Freeman C, Korones DN, Bernstein M, Friedman H, Blaney S, Hershon L, Zhou T, Chen Z, Kretschmar C (2005) Etoposide, vincristine, and cyclosporin A with standard-dose radiation therapy in newly diagnosed diffuse intrinsic brainstem gliomas: a pediatric oncology group phase I study. *Pediatr. Blood Cancer* 45:644-648.

Hargrave D, Bartels U, Bouffet E (2006) Diffuse brainstem glioma in children: critical review of clinical trials. *Lancet Oncol.* 7:241-248.

Hawkins C, Walker E, Mohamed N, Zhang C, Jacob K, Shirinian M, Alon N, Kahn D, Fried I, Scheinemann K, Tsangaris E, Dirks P, Tressler R, Bouffet E, Jabado N, Tabori U (2011) BRAF-KIAA1549 fusion predicts better clinical outcome in pediatric low-grade astrocytoma. *Clin. Cancer Res.* 17:4790-4798.

Helton KJ, Weeks JK, Phillips NS, Zou P, Kun LE, Khan RB, Gajjar A, Fouladi M, Broniscer A, Boop F, Li CS, Ogg RJ (2008) Diffusion tensor imaging of brainstem tumors: axonal degeneration of motor and sensory tracts. *J. Neurosurg. Pediatr.* 1:270-276.

Hoffman HJ, Becker L, Craven MA (1980) A clinically and pathologically distinct group of benign brain stem gliomas. *Neurosurgery* 7:243-248.

Hoffman KE, Yock TI (2009) Radiation therapy for pediatric central nervous system tumors. *J. Child Neurol.* 24:1387-1396.

Horbinski C, Nikiforova MN, Hagenkord JM, Hamilton RL, Pollack IF (2012) Interplay among BRAF, p16, p53, and MIB1 in pediatric low-grade gliomas. *Neuro Oncol.* 14:777-789.

Jakacki RI, Siffert J, Jamison C, Velasquez L, Allen JC (1999) Dose-intensive, time-compressed procarbazine, CCNU, vincristine (PCV) with peripheral blood stem cell support and concurrent radiation in patients with newly diagnosed high-grade gliomas. *J. Neurooncol.* 44:77-83.

Jalali R, Raut N, Arora B, Gupta T, Dutta D, Munshi A, Sarin R, Kurkure P (2010) Prospective evaluation of radiotherapy with concurrent and adjuvant temozolomide in children with newly diagnosed diffuse intrinsic pontine glioma. *Int. J. Radiat. Oncol. Biol. Phys.*77:113-118.

Jenkin RD, Boesel C, Ertel I, Evans A, Hittle R, Ortega J, Sposto R, Wara W, Wilson C, Anderson J, et al. (1987) Brain-stem tumors in childhood: a prospective randomized trial of irradiation with and without adjuvant CCNU, VCR, and prednisone. A report of the Childrens Cancer Study Group. *J. Neurosurg.* 66:227-233.

Jennings MT, Sposto R, Boyett JM, Vezina LG, Holmes E, Berger MS, Bruggers CS, Bruner JM, Chan KW, Dusenbery KE, Ettinger LJ, Fitz CR, Lafond D, Mandelbaum DE, Massey V, McGuire W, McNeely L, Moulton T, Pollack IF, Shen V (2002) Preradiation chemotherapy in primary high-risk brainstem tumors: phase II study CCG-9941 of the Children's Cancer Group. *J. Clin. Oncol.* 20:3431-3437.

Joshi BH, Puri RA, Leland P, Varricchio F, Gupta G, Kocak M, Gilbertson RJ, Puri RK (2008) Identification of interleukin-13 receptor alpha2 chain overexpression in situ in high-grade diffusely infiltrative pediatric brainstem glioma. *Neuro Oncol.* 10:265-274.

Kaplan AM, Albright AL, Zimmerman RA, Rorke LB, Li H, Boyett JM, Finlay JL, Wara WM, Packer RJ (1996) Brainstem gliomas in children. A Children's Cancer Group review of 119 cases. *Pediatr. Neurosurg.* 24:185-192.

Kernohan GW, Sayre GS (1952) Tumors of the central nervous system. In: Atlas of Tumor Pathology: Section X. Washington, DC: Armed Forces Institute of Pathology.

Khatib ZA, Heideman RL, Kovnar EH, Langston JA, Sanford RA, Douglas EC, Ochs J, Jenkins JJ, Fairclough DL, Greenwald C, et al. (1994) Predominance of pilocytic histology in dorsally exophytic brain stem tumors. *Pediatr. Neurosurg.* 20:2-10.

Khuong-Quang DA et al. (2012) K27M mutation in histone H3.3 defines clinically and biologically distinct subgroups of pediatric diffuse intrinsic pontine gliomas. *Acta neuropathologica* 124:439-447.

Korinthenberg R, Neuburger D, Trippel M, Ostertag C, Nikkhah G (2011) Long-term results of brachytherapy with temporary iodine-125 seeds in children with low-grade gliomas. *Int. J. Radiat. Oncol. Biol. Phys.* 79:1131-1138.

Korones DN, Fisher PG, Kretschmar C, Zhou T, Chen Z, Kepner J, Freeman C (2008) Treatment of children with diffuse intrinsic brain stem glioma with radiotherapy, vincristine and oral VP-16: a Children's Oncology Group phase II study. *Pediatr. Blood Cancer* 50:227-230.

Krauze MT, Vandenberg SR, Yamashita Y, Saito R, Forsayeth J, Noble C, Park J, Bankiewicz KS (2008) Safety of real-time convection-enhanced delivery of liposomes to primate brain: a long-term retrospective. *Exp. Neurol.* 210:638-644.

Kretschmar CS, Tarbell NJ, Barnes PD, Krischer JP, Burger PC, Kun L (1993) Pre-irradiation chemotherapy and hyperfractionated radiation therapy 66 Gy for children with brain stem tumors. A phase II study of the Pediatric Oncology Group, Protocol 8833. *Cancer* 72:1404-1413.

Laske DW, Morrison PF, Lieberman DM, Corthesy ME, Reynolds JC, Stewart-Henney PA, Koong SS, Cummins A, Paik CH, Oldfield EH (1997) Chronic interstitial infusion of protein to primate brain: determination of drug distribution and clearance with single-photon emission computerized tomography imaging. *J. Neurosurg.* 87:586-594.

Leach PA, Estlin EJ, Coope DJ, Thorne JA, Kamaly-Asl ID (2008) Diffuse brainstem gliomas in children: should we or shouldn't we biopsy? *British journal of neurosurgery* 22:619-624.

Lonser RR, Walbridge S, Garmestani K, Butman JA, Walters HA, Vortmeyer AO, Morrison PF, Brechbiel MW, Oldfield EH (2002) Successful and safe perfusion of the primate brainstem: in vivo magnetic resonance imaging of macromolecular distribution during infusion. *J. Neurosurg.* 97:905-913.

Lonser RR, Schiffman R, Robison RA, Butman JA, Quezado Z, Walker ML, Morrison PF, Walbridge S, Murray GJ, Park DM, Brady RO, Oldfield EH (2007) Image-guided, direct convective delivery of glucocerebrosidase for neuronopathic Gaucher disease. *Neurology* 68:254-261.

Louis DN, Rubio MP, Correa KM, Gusella JF, von Deimling A (1993) Molecular genetics of pediatric brain stem gliomas. Application of PCR techniques to small and archival brain tumor specimens. *J. Neuropathol. Exp. Neurol.* 52:507-515.

Luther N, Cheung NK, Dunkel IJ, Fraser JF, Edgar MA, Gutin PH, Souweidane MM (2008) Intraparenchymal and intratumoral interstitial infusion of anti-glioma monoclonal antibody 8H9. *Neurosurgery* 63:1166-1174; discussion 1174.

Luther N, Cheung NK, Souliopoulos EP, Karempelas I, Bassiri D, Edgar MA, Guo HF, Pastan I, Gutin PH, Souweidane MM (2010) Interstitial infusion of glioma-targeted recombinant immunotoxin 8H9scFv-PE38. *Mol. Cancer Ther.* 9:1039-1046.

Mauffrey C (2006) Paediatric brainstem gliomas: prognostic factors and management. J Clin Neurosci 13:431-437.

Murad GJ, Walbridge S, Morrison PF, Szerlip N, Butman JA, Oldfield EH, Lonser RR (2007) Image-guided convection-enhanced delivery of gemcitabine to the brainstem. *J. Neurosurg.* 106:351-356.

Murad GJ, Walbridge S, Morrison PF, Garmestani K, Degen JW, Brechbiel MW, Oldfield EH, Lonser RR (2006) Real-time, image-guided, convection-enhanced delivery of interleukin 13 bound to pseudomonas exotoxin. *Clin. Cancer Res.* 12:3145-3151.

Nguyen TT, Pannu YS, Sung C, Dedrick RL, Walbridge S, Brechbiel MW, Garmestani K, Beitzel M, Yordanov AT, Oldfield EH (2003) Convective distribution of macromolecules in the primate brain demonstrated using computerized tomography and magnetic resonance imaging. *J. Neurosurg.* 98:584-590.

Okada H, Low KL, Kohanbash G, McDonald HA, Hamilton RL, Pollack IF (2008) Expression of glioma-associated antigens in pediatric brain stem and non-brain stem gliomas. *J. Neurooncol.* 88:245-250.

Ostrom QT, Gittleman H, Farah P, Ondracek A, Chen Y, Wolinsky Y, Stroup NE, Kruchko C, Barnholtz-Sloan JS (2013) CBTRUS statistical report: Primary brain and central nervous system tumors diagnosed in the United States in 2006-2010. *Neuro Oncol.* 15 Suppl 2:ii1-56.

Panitch HS, Berg BO (1970) Brain stem tumors of childhood and adolescence. *American journal of diseases of children* 119:465-472.

Paugh BS, Broniscer A, Qu C, Miller CP, Zhang J, Tatevossian RG, Olson JM, Geyer JR, Chi SN, da Silva NS, Onar-Thomas A, Baker JN, Gajjar A, Ellison DW, Baker SJ (2011) Genome-wide analyses identify recurrent amplifications of receptor tyrosine kinases and cell-cycle regulatory genes in diffuse intrinsic pontine glioma. *J. Clin. Oncol.* 29:3999-4006.

Paugh BS, Qu C, Jones C, Liu Z, Adamowicz-Brice M, Zhang J, Bax DA, Coyle B, Barrow J, Hargrave D, Lowe J, Gajjar A, Zhao W, Broniscer A, Ellison DW, Grundy RG, Baker SJ (2010) Integrated molecular genetic profiling of pediatric high-grade gliomas reveals key differences with the adult disease. *J. Clin. Oncol.* 28:3061-3068.

Pierre-Kahn A, Hirsch JF, Vinchon M, Payan C, Sainte-Rose C, Renier D, Lelouch-Tubiana A, Fermanian J (1993) Surgical management of brain-stem tumors in children: results and statistical analysis of 75 cases. *J. Neurosurg.* 79:845-852.

Pincus DW, Richter EO, Yachnis AT, Bennett J, Bhatti MT, Smith A (2006) Brainstem stereotactic biopsy sampling in children. *J. Neurosurg.* 104:108-114.

Pirotte BJ, Lubansu A, Massager N, Wikler D, Goldman S, Levivier M (2007) Results of positron emission tomography guidance and reassessment of the utility of and indications for stereotactic biopsy in children with infiltrative brainstem tumors. *J. Neurosurg.* 107:392-399.

Pollack IF, Hoffman HJ, Humphreys RP, Becker L (1993) The long-term outcome after surgical treatment of dorsally exophytic brain-stem gliomas. *J. Neurosurg.* 78:859-863.

Pollack IF, Jakacki RI, Butterfield LH, Okada H (2013) Peptide vaccine therapy for childhood gliomas. *Neurosurgery* 60 Suppl 1:113-119.

Porto L, Hattingen E, Pilatus U, Kieslich M, Yan B, Schwabe D, Zanella FE, Lanfermann H (2007) Proton magnetic resonance spectroscopy in childhood brainstem lesions. *Childs Nerv. Syst.* 23:305-314.

Puget S, Philippe C, Bax DA, Job B, Varlet P, Junier MP, Andreiuolo F, Carvalho D, Reis R, Guerrini-Rousseau L, Roujeau T, Dessen P, Richon C, Lazar V, Le Teuff G, Sainte-Rose C, Geoerger B, Vassal G, Jones C, Grill J (2012) Mesenchymal transition and PDGFRA amplification/mutation are key distinct oncogenic events in pediatric diffuse intrinsic pontine gliomas. *PloS one* 7:e30313.

Robertson PL, Muraszko KM, Brunberg JA, Axtell RA, Dauser RC, Turrisi AT (1995) Pediatric midbrain tumors: a benign subgroup of brainstem gliomas. *Pediatr. Neurosurg.* 22:65-73.

Roujeau T, Machado G, Garnett MR, Miquel C, Puget S, Geoerger B, Grill J, Boddaert N, Di Rocco F, Zerah M, Sainte-Rose C (2007) Stereotactic biopsy of diffuse pontine lesions in children. *J. Neurosurg.* 107:1-4.

Sandberg DI, Edgar MA, Souweidane MM (2002) Convection-enhanced delivery into the rat brainstem. *J. Neurosurg.* 96:885-891.

Sandri A, Sardi N, Genitori L, Giordano F, Peretta P, Basso ME, Bertin D, Mastrodicasa L, Todisco L, Mussa F, Forni M, Ricardi U, Cordero di Montezemolo L, Madon E (2006)

Diffuse and focal brain stem tumors in childhood: prognostic factors and surgical outcome. Experience in a single institution. *Childs Nerv. Syst.* 22:1127-1135.

Sanghavi SN, Needle MN, Krailo MD, Geyer JR, Ater J, Mehta MP (2003) A phase I study of topotecan as a radiosensitizer for brainstem glioma of childhood: first report of the Children's Cancer Group-0952. *Neuro Oncol.* 5:8-13.

Schild SE, Stafford SL, Brown PD, Wood CP, Scheithauer BW, Schomberg PJ, Wong WW, Lyons MK, Shaw EG (1998) The results of radiotherapy for brainstem tumors. *J. Neurooncol.* 40:171-177.

Schindler G, Capper D, Meyer J, Janzarik W, Omran H, Herold-Mende C, Schmieder K, Wesseling P, Mawrin C, Hasselblatt M, Louis DN, Korshunov A, Pfister S, Hartmann C, Paulus W, Reifenberger G, von Deimling A (2011) Analysis of BRAF V600E mutation in 1,320 nervous system tumors reveals high mutation frequencies in pleomorphic xanthoastrocytoma, ganglioglioma and extra-cerebellar pilocytic astrocytoma. *Acta neuropathologica* 121:397-405.

Schwartzentruber J et al. (2012) Driver mutations in histone H3.3 and chromatin remodelling genes in paediatric glioblastoma. *Nature* 482:226-231.

Sethi R, Allen J, Donahue B, Karajannis M, Gardner S, Wisoff J, Kunnakkat S, Mathew J, Zagzag D, Newman K, Narayana A (2011) Prospective neuraxis MRI surveillance reveals a high risk of leptomeningeal dissemination in diffuse intrinsic pontine glioma. *J. Neurooncol.* 102:121-127.

Skowronska-Gardas A (2003) Evaluation of radiotherapy for pediatric CNS tumors. *Expert review of neurotherapeutics* 3:491-500.

Smith MA, Freidlin B, Ries LA, Simon R (1998) Trends in reported incidence of primary malignant brain tumors in children in the United States. *Journal of the National Cancer Institute* 90:1269-1277.

Souweidane MM, Occhiogrosso G, Mark EB, Edgar MA (2004a) Interstitial infusion of IL13-PE38QQR in the rat brain stem. *J. Neurooncol.* 67:287-293.

Souweidane MM, Occhiogrosso G, Mark EB, Edgar MA, Dunkel IJ (2004b) Interstitial infusion of carmustine in the rat brain stem with systemic administration of O6-benzylguanine. *J. Neurooncol.* 67:319-326.

Szerlip NJ, Walbridge S, Yang L, Morrison PF, Degen JW, Jarrell ST, Kouri J, Kerr PB, Kotin R, Oldfield EH, Lonser RR (2007) Real-time imaging of convection-enhanced delivery of viruses and virus-sized particles. *J. Neurosurg.* 107:560-567.

Thakur SB, Karimi S, Dunkel IJ, Koutcher JA, Huang W (2006) Longitudinal MR spectroscopic imaging of pediatric diffuse pontine tumors to assess tumor aggression and progression. *AJNR Am. J. Neuroradiol.* 27:806-809.

Ueoka DI, Nogueira J, Campos JC, Maranhao Filho P, Ferman S, Lima MA (2009) Brainstem gliomas--retrospective analysis of 86 patients. *Journal of the neurological sciences* 281:20-23.

Ullrich NJ, Raja AI, Irons MB, Kieran MW, Goumnerova L (2007) Brainstem lesions in neurofibromatosis type 1. *Neurosurgery* 61:762-766; discussion 766-767.

Walker DA, Punt JA, Sokal M (1999) Clinical management of brain stem glioma. *Archives of disease in childhood* 80:558-564.

Walter AW, Gajjar A, Ochs JS, Langston JW, Sanford RA, Kun LE, Heideman R (1998) Carboplatin and etoposide with hyperfractionated radiotherapy in children with newly diagnosed diffuse pontine gliomas: a phase I/II study. *Med. Pediatr. Oncol.* 30:28-33.

Warren K, Bent R, Wolters PL, Prager A, Hanson R, Packer R, Shih J, Camphausen K (2012) A phase 2 study of pegylated interferon alpha-2b (PEG-Intron((R))) in children with diffuse intrinsic pontine glioma. *Cancer* 118:3607-3613.

Weiner HL, Freed D, Woo HH, Rezai AR, Kim R, Epstein FJ (1997) Intra-axial tumors of the cervicomedullary junction: surgical results and long-term outcome. *Pediatr. Neurosurg.* 27:12-18.

Wilkinson R, Harris J (2008) Moral and legal reasons for altruism in the case of brainstem biopsy in diffuse glioma. *British journal of neurosurgery* 22:617-618.

Wolff JE, Westphal S, Molenkamp G, Gnekow A, Warmuth-Metz M, Rating D, Kuehl J (2002) Treatment of paediatric pontine glioma with oral trophosphamide and etoposide. *Br. J. Cancer* 87:945-949.

Wolff JE, Classen CF, Wagner S, Kortmann RD, Palla SL, Pietsch T, Kuhl J, Gnekow A, Kramm CM (2008) Subpopulations of malignant gliomas in pediatric patients: analysis of the HIT-GBM database. *J. Neurooncol.* 87:155-164.

Wolff JE, Driever PH, Erdlenbruch B, Kortmann RD, Rutkowski S, Pietsch T, Parker C, Metz MW, Gnekow A, Kramm CM (2010) Intensive chemotherapy improves survival in pediatric high-grade glioma after gross total resection: results of the HIT-GBM-C protocol. *Cancer* 116:705-712.

Wu G et al. (2012) Somatic histone H3 alterations in pediatric diffuse intrinsic pontine gliomas and non-brainstem glioblastomas. *Nat. Genet.* 44:251-253.

Yen CP, Sheehan J, Steiner M, Patterson G, Steiner L (2007) Gamma knife surgery for focal brainstem gliomas. *J. Neurosurg.* 106:8-17.

Young Poussaint T, Yousuf N, Barnes PD, Anthony DC, Zurakowski D, Scott RM, Tarbell NJ (1999) Cervicomedullary astrocytomas of childhood: clinical and imaging follow-up. *Pediatric radiology* 29:662-668.

Yu J, Deshmukh H, Gutmann RJ, Emnett RJ, Rodriguez FJ, Watson MA, Nagarajan R, Gutmann DH (2009) Alterations of BRAF and HIPK2 loci predominate in sporadic pilocytic astrocytoma. *Neurology* 73:1526-1531.

Zarghooni M, Bartels U, Lee E, Buczkowicz P, Morrison A, Huang A, Bouffet E, Hawkins C (2010) Whole-genome profiling of pediatric diffuse intrinsic pontine gliomas highlights platelet-derived growth factor receptor alpha and poly (ADP-ribose) polymerase as potential therapeutic targets. *J. Clin. Oncol.* 28:1337-1344.

Zhang S, Feng X, Koga H, Ichikawa T, Abe S, Kumanishi T (1993) p53 gene mutations in pontine gliomas of juvenile onset. *Biochem. Biophys. Res. Commun.* 196:851-857.

In: Gliomas: Classification, Symptoms, Treatment and Prognosis ISBN: 978-1-63117-868-9
Editor: David Cory Adamson

Chapter 3

Pediatric Gliomas: Classification, Biology, Treatment and Prognosis

***Eugene I. Hwang*[1], *Lindsay B. Kilburn*[1] *and Katherine E. Warren*[2*]**
[1]Children's National Medical Center, Washington, DC;
[2]National Cancer Institute, Bethesda, Maryland, US

Abstract

The majority of central nervous system (CNS) tumors in children are gliomas. Unlike adults in whom the majority of gliomas are glioblastomas, pediatric gliomas vary tremendously in their grading, histologic appearance, biology, treatment approach, and prognosis. Historically, treatment of gliomas has been determined by tumor grade based upon histologic appearance and WHO classification, with WHO grades I-II tumors considered low-grade neoplasms, and WHO grades III-IV tumors considered high-grade, malignant neoplasms. Treatment of gliomas incorporates surgery, chemotherapy, and, in some cases, radiation therapy. Cytotoxic chemotherapeutic agents are non-specific; although they play a significant role in the treatment of gliomas, their role in high-grade gliomas is not clearly defined. Recent clinical trials have incorporated therapeutic agents with a more biologic rationale, targeting specific changes that distinguish tumor cells from normal cells. However, it is becoming clearer that pediatric gliomas differ biologically from their adult counterparts despite similar histologic appearance, and can also differ biologically depending on tumor location. Recently, certain molecular and cell pathway aberrations have been identified in subsets of tumors, including pediatric gliomas. The objective of this review is to summarize classification, treatment, and prognosis for pediatric gliomas, and discuss recent insights into biology that may lead to potential new therapeutic options.

* Corresponding Author: Katherine E. Warren, M.D., National Cancer Institute, Pediatric Oncology Branch, Building 10 CRC, Room 1-5750, Bethesda, Maryland 20892-1104, Telephone: (301) 435-4683, FAX: (301) 480-2308, Email: warrenk@mail.nih.gov.

Introduction

Tumors of the central nervous system (CNS) are the most common solid tumors in children. These tumors are heterogeneous, representing a number of different disease entities that can vary considerably in their histologic appearance, biology and prognosis. Although overall five-year survival rates for children with CNS tumors is greater than 70%, CNS tumors represent the most common cause of death from solid tumors in children [1]. Progress has been made in improving the prognosis of children with some CNS tumor types, yet the outcome of others, particularly those with glioblastoma and diffuse intrinsic pontine gliomas (DIPG), remains unchanged despite numerous clinical investigations of new agents and therapeutic modalities. Additionally, long term toxicities, including neurotoxicity, remain a major issue.

Historically, the designation and classification of CNS tumors depend on tumor cell type, degree of differentiation, and/or tumor location. Gliomas, particularly astrocytomas, are the most common type of CNS tumor in children. Histologic grading of gliomas is most commonly used to predict biologic behavior, prognosis, and determine subsequent treatment recommendations accordingly. Several different grading systems have been used to histologically classify gliomas, but the World Health Organization (WHO) tumor classification system is the most widely utilized. This system categorizes gliomas to one of four grades (I-IV) based on degree of malignancy, taking into account tumor tissue characteristics such as cellularity, nuclear atypia, mitoses, infiltrative patterns, vascular proliferation and necrosis [2]. (Figure 1) Tumors classified as WHO Grades I and II have a relatively low proliferative index and are considered low-grade lesions. While Grade I tumors typically have clear margins and can be surgically resected, Grade II tumors appear more infiltrative and have a higher rate of recurrence. Grade III and IV tumors are considered high-grade lesions; Grade III astrocytic tumors have anaplasia and increased mitotic activity while Grade IV tumors also show tumor necrosis and/or microvascular endothelial proliferation. The more common pediatric astrocytic tumors are listed by WHO grade in Table 1.

The clinical presentation of children with CNS tumors depends on a number of factors including tumor type, location, and growth rate. In addition, the method of expansion (i.e., invasion versus compression of surrounding tissues), associated edema and mass effect, and age of the child (*e.g.,* open or closed fontanel) determine presenting symptoms. Symptoms may be specific to the location of the tumor or more generalized. For example, headache, nausea, and emesis may be the result of increased intracranial pressure. Children with slow growing tumors may present with seizures. Children with tumors in the posterior fossa may have localized symptoms such as cranial neuropathies and ataxia, along with symptoms of increased intracranial pressure resulting from cerebrospinal (CSF) obstruction. The diagnosis of CNS tumors ultimately depends on a thorough neurologic examination combined with adequate imaging, typically an MRI scan performed with and without intravenous contrast administration. With the exception of DIPG and some optic pathway gliomas, the final diagnosis is made by histologic examination of tissue. For a small number of tumors that are historically difficult to classify histologically, diagnostic markers may be utilized (e.g., INI1 for atypical teratoid/rhabdoid tumors [3] or LIN28A immunoreactivity for embryonal tumor with multilayered rosettes, also known as ETMR [4]).

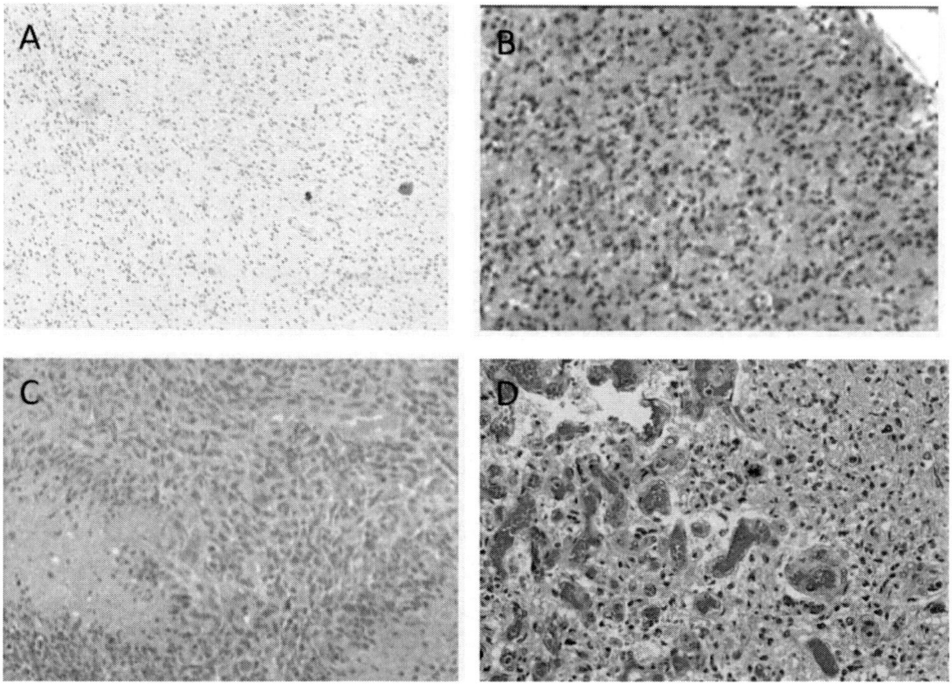

Figure 1. Histologic representation of different grades of glioma. A) WHO Grade II demonstrating increased cellularity; B. WHO Grade III with increased cellularity and some atypia; C) WHO Grade IV glioma with increased cellularity, nuclear atypia, increased mitoses and palisading necrosis; D) WHO Grade IV glioma with increased cellularity, nuclear atypia, increased mitoses and increased vascular proliferation.

Table 1. Common Pediatric Astrocytic Tumors by WHO Grading

WHO Grade	Tumor Type
I	Pilocytic Astrocytoma
	Subependymal Giant Cell Astrocytoma
II	Diffuse Astrocytoma
	Pleomorphic Xanthoastrocytoma
III	Anaplastic Astrocytoma
IV	Glioblastoma
(II-IV)	Gliomatosis cerebri

In general, the initial treatment of children with CNS tumors depends on presenting signs and symptoms, as well as suspected tumor type. Immediate therapy involves patient stabilization with anticonvulsants if necessary for seizures, steroids to decrease tumor associated edema, and surgery for prompt CSF diversion in cases of obstruction. Those with suspected embryonal tumors, ependymomas or germinomas, as well as those with symptoms localized to the spinal cord, require staging. Surgery is used to establish a histologic diagnosis, reduce tumor bulk, and in some cases, such as low-grade gliomas, may be curative. Radiation is generally reserved for those with malignant tumors or those with rapid tumor growth and impending loss of function, such as vision loss. Chemotherapeutic regimens are commonly utilized as adjuvant therapies for several tumor types including malignant gliomas; chemotherapy is also the mainstay of therapy for those with low-grade gliomas. Given the variability in prognosis and high incidence of neurotoxicity noted in long term survivors, a major goal in managing children with gliomas is to reduce the potential of long term toxicities in those with tumor types associated with high survival rates while aggressively treating those with low predicted survival in an effort to eradicate the tumor. Tumor classification systems that are predictive of behavior are therefore critical.

In addition to histologic grade, prognostic factors for pediatric gliomas include clinical features such as age at diagnosis, extent of tumor resection, and tumor location. Some of these factors have been incorporated into clinical trials to stratify high risk versus average risk patients. While histologic grading and some clinical features may prove to be prognostic, additional features (molecular, genetic, chromosomal) within and between glioma subgroups are being identified. Perhaps the most widely used prognostic and predictive feature, particularly in adult neuro-oncology, is loss of heterozygosity of chromosomes 1p and 19q observed in some oligodendroglial tumors and its association with a markedly better response to therapy [5]. More recently, adult gliomas are being classified using gene signatures, where identified prognostic molecular abnormalities involving methylguanine methyltransferase (*MGMT*), isocitrate dehydrogenase 1 (*IDH1*), and *TP53,* for example, are incorporated into the information dataset used to determine treatment [6]. The clinical significance of prognostic factors identified in adults may differ for pediatric gliomas.

As we learn more about the biology of these tumors, factors that may better predict tumor behavior are being identified. Information gained from molecular and –omics studies (i.e., proteomics, genomics) may be useful to identify pathways involved in tumor pathogenesis, aid in diagnosis, subclassify patients by risk (i.e., prognostic), discover therapeutic targets, or predict response to therapy. Here, we broadly classify pediatric gliomas as low-grade versus high-grade tumors to discuss biology, treatment, and prognosis by group. Specific glioma subtypes, particularly those for which biology is known and that may impact prognosis or therapeutic choices, are described in more detail. Of note, a key feature of pediatric neuro-oncology is that tissue is not obtained for all tumors at diagnosis. Some tumors, such as diffuse intrinsic pontine gliomas (DIPG) and some optic pathway gliomas (OPG), are diagnosed based on clinical and radiographic presentation, and no tissue may ever be obtained throughout the course of the patient's illness. This limits our ability to subclassify each pediatric brain tumor based on biology and hinders choice of treatment based on biologic rationale.

I. Low-Grade Gliomas

Pediatric low-grade gliomas (PLGG) encompass a relatively diverse group of slow-growing CNS tumors. Together, they are the most common pediatric primary CNS neoplasms, accounting for more than a third of brain tumors diagnosed in children [7]. As a group, PLGGs tend to be relatively well circumscribed and often have an indolent course, although they may cause significant morbidity or, even, mortality. Although pediatric low-grade gliomas are all neuroepithelial tumors sharing many characteristics, each tumor type has discrete histopathological and molecular aspects that inform outcomes and influence clinical care.

Epidemiology

Sporadic low-grade gliomas arise most frequently in children in the 5- to 9-year age range; however, almost a quarter of newly symptomatic patients are older than 11 years of age [8]. In children with neurofibromatosis type I (NF1), who have a predilection towards development of low-grade gliomas, tumors more typically occur at a younger age. Other genetic predisposition syndromes, including tuberous sclerosis complex (TSC) types 1 and 2, are evident in a small subset of children who develop these tumors. Gender distribution is roughly equivalent.

Clinical Presentation

The clinical presentation of a child with a low-grade glioma is determined largely by the location of the tumor. Pediatric low-grade gliomas (PLGGs) can present with focal neurologic symptoms such as visual impairment or proptosis (optic nerve) [9], ataxia and nausea (cerebellum/brainstem) [10][13], or endocrinopathies (hypothalamic-chiasmatic) [11]. Other symptoms such as seizures, failure to thrive and cranial nerve palsies are less common but occur with particular tumor locations. Although some low-grade gliomas are known to cause seizures [10], pilocytic astrocytomas typically do not, likely because of their predominantly infratentorial site of origin. Non-specific symptoms such as headache, nausea, or fatigue may also form part of the presentation if tumor obstructs CSF flow and increases intracranial pressure.

PLGGs are most commonly located in the cerebellum, although may be found anywhere in the CNS. This includes the brainstem, where pilocytic astrocytomas, pilomyxoid tumors, and grade II gliomas may be distinguished radiographically from their higher grade cousins (diffuse intrinsic pontine gliomas) by their focal, dorsally exophytic nature [12]. The majority of LGG associated with NF1 are optic pathway gliomas (OPGs), although NF1-associated PLGGs may also arise elsewhere within the CNS.

While PLGG are not considered to have high metastatic potential, dissemination on presentation or with progression may occur. This was prospectively examined in the *Hirntumorstudien* (HIT)-LGG 1996 trial, which had a total accrual of 1181 children [13]. In this patient population, 2.8% of children had metastatic disease present at initial diagnosis, and 5.2% of patients eventually were diagnosed with dissemination. Infants with hypothalamic/chiasmatic gliomas and associated diencephalic syndrome had a particularly high rate of dissemination at 16% [13]. Although dissemination along the neuraxis is not common, in situations with intracranial metastatic disease or in the context of clinical suspicion, spinal MRI and CSF sampling should be considered.

Diagnosis

Magnetic resonance imaging (MRI) is the preferred modality to establish the radiographic signature of PLGGs. In general, low-grade gliomas are hypointense on T1-weighted images and hyperintense on T2-weighted images when compared with surrounding brain. Some PLGGs have characteristic radiographic features, although these may be non-specific. Pilocytic astrocytomas are usually well demarcated with significant contrast enhancement. The presence of a cystic component with an enhancing mural nodule is characteristic of pilocytic astrocytomas, although not specific or observed in all cases. Pleomorphic xanthochromic astrocytomas (PXA) also often involve cystic changes and usually are found at the surface of the cortex. Subependymal giant cell astrocytomas (SEGA) typically are found near the foramen of Monro and may display calcification. Diffuse astrocytomas such as fibrillary gliomas have less well-defined margins and often do not demonstrate significant contrast enhancement.

Histologically, PLGGs include all 'low' grade gliomas. However, this attribution can sometimes be difficult to make, may be heterogeneous within a given tumor, and disagreement amongst pathologists can render the grading distinction somewhat unpredictable [14]. In one retrospective, centrally-reviewed clinical trial, original grading assessments were significantly altered in 28% of the cases [15]. Histological characteristics are discussed with each tumor subtype later in this chapter.

Given the non-specific radiographic features, tissue diagnosis is undertaken for suspected PLGGs with a few exceptions. Ideally, complete resection of the tumor is attempted at the time of tissue acquisition for diagnosis when the risk for significant morbidity is low. Conversely, in cases where children are asymptomatic and radiographically diagnosed tumors are not progressive, surgical approaches should be cautious, especially when biopsy or resection has a high risk of morbidity. For example, some intrinsic optic pathway gliomas (OPG) have archetypal imaging and demographic characteristics, and in these situations, therapy may be initiated without upfront tissue confirmation. In NF1 patients who have OPG, biopsy is infrequently undertaken unless atypical features raise clinical concerns or response to treatment is unusual.

Treatment

Surgery

In general, gross total resection (GTR), confirmed by both the neurosurgeon's postoperative assessment as well as an MRI scan obtained within the first 48 hours after surgery, can be curative for children with low-grade gliomas. In a large study of 518 evaluable children with low-grade gliomas managed by primary surgery and subsequent observation, outcome was generally good and appeared related to both histology and tumor location [16]. For children with pilocytic astrocytomas, 8-year progression-free survival (PFS) with GTR alone was 95% with 100% overall survival (OS). In children with non-pilocytic low-grade gliomas, GTR was slightly less efficacious but continued to confer an excellent prognosis, with 8-year PFS of 89% and OS of 98%. Thus, when GTR is attained, suggested care consists of close clinical and radiographic monitoring only. If GTR cannot be obtained, children with pilocytic astrocytomas still maintain an excellent 8-year OS of 100%, but PFS is 41% for midline/chiasmatic pilocytic astrocytomas and 58% for those located in the cerebellum and cerebral cortex. For children with non-pilocytic gliomas who do not attain a GTR, 8-yr PFS is similar at 54-56% [16]. These results inform the prognostic significance of extent of resection. The differences in location-based outcomes may in part reflect the discrepancy in ability to attain GTR in specific regions of the brain [17]. Regardless, patients with GTR of a PLGG may be observed closely without additional therapy until signs of tumor recurrence. Children with PLGGs and limited residual disease or near-total resection may also be observed. A large prospective study quantified the relative risk of progression in children with residual tumor <1.5 cm^2 to be 6.0 [16]. If the amount of residual disease is >1.5 cm^2 after resection, relative risk increased to 7.9. Five-year event-free survival (EFS) for these patients with residual disease was only 56% [16]. Despite the clearly increased risk for recurrence or progression in patients with residual disease, a significant number may not require further therapy and a few tumors may regress. Overall survival in this group remains quite high at greater than 90% at 8 years [13]. Therefore, unless impending neurologic deterioration is of concern, close clinical and radiographic monitoring for tumor progression in children with PLGG and limited residual disease is often undertaken without other therapy [18]. In fact, in the recent large HIT-LGG-1996 protocol, observation was recommended for any patient with newly diagnosed LGG without 'threatening' symptoms. Radiation or chemotherapy was only offered to children with clear disease progression or clinical deterioration, and outcomes were similar to US-based treatment protocols, namely, 10-year OS of 94% and 10-year EFS of 47% [13]. Additionally, in selected cases where the risk for morbidity is considered low, GTR may be achieved at second look surgery and should be considered, especially in cases of sub-total initial resection [19]. Unfortunately, many PLGGs cannot safely attain near or total resection and thus require non-surgical adjuvant therapy, whether chemotherapy or radiation-based [20].

Radiation Therapy

Radiation therapy is effective in treating children with PLGGs [21]. Multiple institutional studies have demonstrated an improvement in PFS in children with subtotally-resected PLGG when adjuvant focal radiation is administered, typically at doses of 45 to 54 Gy [20]. A significant proportion of irradiated PLGGs decrease in size [22], and in some series, over half of patients did not progress after radiation therapy [20]. This results in approximately 75% 8-10 year EFS and 85% OS [21, 23, 24]. In older children without NF-1, irradiation may be the treatment of choice given the relatively good survival as well as the truncated period of therapy required. However, radiation is accompanied by a high risk of significant morbidity, including cognitive deficits, risk for secondary malignancy, vasculopathy, and other long-term adverse consequences. Patients with NF1 have a particular high risk of cognitive and other radiation-induced insufficiencies [23]. Young children are also at greater risk for more profound adverse events likely because of the susceptibility of the maturing CNS to therapeutic doses of irradiation. Given the many confirmed potential adverse effects of CNS radiation, studies have been undertaken to examine the possibility of reducing the historical radiation margin from 1 cm to 0.5cm [25]. Therefore, despite the demonstrated efficacy of radiotherapy for tumor control, immediate radiation of sub-totally resected PLGGs is somewhat controversial and some studies even describe no benefit to overall survival [26].

Chemotherapy

Chemotherapy, including cytotoxic agents and, more recently, molecularly targeted agents, can be utilized to stabilize PLGGs in an effort to delay or even obviate the need for radiation. When low-grade glioma is clinically symptomatic, progresses radiographically, or the risk for significant clinical symptoms is high, chemotherapy is often preferred as front-line therapy. This is especially true for young patients and those with NF1. Although there is some concern that tumor progression may increase the size of the radiation field if initial chemotherapy is ineffective, careful analysis has demonstrated that tumor size at the time of radiation in children who initially received chemotherapy was not significantly larger than at presentation [17]. Chemotherapy use has also been associated with symptomatic improvement, even in the absence of significant radiographic improvement. In a series of adult patients with seizures secondary to LGG, temozolomide use led to improvement in seizure frequency in 59% of patients compared to 13% in those patients who did not receive temozolomide [27]. Of note, although chemotherapeutic treatment may lead to prolonged disease stability and symptomatic improvement, the majority of children with PLGGs treated with chemotherapy will eventually recur or progress.

Several different chemotherapy regimens have proven effective in the context of either newly diagnosed or progressive PLGGs. (Table 2) The combination of carboplatin and vincristine, administered either weekly or monthly, is a frequently used chemotherapy regimen for PLGGs. Using this treatment, 5-year EFS and OS are 39±4% and 86±3%, respectively [28]. Half of these tumors displayed radiographic response. When compared against an alternate regimen that includes thioguanine, procarbazine, lomustine, and vincristine (also known as the TPCV regimen), both EFS and OS at the 5-year benchmark were similar [28]. Other chemotherapy regimens have been used primarily in the recurrent setting, although smaller trials have evaluated treatments such as vinblastine in an upfront setting with early results that are comparable to these more commonly used initial therapeutic regimens [28]. A recent report evaluating bevacizumab plus irinotecan in children with recurrent low-grade gliomas (in which 16 of 35 patients had known pilocytic astrocytoma) demonstrated 2-yr PFS of 47.8% and 20% of patients had prolonged stable disease for a median of 40.1 months at the time of the report [29].

As is evident by the excellent overall survival but the relatively high number of patients with disease progression, children with PLGGs tend to require repeated treatment courses over the evolution of their disease. When PLGGs progress after initial exposure to chemotherapy, repeated treatment may involve either institution of a new regimen or sometimes a return to the original chemotherapy regimen if prior efficacy and tolerability were demonstrated. These repeated courses of chemotherapy often result in 5-year OS and EFS numbers (86±6% and 37±8%, respectively) that are fairly comparable to those achieved with upfront therapy [30]. Thus, given the frequency of relapse and need for multiple treatment regimens, PLGGs is conceptualized as a chronic disease.

Table 2. Commonly used chemotherapeutic regimens for newly diagnosed and progressive pediatric low-grade gliomas

Regimen	n	Objective Response rate	EFS	OS	Reference
Carboplatin/Vincristine[+]	137	50%	5yr 39±4%	5yr 86±3%	Ater [28]
TPCV[+]	137	54%	5yr 52±5%	5yr 87±7%	Ater [28]
Vinblastine[*]	51	36%	5yr 42±7%	5yr 93±4%	Bouffet [188]
Temozolomide[$]	30	15%	4yr 17%	4yr 71%	Gururangan [189]
Carboplatin (monthly)[$]	81	28%	3yr 64%	3yr 84%	Gururangan [190]
Bevacizumab/Irinotecan[*]	10	70%	N/A	N/A	Hwang [191]
Baby SFOP[+^]	85	42%	5yr 34%	5yr 89%	Laithier [192]
Cisplatin/Etoposide[*]	37	65%	3yr 65%	3yr 97%	Massimino [193]

[+] Newly diagnosed tumors.
[*] Recurrent tumors.
[$] Newly diagnosed and recurrent tumors.
[^] Agents include: procarbazine, carboplatin, etoposide, cisplatin, vincristine, cyclophosphamide.

Metronomic therapy is a chronic treatment strategy utilizing relatively lower doses of multiple agents given in a continuous, alternating fashion; this approach is antiangiogenic and also limits significant toxicity in what is often a highly tolerable regimen. This strategy has been more closely explored recently, particularly as the perspective of the natural history of PLGG encompasses more of a chronic disorder. Results from a study utilizing a metronomic regimen consisting of thalidomide, celecoxib, fenofibrate, and alternating etoposide and cyclophosphamide, have recently been reported. This regimen was used in 12 children with recurrent low-grade glioma, resulting in a 33% objective response rate (n=4 partial responses); additionally, 58% of enrolled patients completed the total 27 week course of therapy without progression, demonstrating the efficacy of this approach [31].

Prognosis

The majority of low-grade gliomas in children are indolent, and the overall prognosis for children with PLGGs is relatively good with 15-year overall survival (OS) of greater than 85%, although EFS is only 55% [20, 32]. This is in contrast to adults with low-grade gliomas, which, even with complete resection, often progress or undergo malignant transformation resulting in death for almost half of adult patients [33]. The malignant transformation rate from low-grade to high-grade gliomas is estimated to be >50% in adults compared to <10% in children [34, 35]. Adult LGG differ biologically from PLGG in that they frequently harbor *IDH1* mutations, uncommonly found in PLGGs [36]. Although PLGGs rarely transform to higher-grade tumors, particular subsets of children with PLGGs, including those with unresectable disease, metastases, or with higher-grade histological diagnoses tend to have worse outcomes. Infants less than 6 months of age, especially in the context of diencephalic syndrome, also have inferior outcomes [37], and multiple reports indicate children less than 5 years of age are at higher risk for disease progression [28, 38]. Children with unresectable LGG thus tend to have a natural history of chronic progression and accompanying morbidity, sometimes ending in death; almost half of these children will progress within 5 years and almost 10% will die of their disease within this timeframe [16]. Although metastatic disease is not an independent prognostic factor in multivariate analysis, children with dissemination have a lower OS when compared to those with non-disseminated disease (5-year OS 73% with metastasis vs. 96% without) [39]. Children with NF1 and presumed LGG who are initially observed may not require therapy; however, most of these children will ultimately progress, with 5-year EFS for children with NF1 and LGG only 24% when following this approach [13]. In conjunction with case reports of spontaneous regression in NF1-related LGG, this demonstrates a natural history for NF1-associated PLGGs distinct from that of other PLGGs [8].

Chemotherapy and Toxicity

Chemotherapy may cause significant acute and long-term adverse effects, although the potential cumulative toxicity of repeated therapies in these children is not well characterized. In the most commonly utilized combination of carboplatin and vincristine, up to 40% of children will experience hypersensitivity reactions to carboplatin [40]. While premedication and desensitization may ultimately allow continued use of this agent, in many patients alternative treatment regimens must be used. Peripheral neuropathy, which is not always reversible, is a well-known side effect of vincristine therapy. Cumulative impairment of fertility has been a concern specifically with regards to procarbazine (a component of the TPCV regimen) [41] and bevacizumab, the latter of which caused a significant proportion of adult women to undergo irreversible ovarian failure [42]. This is particularly pertinent as both boys and girls likely to receive chemotherapy in a radiation-delaying strategy are likely to be too young to undergo standard fertility preservation techniques. Secondary malignancy, hearing loss, and other potentially significant long-term adverse consequences also are described after chemotherapy.

Long-term morbidity remains of concern in children who have been treated for LGG. In one large study, significant long-term impairment was noted in several areas [32]. Conditions exhibited by patients 15 years after diagnosis of PLGG included: blindness (18%), hearing loss (22%), obesity (53%), growth hormone deficiency (29%), and adrenocorticotropic hormone (ACTH) deficiency (26%). Approximately one-third of patients had an IQ less than 85, which is below average [32]. Radiation therapy was an independent prognostic indicator of abnormal endocrine function and hearing loss, while tumor location in the diencephalon predicted both hormone dysfunction and blindness. Exposure to chemotherapy was not independently assessed in this study. Because of the chronic nature and prolonged survival of many patients with LGG, increased focus on potential late effects must be considered when administering early treatment.

Cytotoxic chemotherapeutic agents play a major role in the management of children with low-grade gliomas, but these agents are non-specific. In efforts to reduce acute and long-term toxicities associated with therapy, investigations have focused on targeting specific changes that distinguish tumor cells from normal cells.

Biology of Pediatric Low-Grade Gliomas

Our understanding of the biology of PLGGs has recently undergone a transformation, particularly with the knowledge that pediatric low-grade gliomas do not molecularly mirror their adult histologic counterparts. For example, unlike in adults, pediatric LGG have low rates of *TP53* mutations (<10%), *IDH1* mutations, and chromosomes 1p19q alteration [43]. The biology of PLGGs appears to be age and location dependent.

Early understanding of the PLGG molecular phenotype initially arose from observations related to NF1-related low-grade gliomas. In this heritable condition, predisposition to development of PLGGs is related to inactivation of the *NF1* gene [44]. The product of this gene, neurofibromin, is a negative regulator of the RAS pathway and mutation leads to upregulation of the downstream MAP kinase pathway. *NF1*-associated alterations predispose patients towards the development of LGG, especially pilocytic astrocytomas, in as many as 15-20% of patients [45]. Although sporadic (non-NF1 related) pilocytic astrocytomas do not result from a *NF1* gene mutation, most show evidence of activation of the MAPK pathway. Chromosomes 7 and 8 are the most commonly altered chromosomes in sporadic pilocytic astrocytomas.

Recently, it was discovered that many pilocytic astrocytomas have a tandem duplication of chromosome 7q, resulting in a fusion gene (*KIAA1549:BRAF*) which causes constitutive activation of the BRAF/MEK/MAP kinase signaling pathway [46] (Figure 2). Other RAS/RAF pathway mutations have also been identified in pilocytic astrocytomas resulting in activation of the MAP kinase pathway [47].

Activation of the phosphatidylinositol-3 kinase (PI3K) pathway has also been observed in sporadic pilocytic astrocytomas.

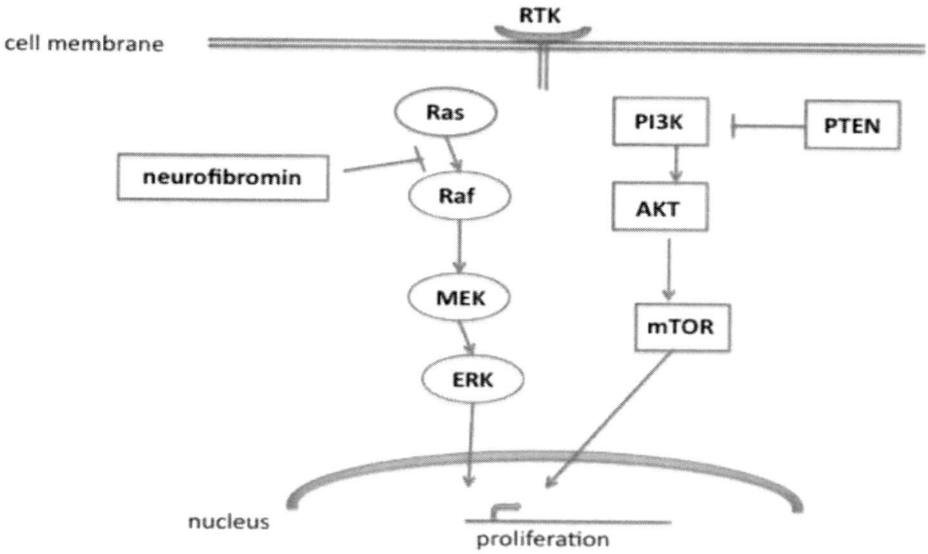

Figure 2. Molecular pathways implicated in the tumorigenesis of PLGGs.

Increased activity of one component of this pathway, the mammalian target of rapamycin (mTOR), was noted by moderate to strong immunostaining for pS6 in 25 of 36 (69%) pilocytic astrocytomas, as well as 2/2 pilomyxoid and 2/2 diffuse astrocytomas [48]. Increased mTOR immunohistochemical signal is also noted in NF1-related pilocytic astrocytomas. In SEGAs, as will be discussed later, mTOR activation is a direct result of the *TSC1* or *2* alterations, and virtually all of these tumors exhibit high mTOR activity. Differential telomere lengths and lack of telomere maintenance have been proposed as possible mechanisms for the spontaneous regression of some PLGGs. In one investigation, tumors with shorter telomere length tended to not recur, providing a potential explanation for the observed phenomenon of tumor senescence in PLGG [49].

In grade II PLGGs, presence of the BRAF fusion protein is less common than in pilocytic astrocytomas; instead, BRAF pathway activation is more often due to a V600E point mutation [50]. Whole genome sequencing also revealed that 24% of diffuse grade II gliomas contain *FGFR1* region duplication, which activates the MAPK/ERK and PI3K pathways [50]. Other genetic events including focal amplification of *MYBL1*, were found only in diffuse grade II astrocytomas [51], although increased protein expression was noted in all LGG subtypes [52]. Further noted was a lack of overlapping mutations, supporting the argument that mutations in *NF1, RAF/RAS, FGFR1*, and *MYB/MYBL1* may be mutually exclusive. This, of course, has implications toward successful potential treatment with direct pathway inhibitors with lessened concern for multiple activating pathways in a given tumor [50].

Genetic analysis of PXAs has been limited given the restricted numbers of patients and existing information showing varying levels of genetic heterogeneity. Chromosomal abnormalities are not unique to PXAs, but loss of chromosome 9 may be seen in almost 50%, and a high proportion of tumors exhibit CDKN2A/p14^{ARF} deletions [53]. Mutations of *TP53* were found in only 6% of cases [54]; similarly, *EGFR*, *MDM2*, and *CDK4* genes were largely unaltered [55]. One recent series additionally demonstrated BRAF V600E mutations in 12 of 20 PXAs (60%), with no BRAF fusion protein abnormalities [56].

Subependymal giant cell astrocytomas (SEGAs) occur in the context of tuberous sclerosis complex (TSC), a multi-system genetic disorder that affects the brain and other organs. The TSC1/2 complex causes inactivation of Ras homolog enriched in brain (Rheb), ultimately leading to overactivation of mTOR, which is the most salient molecular characteristic of this tumor type [57].

Taken collectively, activation of several pro-proliferative pathways may be linked to tumorigenesis in PLGGs. This knowledge may lead to novel targeted therapies. Specific PLGG subtypes are discussed in more detail below.

Pilocytic Astrocytoma

Pilocytic astrocytomas (PAs), which are considered grade I gliomas, account for roughly 18-20% of CNS tumors in childhood and are the most common type of PLGGs [2, 58]. They typically are well circumscribed, exhibit slow growth kinetics and may even spontaneously regress [59]. They have a low likelihood of malignant transformation, although in the context of radiotherapy may very rarely do so [34]. In children, PAs tend to be infratentorial, preferentially arising in the cerebellar hemispheres but may arise anywhere astrocytes are located, including the brainstem and cerebral hemispheres. The most frequent supratentorial locations are the optic chiasm/hypothalamus or the region of the thalamus and basal ganglia [60]. They are also found within the spinal cord, although this is a less common phenomenon [2]. Children with NF1 develop PAs at a rate of close to 15%; these tend to arise more typically in the optic pathway or brainstem [61].

The presentation of children with pilocytic astrocytomas mirrors that of low-grade gliomas in general. Radiographically, PAs are typically well circumscribed, demonstrate contrast enhancement, and frequently have associated cysts that contain proteinaceous fluid with CSF-like signal intensity. PAs usually have higher signal intensity on T2-weighted images, and calcification can be present in 10% of cases. Histologically, PAs are characterized by a biphasic pattern consisting of compacted piloid cells alternating with less-compacted microcystic cellular regions [2]. These tumors are positive for glial fibrillary acid protein (GFAP). PAs contain eosinophilic "corkscrew" fibers known as Rosenthal fibers and other eosinophilic granular bodies; however, there may be considerable heterogeneity in different regions of a given tumor and their presence is not required for a diagnosis of PA. Cells in general have only occasional mitotic activity and notably lack the palisading necrosis or significant nuclear atypia seen in higher grade glial tumors [44]. In peripheral infiltrative portions of the tumor, cells may histologically resemble WHO Grade II astrocytomas [2].

Although benign, PAs may occasionally disseminate despite a low proliferation index; these metastatic lesions usually behave in a benign manner displaying very slow growth kinetics. In general, children with PAs have a very good overall prognosis. With complete or even near-total excision, both OS and PFS approach 100%, although a few patients will recur and require additional therapy [20]. However, PAs in the optic pathway, brainstem, or more central areas are not amenable to complete surgical resection. Without significant resection, survival is negatively impacted despite the use of chemotherapy and/or radiotherapy, with EFS ~74% with the use of radiation [21]. A recent analysis of infants demonstrated that outcomes for infants less than 6 months have a much worse 5-year EFS and OS, at 40% and 84%, respectively [37].

As noted previously, because of the significant toxicities associated with radiation therapy, chemotherapy is often used in an attempt to delay or obviate the need for radiation, especially in more vulnerable populations such as very young children or those with NF1. Chemotherapy for PAs mirrors that of the general PLGG category, with the combination of carboplatin and vincristine commonly used as initial therapy.

Optic Pathway Gliomas

Optic pathway gliomas (OPGs) are low-grade gliomas that arise anywhere within the visual pathway including the optic nerve, chiasm, optic tracts, and posterior visual pathways. Because of their proximity to and frequent involvement of the optic chiasm and pathway, hypothalamic low-grade gliomas are often considered OPGs. Overall, OPGs account for less than 5% of all brain tumors in children. In general, OPGs are PAs with a very small proportion being diffuse fibrillary gliomas [62], although with typical clinical and radiographic findings, many are not initially biopsied for fear of damaging the visual apparatus. OPGs arise predominantly in children with 90% of OPGs found in the first two decades of life and 71% affecting children less than ten years of age. If associated with NF1, OPGs tend to present in children younger than 5 years of age. Children with NF1 have a predilection towards PA development, especially of the optic nerve, and 30-70% of patients with OPG have concomitant NF1 [63, 64]. In general, patients with OPGs have a very good survival outcome; however, OPGs also may cause irreversible visual deterioration so must be managed carefully.

Children with OPGs often present with visual symptoms, including nystagmus, decreased visual acuity, visual field loss, papilledema, or proptosis. Diencephalic syndrome or endocrinopathies, including precocious puberty, may also be present. OPGs that arise from the optic nerve are discrete, focal tumors that do not penetrate the globe itself; however, tumor expansion may impinge on the globe and cause significant proptosis. Radiographic findings and changes do not predict visual deterioration, emphasizing the importance of visual function evaluations and close monitoring. These measures are especially important in children with NF1 and OPGs as only about 50% of these cases will ultimately require therapy.

Treatment is instituted if visual deterioration or radiographic progression occurs. Unless a significant cosmetic deficit already exists, intraorbital optic nerve gliomas are not typically resected as they rarely extend into the chiasm. Debulking other OPGs is likewise avoided except in cases of existent significant visual compromise and tumors that have resisted all other methods of control.

Radiotherapy can be effective in the control of OPG [21, 65], resulting in both radiographic and visual function stabilization in a majority of treated patients; visual function has been reported to improve in up to 40% of patients [65]. The duration of response to radiation is also typically good, with 10-year PFS of 74-89% and 10-year OS of 90-96% [21, 65]. However, because of the relatively young age of most patients who have OPG and the sensitivity of the brain in those with NF1, radiation has become increasingly delayed or avoided in an attempt to mitigate long-term adverse consequences.

Chemotherapy in OPGs has gained increasing acceptance as alternative front-line therapy, and a number of regimens have been employed. In addition to the vincristine/carboplatin and TPCV regimens, there is recent interest in the use of bevacizumab in children with OPGs and declining visual function. Use of bevacizumab in this context appears to achieve rapid, more consistent visual improvement than traditional chemotherapy regimens, although durability of this improvement may not be long [66] and prospective studies in newly diagnosed patients have not been performed. Although a recent report showed encouraging responses in a prospective clinical trial using bevacizumab plus irinotecan in children with recurrent low-grade gliomas, visual outcome measures were not reported [29].

Subependymal Giant Cell Astrocytomas (SEGA)

Subependymal giant cell astrocytomas (SEGA) are slow-growing CNS tumors classified as grade I astrocytic tumors by the WHO classification system. They commonly develop from the wall of the lateral ventricle, often near the foramen of Monro, thereby potentially impeding CSF pathways and causing obstructive hydrocephalus. Children with tuberous sclerosis complex have a 20% increased risk for developing SEGA in the first two decades of life [67]. Tuberous sclerosis complex is an autosomal dominant disorder caused by abnormalities in either the *TSC1* or *TSC2* genes, which usually function as tumor suppressors [68]. Because of the slow growth of this tumor, observation of stable tumors with MRI is standard practice, and a recent consensus statement recommends MRI scans every 6 months for tumors greater than 1 centimeter [69]. If a given SEGA causes symptoms such as obstructive hydrocephalus or neurologic deterioration, or exhibits consistent radiographic worsening, then surgical resection is the therapy of choice. Much like other PLGGs, complete or near total resection can be curative. Focal radiation therapy has been effective in prolonged stabilization.

Because mTOR pathway dysregulation is critical to the pathogenesis of tuberous sclerosis, mTOR inhibition was hypothesized to inhibit SEGA progression. A clinical trial using everolimus, an mTOR inhibitor, was recently completed [70]. In patients (n=28) with TSC-associated SEGA, at least 30% tumor shrinkage was demonstrated in over two-thirds of children. Tumor response remained stable over the median duration of therapy, which was 34.2 months at time of publication, supporting the durability and efficacy of this molecularly targeted approach [70]. Another study of everolimus in young children noted a tumor response of greater than 50% in 6 of 8 enrolled children; there was no evidence of progression over a minimum treatment duration of 33 months, in addition to improvement of intractable seizures [71]. Due to these robust responses, everolimus is now FDA-approved for the treatment of patients with TSC-associated SEGAs, and is frequently the initial treatment in this patient population.

Grade II Low-Grade Gliomas

Grade II LGGs encompass both pleomorphic xanothoastrocytomas (PXAs) and diffuse low-grade astrocytomas (fibrillary, gemistocytic, and protoplasmic astrocytomas). Together, these tumors make up only a small percentage of tumors in children but tend to be more clinically aggressive with poorer outcomes than those tumors already discussed.

Pleomorphic Xanthochromic Astrocytoma (PXA)

Pleomorphic xanthoastrocytomas (PXAs) are grade II gliomas first described in 1979 [72]. They are most often found in older children and adolescents, with a median age of 14 years at presentation, although they may also be found in younger children and the elderly. PXAs only comprise 1-2% of all pediatric CNS neoplasms [54]. Interestingly, PXAs usually involve the superficial aspect of the brain and meninges, most commonly involving the temporal lobe, with only rare cases being described infratentorially [54]. Seizures are more commonly associated with PXA presentation than other PLGGs [56]. Roughly half will display cysts on imaging; other imaging characteristics are similar to those of other low-grade gliomas, i.e., hypointensity on T1-weighted imaging and contrast enhancement of the solid component of the tumor [73].

Histologically, PXAs have a heterogeneous appearance (hence the moniker 'pleomorphic') with spindle elements mixed with large multinucleate astrocytes, the latter being present in over 90% of cases [54]. Granular bodies and xanthomatous (yellowish) cells with significant intracellular lipid droplets are frequent [2]. Tumors are further characterized on silver staining by a rich reticulin fiber network. In general, PXAs do not initially display significant anaplasia, although they may eventually progress to resemble higher-grade gliomas. Further, PXAs may occasionally contain rare Rosenthal fibers [54]. Tumors are positive for GFAP and S-100 protein, demonstrating their glial origin, but also express neuronal markers such as synaptophysin, neurofilament, and MAP2. Mitotic activity is the only histologic feature to be somewhat predictive of outcome [54].

Clinically, PXAs begin as slow-growing lesions; 10-year EFS and OS are 61% and 70%, respectively, in both children and adults [54]. However, up to 15% of PXAs may undergo malignant transformation, although this is more common in adult than pediatric patients [74]. In addition, on recurrence PXAs will often exhibit anaplasia and necrosis [54]. The most significant prognostic factor is the extent of initial resection ($p<0.003$) [54].

Standard treatment for PXAs initially involves complete resection with subsequent careful monitoring. However, in cases of clear anaplasia or incomplete resection, irradiation has been demonstrated to potentially contribute to prolonged tumor control [75]. Upon recurrence, PXAs may exhibit leptomeningeal spread. The role for chemotherapy at either initial presentation or at the time of recurrence has not been well demonstrated and is not frequently utilized [54], although scattered reports of chemotherapeutic use have been reported with mixed results. Given the recent information regarding the high frequency (60%) of the V600E mutation in PXAs as discussed above [56], new V600E or MAPK-targeted therapies may be of benefit [56].

Diffuse Low-Grade Gliomas

Fibrillary astrocytoma is the most common diffuse LGG. Overall, fibrillary astrocytomas tend to arise later in life, with only approximately 10% occurring in patients less than 20 years of age. They are typically found in the supratentorium and, less commonly, brainstem and cervicomedullary junction [63, 76]. Because fibrillary gliomas usually occur in the supratentorial compartment, often favoring the temporal lobe, seizures are not uncommon.

On imaging, fibrillary tumors are poorly demarcated with inconsistent enhancement. Histologically, they are primarily comprised of fibrillary astrocytes without evidence of necrosis or significant mitotic activity, and MIB-1 indices are typically less than 5% [77]. As discussed previously, *BRAF-KIAA1549* fusions are less common but do occur in diffuse LGG, as do V600E point mutations [50]. Activation of the mTOR/PI3K pathway is also evident in some diffuse grade II gliomas.

As with all low-grade gliomas, extent of resection is a predictive factor. In at least one series, when complete resection was achieved, long-term survival was similar to that for children with pilocytic astrocytomas [20], although reports are not consistent [26]. Unfortunately, given the predilection of fibrillary tumors to arise in critical areas of the brain, as well as the infiltrative nature of the tumor, GTR is not easily or commonly achieved [20]. Thus, children with fibrillary LGG have a poorer outcome than those with PA, with increased incidences of recurrence and progression [15, 26]. Treatment consists of surgical, radiation or chemotherapy options as outlined previously.

Pilomyxoid LGG

Pilomyxoid astrocytoma (PMA) was recently included as a new entity in the 2007 WHO classification of tumors [77]. These tumors, originally included in the PA category, represent a more aggressive clinical phenotype associated with specific histologic features, prompting its classification into a separate group [77]. In pediatric patients, pilomyxoid astrocytomas are more common in infants with a mean age of less than 2 years [78] and typically arise in the hypothalamic/chiasmatic region, although they may be observed in older children and other regions of the brain [79]. PMAs are Grade II gliomas that have fewer Rosenthal fibers and hyaline droplets (which are more typically characteristic of PAs), and instead are identified by an angiocentric arrangement of bipolar, monomorphic tumor cells and a prominent mucoid matrix [77].

Pilomyxoid astrocytomas are more aggressive than PA tumors, and more commonly disseminate. Overall prognosis is worse, with 1-year PFS of 37.8% [80]. Radiographically, greater portions of PMAs exhibit non-enhancing components, although PAs may also lack contrast enhancement [81]. PMAs have a greater incidence of leptomeningeal dissemination. Nevertheless, treatment for PMA mirrors that of PA, i.e., surgical resection with potential irradiation and chemotherapy. Notably, BRAF fusion proteins have also been identified in a portion of PMAs [82, 83], however, the numbers of PMA tumors in the analyses remains too small to make definitive conclusions regarding therapy.

Future Directions

Predicting the behavior of PLGGs is clinically important so as to reduce long-term toxicities; there has been interest in incorporating various imaging modalities to improve our current ability to do this, particularly for diffuse gliomas. Because of the chronic nature of PLGGs and the possibility of long periods of minimal growth even with treatment, tools that may predict tumor behavior would be extraordinarily helpful in clinical management. Radiographic features such as cerebral blood volume measurements [84], contrast enhancement [85], spectroscopy findings [86], and FDG PET uptake have all demonstrated mixed results, with some studies showing predictive utility to each of these imaging modalities while other studies show the converse. Also of potential predictive value would be a more accurate assessment of the initiation and trajectory of visual deterioration from optic pathway gliomas. The challenges of accurate, reproducible, and predictive visual assessments in young children are myriad; however, newer techniques such as Optical Coherence Tomography (OCT) are currently being investigated as possible solutions to these issues [87].

Exciting preclinical and early clinical evidence for molecular targeting of low-grade gliomas has recently emerged. As discussed, the majority of PAs exhibit activation of the MAPK pathway, many via the BRAF fusion protein or V600E point mutation. Pre-clinical work has demonstrated the efficacy of pathway inhibition using a variety of MEK and V600E inhibitors, either singly or in combination; this appears moderately effective, at least preliminarily, in early clinical trials. Targeted therapy has become standard treatment in

SEGAs, which frequently harbor BRAF pathway abnormalities. Blockade of this pathway also seemed effective in a retrospective series using vemurafenib-targeting of the V600E mutation in PXA [88]. Combination with mTOR inhibitors have had some preclinical efficacy via putative cross-talk between the mutant BRAF V600E enzyme and the PI3K/mTOR pathway and are also in clinical trials for PLGG [89]. However, as investigation continues in directed molecular therapy, a more complete understanding of these pathways is important. For instance, inadvertent activation of tumor growth was seen pre-clinically when using an inhibitor targeting the V600E mutation in the context of BRAF fusion protein-driven pathway activation [90]. Further investigations to determine the optimal treatment regimen, potential combinations, and long-term adverse effects of these newer therapeutic strategies are ongoing.

II. High-Grade Gliomas

The term pediatric high-grade gliomas (PHGG) is used here to include tumors of glial lineage (with the exception of ependymoma) that are categorized by WHO as grades III and IV tumors. Gliomatosis cerebri and diffuse intrinsic pontine gliomas (DIPG) occasionally reveal Grade II histology, but due to their aggressive clinical picture, they are often discussed in the context of high-grade gliomas and will also be included in this section. Although the same histologic criteria are used to classify adult and pediatric gliomas (i.e., cellularity, nuclear atypia, mitoses, infiltrative patterns, vascular proliferation and necrosis), CBTRUS registry data suggest that high-grade gliomas may be more difficult to classify in children as a majority are reported as malignant glioma *NOS* (not otherwise specified) [91].

Epidemiology

High-grade gliomas, which represent 80% of adult malignant brain tumors, are relatively rare in children, representing 15-20% of all childhood CNS tumors [91]. In general, they are evenly distributed between male and female children [92] and peak in adolescence [93]. The majority of PHGGs are sporadic, although a small number are associated with prior radiation therapy or a known tumor predisposition syndrome. Germline mutations in patients with tumor predisposition syndromes can result in abnormalities in specific signaling pathways that play key roles in gene regulation, cell proliferation, and apoptosis, and identification of these abnormalities have contributed to a better understanding of the pathogenesis of some PHGGs. Patients with neurofibromatosis type 1 (NF-1), which more typically predisposes patients to the development of benign lesions or low-grade gliomas, also carry an increased risk for development of high-grade gliomas. Patients with Li-Fraumeni syndrome and *TP53* mutations, as well as those with Turcot syndrome and associated defects in mismatch repair genes, also have an increased risk for development of high-grade gliomas [94].

Clinical Presentation

As in low-grade gliomas, the clinical presentation of PHGG may depend more on tumor location and patient age than tumor grade. Duration of symptoms is typically shorter due to more rapid tumor growth, and symptoms related to mass effect, peritumoral edema and increased intracranial pressure are not uncommon. Signs and symptoms can be non-specific and/or focal primarily depending on location. The most common symptoms at presentation are headache, nausea, abnormalities in gait and coordination, and evidence of increased intracranial pressure, such as papilledema or morning emesis [95].

Although PHGGs can occur anywhere within the CNS, they are frequently found in deep grey matter and the brainstem [96]. Most adult high-grade gliomas are glioblastomas and are located supratentorially; although adolescents tend to follow adult patterns, high-grade gliomas in young children are more commonly located infratentorially, particularly in the brainstem and in the thalamus [97]. PHGGs demonstrate evidence of local invasion and edema; however, dissemination is relatively rare at diagnosis with metastatic disease observed in less than 10% of children at the time of presentation [98, 99].

Diagnosis

Neuroimaging evaluation by MRI in patients with HGG typically reveals a lesion that is hypointense on T1-weighted imaging, and hyperintense on T2-weighted and FLAIR imaging, with evidence of surrounding edema generally attributed to rapid growth. High-grade gliomas appear more infiltrative, have increased cerebral blood flow on perfusion imaging, and may have more elevated choline:NAA ratio and the presence of lactate on MR spectroscopy compared to PLGGs. While MR imaging features may be suggestive of HGG, pathologic diagnosis is still required prior to treatment in most cases.

Histologically, infiltrating gliomas have ill-defined borders on both gross and microscopic examination. In children, the majority of HGG are purely astrocytic; glial tumors with oligodendroglial or neuronal components are rare[100]. Anaplastic astrocytomas (AA) demonstrate hypercellularity with nuclear atypia, fibrillary processes and increased mitotic activity, but lack the microvascular proliferation and necrosis (often pseudopalisading necrosis) that defines glioblastoma. Evaluation by immunohistochemistry reveals glial fibrillary acidic protein (GFAP) expression as well as S-100 and vimentin positivity. Demarcating tumor grades, particularly for grades II and III tumors, is often difficult, especially in tumors with significant heterogeneity or those assessed from a small biopsy specimen[101]. In pediatric studies, MIB1 proliferation index is often evaluated and has been correlated with tumor grade and survival. For example, in one study, AA had mean labeling indices of 19% *vs.* 32% for glioblastomas; 5-year survival was 11% versus 33% in patients with indices greater than 36% or less than 18%, respectively [102].

Treatment

Surgery

Surgery is generally the initial definitive treatment of non-brainstem high-grade gliomas and is used to make a histologic diagnosis, decrease tumor burden, and potentially relieve elevated intracranial pressure. Maximum safe surgical resection should be attempted as several studies have documented an association between gross total resection (GTR) and improved survival [103-105]. In one of the early PHGG treatment studies, Children's Cancer Group study CCG943, patients with at least a partial resection had improved survival compared to those undergoing biopsy only [106]. Successor studies confirmed the importance of degree of resection. In CCG945, gross total resection (GTR), defined as greater than 90% resection, was associated with significantly better survival. Five-year PFS was 35% versus 17% in those unable to achieve GTR (p= 0.006), independent of primary tumor location for those located in the cerebral hemispheres [103]. In Children's Oncology Group trial, ACNS0126, children with high-grade glioma were treated with radiation and concurrent temozolomide followed by maintenance temozolomide. Three-year EFS for children in whom a GTR was achieved was 30% compared to 4% ($p < 0.01$) in patients without a GTR [107]. Unfortunately, for patients with thalamic and other midline tumors, the morbidity associated with aggressive resection is significant, often making a safe GTR impossible.

Radiation Therapy

Because complete resection of PHGG is difficult, if not impossible, due to the invasive nature of the tumors, radiation therapy is utilized in an attempt to eradicate remaining tumor cells. Although the benefit of radiation therapy in adults with high-grade gliomas has been demonstrated, no randomized study specifically comparing surgery *vs.* surgery plus radiation has been performed in children with PHGGs. Despite this, focal radiation therapy is the standard backbone therapy for children over 3 years of age with high-grade glioma. Most do not demonstrate evidence of dissemination, and therefore local radiation therapy is utilized for the majority of patients. For those patients with evidence of leptomeningeal disease, craniospinal radiation is generally recommended. Radiation therapy may be delayed or deferred in a subset of patients with increased risk of treatment-related complications, particularly the very young and those with NF-1.

In contrast to children with PLGG in whom there are increasing attempts to delay or avoid radiation given the slow, indolent disease course and long term morbidity associated with radiation in young children, most children with high-grade glioma are treated as aggressively as possible in attempts to halt symptom progression and eradicate disease. Avoiding delays in initiating radiation for children with PHGGs appears to be important. A study incorporating neoadjuvant chemotherapy prior to radiation therapy in children ages 3-17 years suggested that a delay in initiating radiation therapy was associated with earlier disease progression in those with macroscopic residual disease [108]. However, delaying radiation in children less than 3 years may not be detrimental in some cases, as discussed below.

For PHGGs, standard radiation doses of 54-60 Gy are administered locally to the target volume and a surrounding margin, with conformal techniques sometimes utilized to reduce potential toxicity. Studies evaluating higher doses of radiation up to 78 Gy [109] or with addition of radiosensitizers have been performed but none have demonstrated a clear improvement in treatment outcome. (Tables 3 and 4) Intensive high-dose chemotherapy followed by autologous bone marrow rescue administered with adjuvant radiation therapy has also been evaluated [110, 111]. In one study, children with newly diagnosed high-grade glioma (n=11) treated with high-dose thiotepa and cyclophosphamide followed by autologous bone marrow rescue then hyperfractionated (n=9) or conventional radiation therapy (n=2), median PFS was 9 months and OS 14 months, indicating no survival benefit compared to conventional treatment regimens [110].

Interestingly, infants with high-grade gliomas appear to have a slightly improved outcome, and can at times be effectively treated with intensive chemotherapy approaches without the use of radiation therapy [112-114]. This clinical data as well as biologic data demonstrating that infants lack the HOXA9/HOXA10 signature observed in many adolescent and adult HGGs suggest that PHGGs in infants may be biologically distinct from PHGGs in older children [115].

Chemotherapy

Adjuvant chemotherapeutic and biologic therapies have been instituted in efforts to improve survival for children with PHGG. The pCV regimen (prednisone, CCNU or lomustine, and vincristine) is considered by some to be the standard against which other approaches are compared. This regimen was the first to show benefit in a randomized study evaluating the addition of chemotherapy to radiation (Children's Cancer Group study CCG943) [106]. In this study, 58 children were randomly assigned to receive local radiotherapy alone or weekly vincristine with local radiotherapy followed by every 6-week cycles of pCV for up to one year. Those patients receiving concomitant chemotherapy had a significantly better outcome, with 5-year OS of 46% compared to 18% for patients receiving radiotherapy alone. Improvement in outcome was most evident for children with glioblastoma who underwent at least a partial tumor resection [106]. Radiation therapy and adjuvant chemotherapy became the standard of care; however, subsequent studies have not been able to duplicate the degree of improvement seen in this study with the addition of chemotherapy.

Even with the inability to reproduce the degree of benefit observed in the CCG943 study, there appears to be some benefit, albeit modest, from the addition of chemotherapy for children with PHGGs. The large successor study, Children's Cancer Group study CCG945, compared radiation therapy plus pCV to an "8 drugs in 1 day" regimen [116]. Patients on the "8-in-1" arm received 2 cycles of pre-radiation chemotherapy with lomustine, vincristine, hydroxyurea, procarbazine, cisplatin, cytarabine, and dacarbazine and methylprednisone, followed by radiation therapy then maintenance therapy with the "8-in-1" regimen. On this study, the 5-year OS for patients treated with pCV was 26%; no difference in 5-year PFS was observed between the two chemotherapy regimens in this trial. Of note, subsequent analysis after central pathology review resulted in revised 5-year survival estimates to 19±5% for those treated with pCV and 23±5% for those treated with the 8-in-1 regimen. The probability of long-term survival was less than 10% for those with a consensus diagnosis of glioblastoma [100].

Despite the modest benefit in survival afforded by adjuvant chemotherapy, there is no clear current standard of care in treating children with PHGGs unlike adults [117]. Many children with PHGGs enroll on investigational trials, the majority of which are single arm, phase I or phase II, non-randomized studies. (Tables 3 & 4) A significant number have evaluated the use of temozolomide attempting to demonstrate similar benefit to that observed in adults with high-grade glioma. In the initial large adult trial, a statistically significant improvement in survival was observed in patients with glioblastoma treated with concomitant radiotherapy and continuous temozolomide followed by adjuvant temozolomide for 5 days per 28 day cycle [118]. Patients treated with temozolomide had a 14.6 month median survival and 26.5% 2-year OS compared to 12.1 months median survival and 10.4% 2-year OS with radiation alone. In the Children's Oncology Group (COG) single arm study (ACNS0126) which enrolled 90 eligible pediatric patients with PHGGs, patients received temozolomide at a dose of 90 $mg/m^2/d$ during radiation therapy followed by adjuvant temozolomide maintenance at a dose of 200 $mg/m^2/d$ for 5 days on a 28-day cycle, and survival was compared to a historical control of patients treated on CCG945 [107]. The 3-year EFS and OS were 11% and 22%, which were not statistically different than the historical control even in subset analyses by histology, indicating that temozolomide conferred no significant survival advantage over the pCV or 8-in-1 chemotherapy regimens. Similar to adult studies, expression of the DNA repair protein, methylguanine methyltransferase (MGMT) as determined by immunohistochemical analysis was correlated with poor survival; those patients without MGMT overexpression had better 2-year EFS (17% *vs.* 5% in those with overexpression) [107].

Several studies have investigated the use of high dose chemotherapy in both the upfront and recurrent setting in children with high-grade glioma [110, 119-122]. The CCG9933 study evaluated children with high-grade astrocytomas who received four courses of high dose chemotherapy prior to radiotherapy. Patients were randomized between three chemotherapy arms (carboplatin/etoposide, ifosfamide/etoposide, or cyclophosphamide/etoposide), followed by focal radiation therapy, and then by lomustine and vincristine. Of the 76 evaluable patients, 30 patients recurred or progressed during chemotherapy and an additional 11 patients did not complete the planned 4 courses due to toxicity. Response rates between arms were not statistically different. Overall survival at 5 years was 24%, indicating that the use of high dose chemotherapy did not provide additional benefit in the initial treatment of PHGG [119].

Prognosis

Outcomes for children with PHGG is poor, with 70-90% surviving less than 2 years from diagnosis [93, 123]. As mentioned, prognosis is related to the extent of surgical resection as well as the histologic grade of the tumor [116]. After recurrence, patients have a dismal prognosis; the majority of clinical trials involving children with disease progression demonstrate further disease progression within a few months, and most die within 1 year [93, 124-127]. For patients who had minimal residual disease at recurrence, high-dose chemotherapy with stem cell rescue appeared to offer some advantage over conventional chemotherapy based on historical data, although the number of enrolled patients and number of patients demonstrating benefit was small (n=5/27) [124, 127].

A number of recent trials are based on a biologic rationale as determined by data obtained from adult glioblastoma. These studies, such as those evaluating tipifarnib or gefitinib, include inhibitors of specific targets and pathways upregulated in adult GBM. (Tables 4, 5) However, none have demonstrated significant efficacy. Recent advances in understanding tumor biology specifically in PHGG and DIPG, as discussed below, will hopefully allow us to further refine our approach to treating these difficult tumors.

Biology of Pediatric High-Grade Gliomas

Pediatric high-grade gliomas are now considered distinct entities from adult high-grade gliomas. As discussed, therapeutic approaches for PHGGs were historically often inferred from adult data. Over the past decade, however, it has become very clear that adult and pediatric gliomas are separate, albeit related entities, differing in location, biology, pathogenesis, and molecular characterizations. For example, PHGGs have fewer DNA copy number aberrations than adult HGGs [128-130]. Genomic analysis and gene expression studies in HGG confirm significant differences in copy number alterations between adult and pediatric patients with gain of chromosome 7 and loss of chromosome 10q occurring in 74% and 80% of adult HGG, respectively, but at a much lower frequency in children [128, 129, 131]. PHGGs also display more frequent gain of chromosome 1q compared to adults [129]. While *TP53*, *CDKN2A* and *PIK3CA* mutations are common in both populations [132-134], significant differences are noted in the frequency of other aberrations. Mutations in *PTEN* and amplification of *EGFR*, which are common in adults with HGG, are found less frequently in PHGGs [133-135]. Also, notably, PHGGs have more frequent changes involving PDGFRA (chromosome 4q) compared to adults [136]. Although this work highlights differences in PHGGs and adult HGGs, it also demonstrates that no one mutation or alteration appears to be accountable or representative of PHGGs.

Recent work has identified mutations in histone and chromatin remodeling genes in PHGGs; in fact, PHGGs were the first human disease to be associated with mutations in histones [137]. Mutations in *H3F3A,* which encodes H3.3, are present in over 30% of pediatric GBMs and seem specific to this cancer as they are not found in other tumor types or in adult HGG datasets [43, 137-140]. The *H3F3A* mutations involve either the lysine residue at position 27 (K27M) or the glycine residue at position 34 (G34R/V). Methylation of H3K27 is associated with transcription silencing; *H3F3A* K27M mutations are thought to contribute to carcinogenesis via altering methylation at H3K27, which can subsequently affect differentiation pathways [141]. Brainstem and thalamic tumors are biologically similar, yet distinct from high-grade hemispheric tumors, indicating potential key biologic differences associated with location and microenvironment. H3.3 K27M mutations were primarily found in younger pediatric patients (median age 11 yrs.) and those with thalamic GBM while the G34R/V mutations were primarily found in older patients (median age 20 yrs.) and cortical GBM [137, 139]. Further, K27M-H3.3 and G34R/V-H3.3 mutations overlap with *TP53* mutations in patients with both thalamic glioblastoma and DIPG, and with *ATRX* alterations in thalamic glioblastoma [137, 140]. The H3.3 mutations lead to alterations in histone methylation and *ATRX* mutations are associated with alternative lengthening of telomeres. Upregulation of MYCN has also been seen in H3.3 G34R/V mutant GBM [142].

Given this recent influx of exciting biologic information and its likely role in PHGG tumorigenesis, there is a groundswell of interest in targeting chromatin remodeling as a means of eradicating these tumors. However, a number of key questions such as assessing epigenetic changes remains to be addressed before we have adequate understanding to target these in the clinic.

Glioblastoma

Glioblastomas (GBM) are WHO Grade IV neoplasms accounting for approximately 3% of CNS tumors in childhood [91], although they are by far the majority of malignant gliomas in adults. Because of the small numbers of patients, they are frequently combined with other high-grade gliomas including anaplastic astrocytoma, for clinical trials. Histologically, GBM are defined by the presence of vascular proliferation and/or necrosis. Radiographically, they appear as invasive lesions with poorly demarcated edges, variable enhancement, and peritumoral edema. Elevated perfusion reflecting increased blood flow, and a high choline: N-acetyl aspartate ratio on MR spectroscopy indicating increased cell density and cell turnover, are typically noted.

Glioblastomas can occur throughout the CNS and, in children, are frequently found in the brainstem; the most common location of non-brainstem glioblastomas is the cerebral hemispheres [143]. Children with GBM typically present with a short duration of symptoms. As with other PHGGs, symptoms may be localizing, such as focal motor deficits, or generalized, such as headache and morning emesis, indicative of increased intracranial pressure [143]. Primary tumor dissemination at diagnosis is rare, present in <5% of patients [99].

Table 3. Trials of Chemotherapy in Newly Diagnosed PHGG

Regimen	n	PFS/EFS	OS	Reference
TMZ + RT, then TMZ	90	11% (3yr)	22% (3y)	Cohen [107]
vcr/cispl/E, then PEI + RT, then PEI, then valproic acid	97	13% (5yr)*	19± 4% (5y) 63% 5y for GTR group	Wolff [108]
HD Chemo then RT (carbo/E or I/E or cyclo/E)	76	8 ± 3% (5yr)	24±5% (5y)	MacDonald [119]
pCV vs "8-in-1"	85 (PCV) 87 (8 in 1)	26% (5yr) 33 %(5yr)	19±5% PCV 23±5 8-in-1	Finlay [116]
pCV vs RT	58		46% PCV (5yr) 18% RT (5yr)	Sposto [106]

RT = radiation therapy.
TMZ = temozolomide.
vcr = vincristine.
cispl = cisplatin.
E = etoposide, carbo=carboplatin.
PEI = cisplatin, etoposide, ifosfamide.
pCV = prednisone, CCNU (lomustine), vincristine.
cyclo = cyclophosphamide.
*includes DIPG.

Standard therapy for children with GBM consists of maximum surgical resection followed by radiation therapy and chemotherapy. A number of clinical trials evaluating the addition of various chemotherapy regimens have been evaluated. (Table 3) Many chemotherapeutic agents assessed to date are non-specific cytotoxic agents. Although most agree that chemotherapy is beneficial in this population, the degree of benefit for children with GBM is unclear and prognosis remains poor with 5-year OS rates of <10% [144].

Agents that show apparent benefit in adults with glioblastoma may not demonstrate the same benefit in children with glioblastoma. Approximately 45% of adults with GBM will have promoter methylation of the DNA repair protein, O^6-methylguanine methyltransferase (MGMT), resulting in inability to repair DNA damage induced by temozolomide, and thus increased sensitivity of the tumor to temozolomide's effects [145, 146]. The frequency of MGMT promoter methylation in children varies in different reports from 16-50% of cases [147, 148], and it remains unclear if this biomarker is predictive of response to temozolomide in the pediatric population. Similarly, the combination of bevacizumab and irinotecan was evaluated based on the association of increased angiogenesis in malignant gliomas and clinical benefit in adults with recurrent glioblastoma [149] However, the phase II study in children with recurrent or refractory high-grade glioma and brainstem gliomas failed to demonstrate significantly improved outcomes [149]. Other targeted agents such as the farnesyl transferase inhibitor, tipifarnib, have also been evaluated based on preclinical data suggesting its role as a radiation sensitizer and having anti-glioma efficacy, but with no evidence of significant efficacy in the recurrent setting [150].

As noted, the DNA repair protein, O^6-methylguanine methyltransferase (MGMT) is present in a number of gliomas, and thought to confer resistance to temozolomide. Again based on excitement from adult data about the therapeutic potential for temozolomide in the treatment of glioma and the potential to block the DNA repair protein, MGMT, with the agent O6-benzylguanine (O^6-BG), a study of temozolomide given in conjunction with O^6-BG in children with brain tumors was performed; however, only one objective response was observed and survival was not significantly improved [126]. New approaches to therapy for glioblastoma and other PHGGs are clearly needed, and those that translate the recent advances in our understanding of the unique biology of PHGG to the clinic will hopefully provide new, more effective treatment options for this population.

Gliomatosis Cerebri

Gliomatosis cerebri, or gliomatosis, is defined as a highly invasive, neuroepithelial neoplasm involving at least three cerebral lobes, with or without a discrete mass [77]. Gliomatosis is not a distinct histopathologic entity, but rather defined by low cellular density and an extraordinary invasive growth pattern [151, 152]. Histologically, tissue from biopsies of patients with gliomatosis often reveals a WHO Grade III astrocytoma, although oligodendrogliomas also occur [151, 153]. The neoplastic cells are frequently GFAP positive, and appear as small astrocytes with hyperchromatic, elongated, naked nuclei within brain parenchyma with perineuronal and perivascular satellitosis [153]. Some have prominent microglia. Characteristics of higher grade lesions such as neovascularization, necrosis, and high mitotic activity are typically absent [153].

Gliomatosis can occur at any age. Although reported cases are relatively rare, there appears to be a peak in adults at 40-50 years [151]; pediatric cases generally peak in the second decade at age 12-13 years [153]. Males are affected more commonly than females. Because gliomatosis is associated with low cellular density, destruction of structures may not be present until late in the course of the disease and neurologic function is often preserved for a long period of time. Symptoms at presentation are therefore frequently non-specific. The most common presenting symptom of gliomatosis cerebri is seizures (38%), which are frequently intractable [153]. Other reported symptoms include lethargy, altered mental status, cranial nerve deficits, hemiparesis and intention tremor [151, 153]. Median time from symptom onset to diagnosis is generally measured in months [153, 154]. As with other CNS tumors, diagnosis is generally made radiographically and confirmed histologically. Lesions appear hyperintense on T2-weighted or FLAIR MRI scans, may appear as thickening of the gyri, and typically do not enhance [151]. (Figure 3) Interestingly, one review found gliomatosis more frequently affected the right side of the brain [151, 154].

Very little data is available regarding the biology of gliomatosis cerebri. The tumors are characterized primarily by their invasiveness. Histologically, they resemble other astrocytic or oligodendroglial lesions. Although there may be intratumoral heterogeneity, they are considered genetically similar to diffuse atrocytomas, with some evidence of *TP53* alterations, although the frequency is low and results are inconsistent [152]. Although the neural cell adhesion molecule, L1, has been correlated with extensive invasive potential [155], there is no evidence for unique alterations although this may be due to the limited tissue availability and few studies [156]. Patients are generally treated as are those with unresectable high-grade gliomas.

The majority of patients with gliomatosis are treated with radiotherapy [153]. Many children also receive adjuvant chemotherapy, although there is no standard regimen [153]. Reduction in tumor volume is rare in pediatric patients with gliomatosis, and most patients have radiographically stable disease following therapy until progression.

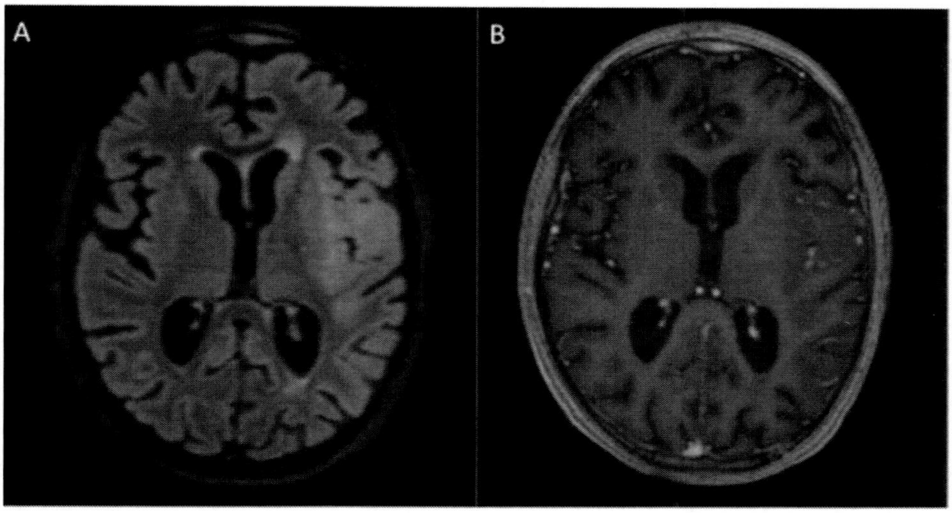

Figure 3. Axial FLAIR (A) and T1-weighted post-contrast (B) magnetic resonance images from a patient with gliomatosis cerebri. Note extensive involvement of multiple lobes, with some bilateral involvement, and lack of contrast enhancement.

Although there appears to be a benefit with therapy overall, approximately 50% of patients will progress within a year of diagnosis. Overall long term survival is poor, with ~25% surviving 5 years and no pediatric patients surviving more than 6 years in a relatively large series [151, 153]. The presence of enhancement on MRI at diagnosis and younger age appear to be associated with worse prognosis.

Diffuse Intrinsic Pontine Gliomas

DIPG are the most common brainstem tumors in children and represent about 10-15% of all brain tumors in children. These tumors are typically malignant astrocytic neoplasms, histologically classified as WHO Grades II-IV [157], although tissue is not obtained at diagnosis in the majority of patients. DIPGs primarily affect children in middle childhood, generally between the ages of 5-10 years, although children of all ages may be affected.

Patients classically present with a short history (<1 month) of cranial nerve deficits, most commonly involving the abducens and facial nerves, as well as ataxia and long-tract signs (hyperreflexia, and increased tone). Characteristic MRI appearance of DIPG reveals a T2 hyperintense expansile lesion centered in and involving greater than two-thirds of the pons, often with encasement of the basilar artery. The diagnosis of DIPG is based on characteristic magnetic resonance imaging in the context of a typical clinical presentation. Enhancement is typically absent or focal, and its presence may suggest a poorer prognosis [158, 159]. Most patients in the United States are not biopsied at presentation, although children with an atypical presentation, uncharacteristic radiographic findings or enrolled on investigational trials are biopsied with increasing frequency based on demonstrated safety of stereotactic biopsy using modern techniques [160-162].

The only therapeutic intervention ever found to be of significant benefit for these children is radiation therapy [163-166]. Radiation therapy prolongs both progression free and overall survival, and often provides symptomatic improvement. Standard treatment for children with DIPG therefore includes involved field radiation therapy at doses of 54-60 Gy, with a margin to cover microscopic disease [167]. However, radiation therapy is considered by most to be a palliative therapy as median survival remains at less than one year [167].

A number of studies have attempted to improve outcome by further intensifying radiation therapy through hyperfractionated techniques delivering doses up to 78 Gy. Although pilot data suggested improvement in survival using higher doses, subsequent studies did not confirm this finding [168-171]. More recently, an approach of hypofractionated therapy to a total dose of 45 Gy administered over 3 weeks has been reported. This shortened treatment approach resulted in PFS of 5.7 months and OS of 7.6 months [172].

Given the apparent benefit, albeit temporary, of radiation, studies have attempted to improve the outcome of radiation alone using a number of approaches including radiosensitizers, addition of chemotherapy to radiation therapy followed by maintenance chemotherapy, pre-radiation chemotherapy, and increased intensity chemotherapy and/or radiation [168, 173-178]. (Table 4) None have resulted in significantly improved outcome. As in non-brainstem PHGGs, a relatively large number of clinical trials have utilized temozolomide based on the encouraging data from adult patients with glioblastoma. However, no significant efficacy for temozolomide has been observed in children with DIPG using the standard 5-day schedule [107, 179], a dose dense regimen [180], or the addition in maintenance of Irinotecan and bevacizumab [181]. The largest of these studies was the ACNS0126 study where patients received continuous temozolomide during RT, followed by the 5 days per month maintenance approach similar to the adult regimen. Median time to progression was 6.1 months and median survival was 9.6 months [107]. A number of phase II studies have also been performed for children with DIPG, but these have all been single arm, non-randomized studies involving a small number of patients, outcome is not significantly different from historical controls, and therefore clinical benefit is difficult to assess. The outcome for children with DIPG has not appreciably changed over the past three decades.

Until recently our attempts at therapy have been focused on intensifying the effects of radiotherapy or based on biologic data mostly extrapolated from adult patients with supratentorial glioblastoma. However over the past few years there have been significant breakthroughs in our understanding of the biology of DIPG through evaluation of both autopsy and biopsy specimens.

Tumor Biology

While similar in histologic appearance to infiltrating gliomas in other locations, DIPGs seem to be biologically distinct. As with non-brainstem HGG, molecular characteristics of DIPG differ from those found in adult HGG, with PDGFR and PI3 Kinase pathways, as well as epigenetic modifiers, as emerging therapeutic targets [182].

In contrast to PHGGs, there are more reported focal amplifications and deletions in DIPG. The majority of specimens evaluated by comparative genomic hybridization demonstrate one or more abnormalities related to a known cancer gene [183]. Early evaluation of autopsy and biopsy specimens revealed amplification of platelet-derived growth factor receptor alpha (PDGFR-a) [139, 184] and poly (ADP-ribose) polymerase (PARP) [185]. In an early analysis of 9 specimens obtained through biopsy at diagnosis, Grill et al. describe frequent mutations in TP53 (40%) and in the PI3K/AKT/mTOR pathway [186]. Additional tyrosine kinase amplifications including MET, IGFR and ERBB4 have also been reported, often in combination with PDGFR amplification [115].

Table 4. Clinical Trials of Chemotherapy in Newly Diagnosed DIPG

Regimen	n	PFS (1yr)	OS (1 yr)	Reference
Motexafin-Gadolinium plus RT	60	18±5%	53 ± 7%	Bradley [178]
TMZ plus RT then TMZ	63	14 ± 4.5%	40 ± 6.5%	Cohen [107]
TMZ plus RT then TMZ	21	33%	50%	Chassot [194]
RT then PEG-Intron	32	NA	46 ± 9%	Warren[195]
Gefitinib plus RT then Gefitinib	43	21±6%	57 ± 8%	Pollack[196]
Tipifarnib plus RT	40	13±5%	34 ± 7%	Haas-Kogan [197]
TMZ and thalidomide plus RT then TMZ and thalidomide	17	17%	58% 25% (2yr)	Kim [198]
Tamoxifen plus RT	31	3.2%	16%	Michalski [199]
TMZ plus RT then metronomic TMZ	15	7 ± 6%	20 ± 10%	Sharp [200]
TMZ plus RT then TMZ	20	NA	9 mo (mOS)	Jalali [179]
vcr/cispl/E then cispl/E/I plus RT then cispl/E/I then valproic acid	37	40 ± 7%	14mo (mOS)	Wolff[201]
vcr/E (po) plus RT then vcr/E	30	5mo (mEFS)	27 ± 7% 3 ± 2% (2yr)	Korones [202]
TMZ plus RT then TMZ plus cis-retinoic acid	12	42 ± 14%	58 ± 14%	Sirachainan [203]
Tamoxifen, BCNU, cispl then HD methotrexate, then RT	23		17mo (mOS)	Frappaz [204]
Thalidomide plus RT then Thalidomide	12	5mo (mPFS)	9mo (mOS)	Turner [205]
Topotecan plus RT	32		26 ± 8%	Bernier-Chastagner [175]
vcr/E/carbo then RT vs vcr/E/cispl/cyclo then RT	32 31	17 ± 5% (no difference between arms)	~30%	Jennings [206]
RT then HD busulfan and thiotepa	36		10mo (mOS)	Bouffet [176]
Cispl/cyclo then Hyperfractionated RT	32		9mo (mOS)	Kretschmar [111]
RT then PCV vs RT alone	39 (PCV) 35 (RT)	8mo mPFS 7mo mPFS	35% (18mo) 26% (18mo) (difference not significant)	Jenkin[207]
5-FU, CCNU then hydroxyurea and misonidazole plus RT	28	32 weeks (mPFS)	44 weeks (mOS)	Levin [208]

Table 5. Select Phase II studies in Recurrent PHGG

Phase II Regimen	n	OR	Outcome	Reference
Temozolomide, O-6-Benzylguanine	25 HGG 16 BSG	1 PR 0	16±7% (6mo PFS) 0% (6mo PFS)	Warren [126]
Temsirolimus	17 HGG	0	2mo (mPFS)	Geoerger [209]
Metronomic Topotecan (p.o.)	6 HGG 13 BSG	0 0	Median 1.9mo cycles completed*	Minturn [210]
Bevacizumab and Irinotecan	18 HGG 17 BSG	0 0	4.2mo (PFS)* 42% 6mo PFS*	Gururangan [149]
Temozolomide	23 HGG 15 BSG	1 PR 0	26% SD ≥ 4 cycles 0% 6mo PFS	Nicholson [211]
Tipifarnib	38 HGG 35 BSG	1 PR 1 PR	10% SD ≥ 4 cycles 11% SD ≥ 4 cycles	Fouladi [150]
Temozolomide	24 HGG	0	3mo (mPFS)	Ruggiero [212]
Oral Topotecan	14 HGG 18 BSG	1 PR, 1 PR	4.1mo (mTTP)* 3.6mo mOS*	Wagner [125]

* For all patients

Subsequent analysis of a larger series of specimens obtained at diagnosis suggested two subgroups of DIPG, one aggressive group with shorter survival that was oligodendroglial, driven by PDGFRA through amplification or mutation, and a second group described as a mesenchymal group with pro-angiogenic and stem cell markers [187]. Copy number analysis of DIPG autopsy samples found common mutations of 1q and 4q gain as well as 10q loss further supporting the importance of the PI3 kinase and EGFR/PDGFR pathways[183]. Others have demonstrated copy number gains in chromosomes 2, 8q and 9q and losses in 16q, 17p and 20p [115]. Further alterations that target the Rb pathway are also reported in patients with DIPG [184]. TP53 mutations have also been noted at higher frequency in DIPG than in PHGG.

Pediatric gliomas are increasingly being viewed as a disease of the epigenome. Mutations in epigenetic regulation were initially described in DIPG, and point mutations in histone H3 genes are found in the majority of DIPGs, resulting in global disruption of epigenetic regulation [138, 139]. K27M mutations in genes that encode both H3.3 and H3.1 were found in 60% and 18% of samples in one study of DIPGs [138]. Another study noted H3.3 mutations in 71% of cases as well as TP53 mutations in 77% and ATRX mutations in 9% with ATRX mutations more common in older children [139]. The H3.3 mutation was associated with shorter survival when compared to wildtype [139]. Interestingly the H3F3A G34R/V mutations seen in pediatric HGG are absent (or at least not seen with the same frequency, given the relatively small numbers of tumors assessed) in DIPG.

Future Directions

PHGGs, including gliomatosis cerebri and DIPG, represent challenging diagnoses for pediatric neuro-oncologists, with minimal improvement in outcome over the past 30 years despite a myriad of studies and investigational therapeutic approaches. However, significant advances have occurred over the last decade with regards to our understanding of the biology that potentially drives PHGGs. Importantly, there are now major international collaborative efforts underway to further our understanding of the biology particularly of pediatric glioblastoma and DIPG. These collaborative efforts have resulted in whole genome sequencing and RNAseq of a number of autopsy and biopsy specimens leading to therapeutic proposals based on biologic rationale, and the generation of established cell lines and mouse models of DIPG which can be utilized for drug screening. New pre-clinical models will allow for more efficient evaluation of therapeutic approaches including combination of novel agents, and therapies that target histones, PDGFR and PI3K pathways already being evaluated clinically in trials of PHGGs. New approaches to therapy that build on these results as well as further advances in understanding the biology of these tumors will hopefully improve survival for children with these diagnoses.

Conclusion

In pediatric neuro-oncology, we are faced with the challenge of treating children aggressively enough to eradicate all tumor cells yet avoiding toxicities, particularly long-term neurotoxicities, in a developing brain. Treatment decisions for children with gliomas have been based on the premise that biological and clinical behavior is related to histology, but overall survival of children with PHGGs and outcome for children with PLGGs has essentially plateaued. The historical approach of incorporating histologic subclassification of pediatric gliomas to predict tumor behavior and select therapeutic management is now insufficient. With the relatively recent incorporation of molecularly targeted therapies into the therapeutic armamentarium, our goal is to classify pediatric gliomas into meaningful subgroups to be able to treat with more effective, less toxic therapy. However, it is evident that additional tools to identify therapeutic targets, predict tumor behavior, estimate prognosis, and assess response to therapy are crucial if we are to improve the outcome for children with gliomas.

There has been a relatively rapid increase in biologic information regarding pediatric gliomas. A major advance has been the identification of pediatric high-grade and low-grade gliomas as distinct entities from their adult counterparts. Rather than blindly extrapolating tumor biology and clinical trial results from adult to pediatric patients, research into pediatric brain tumors is now distinct. This will hopefully result in pediatric clinical trials with proven, applicable biological rationale.

Even with our increased knowledge of pediatric tumor biology, we are far from a complete understanding of pediatric tumor gliomagenesis, the influence of specific molecular target inhibitors, control of epigenetic phenomena, or assessment of response. Newer agents that target mutations or abnormalities thought to drive tumorigenesis and proliferation are currently undergoing clinical testing with encouraging early results, particularly for those tumors apparently driven by a single mutation for which there is a known inhibitor. With the rapid development of information regarding the underlying biology of pediatric gliomas, more directed and effective therapies continue to be a nearing realization.

A number of obstacles remain. Long-term consequences of pathway blockade remain unknown, especially in the context of a growing child and maturing physiology. We know that histologic, biologic, and genomic inter- and intratumoral heterogeneity exists in gliomas including pediatric gliomas. Determining the tumor characteristics that are representative of the entire tumor or that can allow meaningful classification into prognostic groups will be challenging.

Pediatric gliomas remain understudied and there is insufficient biologic data at present to improve disease management and patient outcomes. Continued emphasis on pediatric gliomas as distinct diseases together with major collaborative efforts amongst researchers should allow for clinical trials using novel therapeutics with a strong scientific rationale and improved clinical outcomes.

References

[1] Smith M, Seibel N, Altekruse S et al.: Outcomes for Children and Adolescents with Cancer: Challenges for the Twenty-First Century. *J. Clin. Oncol.* 28, 2625-2634 (2010).

[2] WHO Classification of Tumours of the Central Nervous System, 4th edition. IARC, Lyon. (2007).

[3] Biegel J: Molecular genetics of atypical teratoid/rhabdoid tumor. *Neurosurg. Focus* 20(1), E11 (2006).

[4] Korshunov A, Ryzhova M, Jones D et al.: LIN28A immunoreactivity is a potent diagnostic marker of embryonal tumor with multilayered rosettes (ETMR). *Acta Neuropathol.* 124(6), 875-881 (2012).

[5] Gladson C, Prayson R, Liu W: The pathobiology of glioma tumors. *Annu. Rev. Pathol.* 5, 33-50 (2010).

[6] Pollo B: Neuropathological diagnosis of brain tumours. *Neurol. Sci.* 32 (Suppl 2), S209-S211 (2011).

[7] Kaderali Z, Lamberti-Pasculli M, Rutka J: The changing epidemiology of paediatric brain tumours: a review from the Hospital for Sick Children. *Childs Nerv. Syst.* 25, 787-793 (2009).

[8] Hernáiz Driever P, Hornstein S, Pietsch T et al.: Natural history and management of low-grade glioma in NF-1 children. *J. Neurooncol.* 100(2), 199-207 (2010).

[9] Avery R, Ferner R, Listernick R, Fisher M, Gutmann D, Liu G: Visual acuity in children with low grade gliomas of the visual pathway: implications for patient care and clinical research. *J. Neurooncol.* 110(1), 1-7 (2012).

[10] Pouratian N, Schiff D: Management of low-grade glioma. *Curr. Neurol. Neurosci. Rep.* 10, 224-231 (2010).

[11] Silva M, Goldman S, Keating G, Marymont M, Kalapurakal J, Tomita T: Optic pathway hypothalamic gliomas in children under three years of age: the role of chemotherapy. *Pediatr. Neurosurg.* 33(3), 151-158 (2000).

[12] Ronghe M, Hargrave D, Bartels U et al.: Vincristine and carboplatin chemotherapy for unresectable and/or recurrent low-grade astrocytoma of the brainstem. *Pediatr. Blood Cancer* 55(3), 471-477 (2010).

[13] Gnekow A, Falkenstein F, Von Hornstein S et al.: Long-term follow-up of the multicenter, multidisciplinary treatment study HIT-LGG-1996 for low-grade glioma in children and adolescents of the German Speaking Society of Pediatric Oncology and Hematology. *Neuro Oncol.*14(10), 1265-1284 (2012).

[14] Gilles F, Tavaré C, Becker L et al.: Pathologist interobserver variability of histologic features in childhood brain tumors: results from the CCG-945 study. *Pediatr. Dev. Pathol.* 11(2), 108-117 (2008).

[15] Fouladi M, Hunt D, Pollack I et al.: Outcome of children with centrally reviewed low-grade gliomas treated with chemotherapy with or without radiotherapy on Children's Cancer Group high-grade glioma study CCG-945. *Cancer* 98(6), 1243-1252 (2003).

[16] Wisoff J, Sanford R, Heier L et al.: Primary neurosurgery for pediatric low-grade gliomas: a prospective multi-institutional study from the Children's Oncology Group. *Neurosurgery* 68(6), 1548-1554 (2011).

[17] Terashima K, Chow K, Jones J et al.: Long-term outcome of centrally located low-grade glioma in children. *Cancer* 119(14), 2630-2638 (2013).

[18] Pollack I: *Supratentorial astrocytomas*. In: *Tumors of the Pediatric Central Nervous System*, Keating R,Goodrich J,Packer R (Eds). Thieme, New York 181-187 (2013).

[19] Khan R, Sanford R, Kun L, Thompson S: Morbidity of second-look surgery in pediatric central nervous system tumors. *Pediatr. Neurosurg.* 35, 225-229 (2001).

[20] Pollack I, Claassen D, Al-Shboul Q, Janosky J, Deutsch M: Low-grade gliomas of the cerebral hemispheres in children: an analysis of 71 cases. *J. Neurosurg.* 82, 536-547 (1995).

[21] Merchant T, Kun L, Wu S, Xiong X, Sanford R, Boop F: Phase II trial of conformal radiation therapy for pediatric low-grade glioma. *J. Clin. Oncol.* 27(22), 3598-3604 (2009).

[22] Fisher B, Bauman G, Leighton C, Stitt L, Cairncross J, Macdonald DR: Low-grade gliomas in children: tumor volume response to radiation. *Neurosurg. Focus* 4(4), e5 (1998).

[23] Packer R: Radiation therapy for pediatric low-grade gliomas: Survival and sequelae. *Curr. Neurol. Neurosci. Rep.* 10, 10-13 (2010).

[24] Paulino A, Mazloom A, Terashima K et al.: Intensity-modulated radiotherapy (IMRT) in pediatric low-grade glioma. *Cancer* 119(14), 2654-2659 (2013).

[25] Children's Oncology Group: Radiation Therapy in Treating Young Patients with Gliomas. *Clinicaltrials. gov*, (2000).

[26] Fisher P, Tihan T, Goldthwaite P et al.: Outcome analysis of childhood low-grade astrocytomas. *Pediatr. Blood Cancer* 51(2), 245-250 (2008).

[27] Sherman J, Moldovan K, Yeoh H et al.: Impact of temozolomide chemotherapy on seizure frequency in patients with low-grade gliomas. *J. Neurosurg.* 114(6), 1617-1621 (2011).

[28] Ater J, Zhou T, Holmes E et al.: Randomized study of two chemotherapy regimens for treatment of low-grade glioma in young children: a report from the Children's Oncology Group. *J. Clin. Oncol.* 30(21), 2641-2647 (2012).

[29] Gururangan S, Fangusaro J, Poussaint T et al.: Efficacy of bevacizumab plus irinotecan in children with recurrent low-grade gliomas- a Pediatric Brain Tumor Consortium study. *Neuro Oncol.*, (2013).

[30] Scheinemann K, Bartels U, Tsangaris E et al.: Feasibility and efficacy of repetaed chemotherapy for progressive pediatric low-grade gliomas. *Pediatr. Blood Cancer* 57(1), 84-88 (2011).

[31] Robison N, Campigotto F, Chi S et al.: A phase II trial of a multi-agent oral antiangiogenic (metronomic) regimen in children with recurrent or progressive cancer. *Pediatr. Blood Cancer*, (2013).

[32] Armstrong G, Conklin H, Huang S et al.: Survival and long-term health and cognitive outcomes after low-grade glioma. *Neuro Oncol.* 13(2), 223-234 (2011).

[33] Mccormack B, Miller D, Budzilovich G, Voorhees G, Ransohoff J: Treatment and survival of low-grade astrocytoma in adults--1977-1988. *Neurosurgery* 31(4), 636-642 (1992).

[34] Broniscer A, Baker S, West A et al.: Clinical and molecular characteristics of malignant transformation of low-grade glioma in children. *J. Clin. Oncol.* 25(6), 682-689 (2007).

[35] Soffietti R, Baumert B, Bello L et al.: Guidelines on management of low-grade gliomas: report of an EFNS-EANO Task Force. *Eur. J. Neurol.* 17, 1124-1133 (2010).

[36] Ichimura K, Pearson D, Kocialkowski S et al.: IDH1 mutations are present in the majority of common adult gliomas but rare in primary glioblastomas. *Neuro Oncol.* 11(4), 341-347 (2009).

[37] Mirow C, Pietsch T, Berkefeld S et al.: Children <1 year show an inferior outcome when treated according to the traditional LGG treatment strategy: A report from the German multicenter trial HIT-LGG 1996 for children with low grade glioma (LGG). *Pediatr. Blood Cancer*, (2013).

[38] Gajjar A, Sanford R, Heideman R et al.: Low-grade astrocytoma: a decade of experience at St. Jude Children's Research Hospital. *J. Clin. Oncol.* 15(8), 2792-2799 (1997).

[39] Von Hornstein S, Kortmann R, Pietsch T et al.: Impact of chemotherapy on disseminated low-grade glioma in children and adolescents: report from the HIT-LGG 1996 trial. *Pediatr. Blood Cancer* 56, 1046-1054 (2011).

[40] Lafay-Cousin L, Sung L, Carret A et al.: Carboplatin hypersensitivity reaction in pediatric patients with low-grade glioma: a Canadian Pediatric Brain Tumor Consortium experience. *Cancer* 112(4), 892-899 (2008).

[41] Toledano H, Ben-Arush M, Yaniv I: Procarbazine and infertility in low-grade gliomas in children. *J. Clin. Oncol.* 30, 4583 (2012).

[42] Roche Pharmaceuticals: Bevacizumab package insert. (2011).

[43] Fontebasso A, Bechet D, Jabado N: Molecular biomarkers in pediatric glial tumors: a needed wind of change. *Curr. Opinion. Oncology* 25(6), 665-673 (2013).

[44] Chen Y-H, Gutmann D: The molecular and cell biology of pediatric low-grade gliomas. *Oncogene*, (2013).

[45] Listernick R, Charrow J, Gutmann D: Intracranial gliomas in neurofibromatosis type 1. *Ann. J. Med. Genet.* 89, 38-44 (1999).

[46] Jones D, Kocialkowski S, Liu L et al.: Tandem duplication producing a novel oncogenic BRAF fusion gene defines the majority of pilocytic astrocytomas. *Cancer Res.* 68(21), 8673-8677 (2008).

[47] Jones D, Kocialkowski S, Liu L, Pearson D, Ichimura K, Collins V: Oncogenic RAF1 rearrangement and a novel BRAF mutation as alternatives to KIAA1549:BRAF fusion in activating the MAPK pathway in pilocytic astrocytoma. *Oncogene* 28(20), 2119-2123 (2009).

[48] Hütt-Cabezas M, Karajannis M, Zagzag D et al.: Activation of mTORC1/mTORC2 signaling in pediatric low-grade glioma and pilocytic astrocytoma reveals mTOR as a therapeutic target. *Neuro Oncol.* 15(12), 1604-1614 (2013).

[49] Tabori U, Vukovic B, Zielenska M et al.: The role of telomere maintenance in the spontaneous growth arrest of pediatric low-grade gliomas. *Neoplasia* 8(2), 136-142 (2006).

[50] Zhang J, Wu G, Miller C et al.: Whole-genome sequencing identifies genetic alterations in pediatric low-grade gliomas. *Nat. Genet.* 45(6), 602-612 (2013).

[51] Ramkissoon L, Horowitz P, Craig J et al.: Genomic analysis of diffuse pediatric low-grade gliomas identifies recurrent oncogenic truncating rearrangements in the transcription factor MYBL1. *Proc. Natl. Acad. Sci. USA* 110(20), 8186-8193 (2013).

[52] Tatevossian R, Tang B, Dalton J et al.: MYB upregulation and genetic aberrations in a subset of pediatric low-grade gliomas. *Acta Neuropathol.* 120(6), 731-743 (2010).

[53] Weber R, Hoischen A, Ehrler M et al.: Frequent loss of chromosome 9, homozygous CDKN2A/p14(ARF)/CDKN2B deletion and low TSC1 mRNA expression in pleomorphic xanthoastrocytomas. *Oncogene* 26(7), 1088-1097 (2007).

[54] Giannini C, Scheithauer B, Burger P et al.: Pleomorphic xanthoastrocytoma: what do we really know about it? *Cancer* 85(9), 2033-2045 (1999).

[55] Kaulich K, Blaschke B, Nümann A et al.: Genetic alterations commonly found in diffusely infiltrating cerebral gliomas are rare or absent in pleomorphic xanthoastrocytomas. *J. Neuropathol. Exp. Neurol.* 61(12), 1092-1099 (2002).

[56] Dias-Santagata D, Lam Q, Vernovsky K et al.: BRAF V600E mutations are common in pleomorphic xanthoastrocytoma: diagnostic and therapeutic implications. *PLoS. One* 6(3), e17948 (2011).

[57] Long X, Lin Y, Portiz-Vega S, Yonezawa K, Avruch J: Rheb binds and regulates the mTOR kinase. *Curr. Biol.* 15, 702-713 (2005).

[58] Dolecek T, Propp J, Stroup N, Kruchko C: CBTRUS Statistical Report: Primary Brain and Central Nervous System Tumors Diagnosed in the United States in 2005-2009. *Neuro-oncology* 14, v1-v49 (2012).

[59] Due-Tønnessen B, Helseth E, Scheie D, Skullerud K, Aamodt G, Lundar T: Long-term outcome after resection of benign cerebellar astrocytomas in children and young adults (0-19 years): report of 110 consecutive cases. *Pediatr. Neurosurg.* 37(2), 71-80 (2002).

[60] Rosemberg S, Fujiwara D: Epidemiology of pediatric tumors of the nervous system according to the WHO 2000 classification: a report of 1,195 cases from a single institution. *Childs Nerv Syst.* 21, 940-944 (2005).

[61] Guillamo J, Créange A, Kalifa C et al.: Prognostic factors of CNS tumours in Neurofibromatosis 1 (NF1): a retrospective study of 104 patients. *Brain* 126(Pt 1), 152-160 (2003).

[62] Sutton L, Molloy P, Sernyak H et al.: Long-term outcome of hypothalamic/chiasmatic astrocytomas in children treated with conservative surgery. *J. Neurosurg.* 83(4), 583-589 (1995).

[63] Sievert A, Fisher M: Pediatric low-grade gliomas. *J. Child. Neurol.* 24, 1397-1408 (2009).

[64] Lewis R, Gerson L, Axelson K, Riccardi V, Whitford R: von Recklinghausen neurofibromatosis. II. Incidence of optic gliomata. *Ophthalmology* 91, 929-935 (1984).

[65] Tao M, Barnes P, Billett A et al.: Childhood optic chiasm gliomas: radiographic response following radiotherapy and long-term clinical outcome. *Int. J. Radiat. Oncol. Biol. Phys.* 39(3), 579-587 (1997).

[66] Packer R, Jakacki R, Horn M et al.: Objective response of multiply recurrent low-grade gliomas to bevacizumab and irinotecan. *Pediatr Blood Cancer* 52(7), 791-795 (2009).

[67] Goh S, Butler W, Thiele E: Subependymal giant cell tumors in tuberous sclerosis complex. *Neurology* 63, 1457-1461 (2004).

[68] Hyman M, Whittemore V: National Institutes of Health consensus conference: tuberous sclerosis complex. *Arch. Neurol.* 57, 662-665 (2000).

[69] Jóźwiak S, Nabbout R, Curatolo P, Management, Participants of the TSC Consensus Meeting for SEGA and Epilepsy Management: Management of subependymal giant cell astrocytoma (SEGA) associated with tuberous sclerosis complex (TSC): Clinical recommendations. *Eur. J. Paediatr. Neurol.* 17, 348-352 (2013).

[70] Krueger D, Care M, Agricola K, Tudor C, Mays M, Franz D: Everolimus long-term safety and efficacy in subependymal giant cell astrocytoma. *Neurology* 80(6), 574-580 (2013).

[71] Kotulska K, Chmielewski D, Borkowska J et al.: Long-term effect of everolimus on epilepsy and growth in children under 3 years of age treated for subependymal giant cell astrocytoma associated with tuberous sclerosis complex. *Eur. J. Paediatr. Neurol.* 17(5), 479-485 (2013).

[72] Kepes J, Rubinstein L, Eng L: Pleomorphic xanthoastrocytoma: a distinctive meningocerebral glioma of young subjects with relatively favorable prognosis. A study of 12 cases. *Cancer* 44, 1839-1852 (1979).

[73] Yu S, He L, Zhuang X, Luo B: Pleomorphic xanthoastrocytoma: MR imaging findings in 19 patients. *Acta Radiol.* 52, 223-228 (2011).

[74] Chakrabarty A, Mitchell P, Bridges L, Franks A: Malignant transformation in pleomorphic xanthoastrocytoma- a report of two cases. *Br. J. Neurosurg.* 13, 516-519 (1999).

[75] Koga T, Morita A, Maruyama K et al.: Long-term control of disseminated pleomorphic xanthoastrocytoma with anaplastic features by means of stereotactic irradiation. *Neuro Oncol.* 11(4), 446-451 (2009).

[76] Fisher P, Breiter S, Carson B et al.: A clinicopathologic reappraisal of brain stem tumor classification. Identification of pilocystic astrocytoma and fibrillary astrocytoma as distinct entities. *Cancer* 89(7), 1569-1576 (2000).

[77] Louis D, Ohgaki H, Wiestler O et al.: The 2007 WHO classification of tumours of the central nervous system. *Acta Neuropathol.* 114(2), 97-109 (2007).

[78] Komotar R, Mocco J, Jones J et al.: Pilomyxoid astrocytoma: diagnosis, prognosis, and management. *Neurosurg Focus* 18(6A), E7 (2005).

[79] Fernandez C, Figarella-Branger D, Girard N et al.: Pilocytic astrocytomas in children: prognostic factors- a retrospective study of 80 cases. *Neurosurgery* 53(3), 544-553 (2003).

[80] Tihan T, Fisher P, Kepner J et al.: Pediatric astrocytomas with monomorphous pilomyxoid features and a less favorable outcome. *J. Neuropathol. Exp. Neurol.* 58(10), 1061-1068 (1999).

[81] Lee I, Kim J, Suh Y et al.: Imaging characteristics of pilomyxoid astrocytomas in comparison with pilocytic astrocytomas. *Eur. J. Radiol.* 79(2), 311-316 (2011).

[82] Lin A, Rodriguez F, Karajannis M et al.: BRAF alterations in primary glial and glioneuronal neoplasms of the central nervous system with identification of 2 novel KIAA1549:BRAF fusion variants. *J. Neuropathol. Exp. Neurol.* 71(1), 66-72 (2012).

[83] Ho C, Bar E, Giannini C et al.: MicroRNA profiling in pediatric pilocytic astrocytoma reveals biologically relevant targets, including PBX3, NFIB, and METAP2. *Neuro Oncol.* 15(1), 69-82 (2013).

[84] Caseiras G, Chheang S, Babb J et al.: Relative cerebral blood volume measurements of low-grade gliomas predict patient outcome in a multi-institution setting. *Eur. J. Radiol.* 73(2), 215-220 (2010).

[85] Chaichana K, Mcgirt M, Niranjan A, Olivi A, Burger P, Quinones-Hinojosa A: Prognostic significance of contrast-enhancing low-grade gliomas in adults and a review of the literature. *Neurol. Res.* 31(9), 931-939 (2009).

[86] Hattingen E, Raab P, Franz K et al.: Prognostic value of choline and creatine in WHO grade II gliomas. *Neuroradiology* 50(9), 759-767 (2008).

[87] Avery R, Liu G, Fisher M et al.: Retinal nerve fiber layer thickness in children with optic pathway gliomas. *Am. J. Ophthalmol.* 151(3), 542-549 (2011).

[88] Chamberlain M: Salvage treatment with BRAF inhibitiors for recurrent pleomorphic xanthoastrocytoma: a retrospective case series. *J. Neurooncol.*114(2), 237-240 (2013).

[89] Sadighi Z, Slopis J: Pilocytic astrocytoma: a disease with evolving molecular heterogeneity. *J. Child Neurol.* 28, 625-632 (2013).

[90] Sievert A, Lang S, Boucher K et al.: Paradoxical activation and RAF inhibitor resistance of BRAF protein kinase fusions characterizing pediatric astrocytomas. *Proc. Natl. Acad. Sci. USA* 110(15), 5957-5962 (2013).

[91] Ostrom Q, Gittleman H, Farah P et al.: CBTRUS Statistical Report: Primary brain and central nervous system tumors diagnosed in the United States in 2006-2010. *Neuro-Oncol* 15(sup 2), ii1-ii56 (2013).

[92] Bunin G: What causes childhood brain tumors? Limited knowledge, many clues. *Pediatr. Neurosurg.* 32(6), 321-326 (2000).

[93] Perkins S, Rubin J, Leonard J et al.: Glioblastoma in children: A single-institution experience. *Int. J. Radiat. Oncol. Biol. Phys.* 80(4), 1117-1121 (2011).

[94] Ohgaki H, Kim Y-H, Steinbach J: Nervous system tumors associated with familial tumor syndromes. *Curr. Opin. Neurol.* 23, 583-591 (2010).

[95] Wilne S, Collier J, Kennedy C, Koller K, Grundy R, Walker D: Presentation of childhood CNS tumours: a systematic review and meta-analysis. *Lancet Oncol.* 8(8), 685-695 (2007).

[96] Cohen B: *Pediatric high-grade glioma.* In: *High-Grade Gliomas: Diagnosis and Treatment*, Barnett G (Eds). Humana Press, Totowa, NJ 45-58 (2007).

[97] Qaddoumi I, Sultan I, Gajjar A: Outcome and prognostic features in pediatric gliomas: a review of 6212 cases from the Surveillance, Epidemiology, and End Results database. *Cancer* 115, 5761-5770 (2009).

[98] Grabb P, Albright A, Pang D: Dissemination of supratentorial malignant gliomas via the cerebrospinal fluid in children. *Neurosurgery* 30, 64-71 (1992).

[99] Benesch M, Wagner S, Berthold F, Wolff J: Primary dissemination of high-grade gliomas in children: experiences from four studies of the Pediatric Oncology Society of the German Language Group (GPOH). *J. Neurooncol.* 72(2), 179-183 (2005).

[100] Broniscer A: Past, present, and future strategies in the treatment of high-grade glioma in children. *Cancer Investigation* 24, 77-81 (2006).

[101] Gilles F, Tavaré C, Becker L et al.: Pathologist interobserver variability of histologic features in childhood brain tumors: results from the CCG-945 study. *Pediatr. Dev. Pathol.* 11(2), 108-117 (2008).

[102] Pollack I, Hamilton R, Burnham J et al.: Impact of proliferation index on outcome of childhood malignant gliomas: results in a multi-institutional cohort. *Neurosurgery* 50(6), 1238-1244 (2002).

[103] Wisoff J, Boyett J, Berger M et al.: Current neurosurgical management and impact of the extent of resection in the treatment of malignant gliomas of childhood: a report of the Children's Cancer Group trial no. CCG-945. *J. Neurosurg.* 89(1), 52-59 (1998).

[104] Campbell J, Pollack I, Martinez A, Shultz B: High-grade astrocytomas in children: radiologically complete resection is asociated with an excellent long-term prognosis. *Neurosurgery* 38(2), 258-264 (1996).

[105] Bucci M, Maity A, Janss A et al.: Near complete surgical resection predicts a favorable outcome inpediatric patients with nonbrainstem, malignant gliomas: results from a single center in the magnetic resonance imaging era. *Cancer* 101(4), 817-824 (2004).

[106] Sposto R, Ertel I, Jenkin R et al.: The effectiveness of chemotherapy for treatment of high grade astrocytoma in children: results of a randomized trial. A report from the Childrens Cancer Study Group. *J. Neurooncol.* 7(2), 165-177 (1989).

[107] Cohen K, Pollack I, Zhou T et al.: Temozolomide in the treatment of high-grade gliomas in children: a report from the Children's Oncology Group. *Neuro Oncol.* 13(3), 317-323 (2011).

[108] Wolff J, Gnekow A, Kortmann R et al.: Preradiation chemotherapy for pediatric patients with high-grade glioma. *Cancer* 94, 264-271 (2002).

[109] Prados M, Wara W, Edwards M, Larson D, Lamborn K, Levin V: The treatment of brain stem and thalamic gliomas with 78 Gy of hyperfractionated radiation therapy. *Int J. Radiat. Oncol. Biol. Phys.* 32(1), 85-91 (1995).

[110] Heideman R, Douglass E, Krance R et al.: High-dose chemotherapy and autologous bone marrow rescue followed by interstitial and external-beam radiotherapy in newly diagnosed pediatric malignant gliomas. *J. Clin. Oncol.* 11(8), 1458-1465 (1993).

[111] Kretschmar C, Tarbell N, Barnes P, Krischer J, Burger P, Kun L: Pre-irradiation chemotherapy and hyperfractionated radiation therapy 66 Gy for children with brain stem tumors. A phase II study of the Pediatric Oncology Group, Protocol 8833. *Cancer* 72(4), 404-413 (1993).

[112] Geyer J, Finlay J, Boyett J et al.: Survival of infants with malignant astrocytomas. A report from the Children's Cancer Group. *Cancer* 75, 1045-1050 (1995).

[113] Duffner P, Krischer J, Burger P et al.: Treatment of infants with malignant gliomas: The Pediatric Oncology Group experience. *J. Neurooncol.* 28, 245-256 (1996).

[114] Dufour C, Grill J, Lellouch-Tubiana A et al.: High-grade glioma in children under 5 years of age: a chemotherapy only approach with the BBSFOP protocol. *Eur. J. Cancer* 42(17), 2939-2945 (2006).

[115] Jones C, Perryman L, Hargrave D: Paediatric and adult malignant glioma: close relatives or distant cousins? *Nat. Rev. Clin. Oncol.* 9(7), 400-413 (2012).

[116] Finlay J, Boyett J, Yates A et al.: Randomized phase III trial in childhood high-grade astrocytoma comparing vincristine, lomustine, and prednisone with the eight-drugs-in-1-day regimen. Childrens Cancer Group. *J Clin Oncol* 13(1), 112-123 (1995).

[117] Fangusaro J, Warren K: Unclear standard of care for pediatric high grade glioma patients. *J. Neurooncol.* 113(2), 341-342 (2013).

[118] Stupp R, Mason W, Van Den Bent M et al.: Radiotherapy plus concomitant and adjuvant temozolomide for glioblastoma. *N. Engl. J. Med.* 352(10), 987-996 (2005).

[119] Macdonald T, Arenson E, Ater J et al.: Phase II study of high-dose chemotherapy before radiation in children with newly diagnosed high-grade astrocytoma: final analysis of Children's Cancer Group Study 9933. *Cancer* 104(12), 2862-2871 (2005).

[120] Massimino M, Cohen K, Finlay J: Is there a role for myeloablative chemotherapy with autologous hematopoietic cell rescue in the management of childhood high-grade astrocytomas? *Pediatr. Blood Cancer* 54(4), 641-643 (2010).

[121] Finlay J, Dhall G, Boyett J et al.: Myeloablative chemotherapy with autologous bone marrow rescue in children and adolescents with recurrent malignant astrocytoma: outcome compared with conventional chemotherapy: a report from the Children's Oncology Group. *Pediatr. Blood Cancer* 51(6), 806-811 (2008).

[122] Guruangan S, Dunkel I, Goldman S et al.: Myeloablative chemotherapy with autologous bone marrow rescue in young children with recurrent malignant brain tumors. *J. Clin. Oncol.* 16(7), 2486-2493 (1998).

[123] Broniscer A, Gajjar A: Supratentorial high-grade astrocytoma and diffuse brainstem glioma: two challenges for the pediatric oncologist. *Oncologist* 9(2), 197-206 (2004).

[124] Finlay J, Goldman S, Wong M et al.: Pilot study of high-dose thiotepa and etoposide with autologous bone marrow rescue in children and young adults with recurrent CNS tumors. The Children's Cancer Group. *J. Clin. Oncol.* 14, 2495-2503 (1996).

[125] Wagner S, Erdlenbruch B, Längler A et al.: Oral topotecan in children with recurrent or progressive high-grade glioma: a Phase I/II study by the German Society for Pediatric Oncology and Hematology. *Cancer* 100(8), 1750-1757 (2004).

[126] Warren K, Gururangan S, Geyer J et al.: A phase II study of 06-benzylguanine and temozolomide in pediatric patients with recurrent or progressive high-grade gliomas and brainstem gliomas: a pediatric Brain Tumor Consortium study. *J. Neurooncol.* 106, 643-649 (2012).

[127] Finlay J: The role of high-dose chemotherapy and stem cell rescue in the treatment of malignant brain tumors: a reappraisal. *Pediatr. Transplant.* 3(Suppl 1), 87-95 (1999).

[128] Barrow J, Adamowicz-Brice M, Cartmill M et al.: Homozygous loss of ADAM3A revealed by genome-wide analysis of pediatric high-grade glioma and diffuse intrinsic pontine gliomas. *Neuro Oncol.* 13(2), 212-222 (2011).

[129] Paugh B, Qu C, Jones C et al.: Integrated molecular genetic profiling of pediatric high-grade gliomas reveals key differences with the adult disease. *J. Clin. Oncol.* 28(18), 3061-3068 (2010).

[130] Qu H, Jacob K, Fatet S et al.: Genome-wide profiling using single-nucleotide polymorphism arrays identifies novel chromosomal imbalances in pediatric glioblastomas. *Neuro Oncol.* 12(2), 153-163 (2010).

[131] Bax D, Mackay A, Little S et al.: A distinct spectrum of copy number aberrations in pediatric high-grade gliomas. *Clin. Cancer Res.* 16(13), 3368-3377 (2010).

[132] Pollack I, Finkelstein S, Burnham J et al.: Age and TP53 mutation frequency in childhood malignant gliomas: results in a multi-institutional cohort. *Cancer Res.* 61(20), 7404-7407 (2001).

[133] Newcomb E, Alonso M, Sung T, Miller D: Incidence of p14ARF gene deletion in high-grade adult and pediatric astocytomas. *Hum. Pathol.* 31(1), 115-119 (2000).

[134] Gallia G, Rand V, Siu I et al.: PIK3CA gene mutations in pediatric and adult glioblastoma multiforme. *Mol. Cancer Res.* 4(10), 709-714 (2006).

[135] Pollack I, Hamilton R, James C et al.: Rarity of PTEN deletions and EGFR amplification in malignant gliomas of childhood: results from the Children's Cancer Group 945 cohort. *J. Neurosurg.* 105(5 Suppl), 418-424 (2006).

[136] Nakamura M, Shimada K, Ishida E et al.: Molecular pathogenesis of pediatric astrocytic tumors. *Neuro Oncol.* 9(2), 113-123 (2007).

[137] Schwartzentruber J, Korshunov A, Liu X et al.: Driver mutations in histone H3.3 and chromatin remodelling genes in paediatric glioblastoma. *Nature* 482(7384), 226-231 (2012).

[138] Wu G, Broniscer A, Mceachron T et al.: Somatic histone H3 alterations in pediatric diffuse intrinsic pontine gliomas and non-brainstem glioblastomas. *Nat. Genet.* 44(3), 251-253 (2012).

[139] Khuong-Quang D, Buczkowicz P, Rakopoulos P et al.: K27M mutation in histone H3.3 defines clinically and biologically distinct subgroups of pediatric diffuse intrinsic pontine gliomas. *Acta Neuropathol.* 124(3), 439-447 (2012).

[140] Sturm D, Witt H, Hovestadt V et al.: Hotspot mutations in H3F3A and IDH1 define distinct epigenetic and biological subgroups of glioblastoma. *Cancer Cell* 22(4), 425-437 (2012).

[141] Venneti S, Garimella M, Sullivan L et al.: Evaluation of Histone 3 Lysine 27 Trimethylation (H3K27m3) and Enhancer of Zest 2 (EZH2) in pediatric glial and glioneuronal tumors shows decreased H3K27me3 in *H3F3A* K27M mutant glioblastomas. *Brain Pathology* 23, 558-564 (2013).

[142] Bjerke L, Mackay A, Nandhabalan M et al.: Histone H3.3 Mutations Drive Pediatric Glioblastoma through Upregulation of MYCN. *Cancer Discovery*, (2013).

[143] Fangusaro J: Pediatric high grade glioma: a review and update on tumor clinical characteristics and biology. *Front. Oncol.* 2(105), (2012).

[144] Gajjar A, Packer R, Foreman N et al.: Children's Oncology Group's 2013 blueprint for research: central nervous system tumors. *Pediatr. Blood Cancer* 60(6), 1022-1026 (2013).

[145] Felsberg J, Thon N, Eigenbrod S et al.: Promoter methylation and expression of MGMT and the DNA mismatch repair genes MLH1, MSH2, MSH6 and PMS2 in paired primary and recurrent glioblastomas. *Int. J. Cancer* 129(3), 659-670 (2011).

[146] Esteller M, Hamilton S, Burger P, Baylin S, Herman J: Inactivation of the DNA repair gene O6-methylguanine-DNA methyltransferase by promoter hypermethylation is a common event in primary human neoplasia. *Cancer Res.* 59(4), 793-797 (1999).

[147] Olson R, Brastianos P, Palma D: Prognostic and predictive value of epigenetic silencing of MGMT in patients with high grade gliomas: a systematic review and meta-analysis. *J. Neurooncol.* 105(2), 325-335 (2011).

[148] Hegi M, Liu L, Herman J et al.: Correlation of O6-methylguanine methyltransferase (MGMT) promoter methylation with clinical outcomes in glioblastoma and clinical strategies to modulate MGMT activity. *J. Clin. Oncol.* 26(25), 4189-4199 (2008).

[149] Gururangan S, Chi S, Young Poussaint T et al.: Lack of efficacy of bevacizumab plus irinotecan in children with recurrent malignant glioma and diffuse brainstem glioma: a Pediatric Brain Tumor Consortium study. *J. Clin. Oncol.* 28(18), 3069-3075 (2010).

[150] Fouladi M, Nicholson H, Zhou T et al.: A phase II study of the farnesyl transferase inhibitor, tipifarnib, in children with recurrent or progressive high-grade glioma, medulloblastoma/primitive neuroectodermal tumor, or brainstem glioma: a Children's Oncology Group study. *Cancer* 110(11), 2535-2541 (2007).

[151] Romeike B, Mawrin C: Gliomatosis cerebri: growing evidence for diffuse gliomas with wide invasion. *Expert. Rev. Neurotherapeutics* 8(4), 587-596 (2008).

[152] Mawrin C: Molecular genetic alteraions in gliomatosis cerebri: What can we learn about the origin and course of the disease? *Acta Neuropathol.* 110, 527-536 (2005).

[153] Armstrong G, Phillips P, Rorke-Adams L, Judkins A, Localio A, Fisher M: Gliomatosis cerebri: 20 years of experience at the Children's Hospital of Philadelphia. *Cancer* 107(7), 1597-1606 (2006).

[154] Vates G, Chang S, Lamborn K, Prados M, Berger M: Gliomatosis cerebri: a review of 22 cases. *Neurosurgery* 53(2), 261-271 (2003).

[155] Suzuki T, Izumoto S, Fujimoto Y, Maruno M, Ito Y, Yoshimine T: Clinicopathological study of cellular proliferation and invasion in gliomatosis cerebri: important role of neural cell adhesion molecule L1 in tumour invasion. *J. Clin. Pathol.* 58(2), 166-171 (2005).

[156] Fuller G, Kros J: *Gliomatosis cerebri.* In: *WHO Classification of Tumours of the Central Nervous System*, Louis D,Ohgaki H,Wiester O,Cavenee W (Eds). IARC, Lyon (2007).

[157] Schumacher M, Schulte-Monting J, Stoeter P, Warmuth-Metz M, Solymosi L: Magnetic resonance imaging compared with biopsy in the diagnosis of braistem diseases of childhood: a multicenter review. *J. Neurosurg.* 106, 111-119 (2007).

[158] Hipp S, Steffen-Smith E, Hammoud D, Shih J, Bent R, Warren K: Predicting outcome of children with diffuse intrinsic pontine gliomas using multiparametric imaging. *Neuro Oncol.* 13(8), 904-909 (2011).

[159] Poussaint T, Kocak M, Vajapeyam S et al.: MRI as a central component of clinical trials analysis in brainstem glioma: a report from the Pediatric Brain Tumor Consortium (PBTC). *Neuro Oncol.* 13(4), 417-427 (2011).

[160] Walker D, Liu J, Kieran M et al.: A multi-disciplinary consensus statement concerning surgical approaches to low-grade, high-grade astrocytomas and diffuse intrinsic pontine gliomas in childhood (CPN Paris 2011) using the Delphi method. *Neuro Oncol.* 15(4), 462-468 (2013).

[161] Roujeau T, Machado G, Garnett M et al.: Stereotactic biopsy of diffuse pontine lesions in children. *J. Neurosurg.* 107(1 Suppl), 1-4 (2007).

[162] Pincus D, Richter E, Yachnis A, Bennett J, Bhatti M, Smith A: Brainstem stereotactic biopsy sampling in children. *J. Neurosurg.* 104(2 Suppl), 108-114 (2006).

[163] Langmoen I, Lundar T, Storm-Mathisen I, Lie S, Hovind K: Management of pediatric pontine gliomas. *Childs Nerv. Syst.* 7(1), 13-15 (1991).

[164] Packer R, Allen J, Goldwein J et al.: Hyperfractionated radiotherapy for children with brainstem gliomas: a pilot study using 7,200 cGy. *Ann Neurol* 27(2), 167-173 (1990).
[165] Whyte T, Colby MJ, Layton DJ: Radiation therapy of brain-stem tumors. *Radiology* 93(2), 413-416 (1969).
[166] Kim T, Chin H, Pollan S, Hazel J, Webster J: Radiotherapy of primary brain stem tumors. *Int. J. Radiat. Oncol. Biol. Phys.* 6(1), 51-57 (1980).
[167] Warren K: Diffuse intrinsic pontine glioma: poised for progress. *Frontiers in Oncology* 2, 1-9 (2012).
[168] Mandell L, Kadota R, Freeman C et al.: There is no role for hyperfractionated radiotherapy in the management of children with newly diagnosed diffuse intrinsic brainstem tumors: results of a Pediatric Oncology Group phase III trial comparing conventional vs. hyperfractionated radiotherapy. *Int. J. Radiat. Oncol. Biol. Phys.* 43(5), 959-964 (1999).
[169] Freeman C, Krischer J, Sanford R et al.: Final results of a study of escalating doses of hyperfractionated radiotherapy in brain stem tumors in children: a Pediatric Oncology Group study. *Int. J. Radiat. Oncol. Biol. Phys.* 27(2), 197-206 (1993).
[170] Packer R, Boyett J, Zimmerman R et al.: Hyperfractionated radiation therapy (72 Gy) for children with brain stem gliomas. A Childrens Cancer Group Phase I/II Trial. *Cancer* 72(4), 1414-1421 (1993).
[171] Packer R, Boyett J, Zimmerman R et al.: Outcome of children with brain stem gliomas after treatment with 7800 cGy of hyperfractionated radiotherapy. A Childrens Cancer Group Phase I/II Trial. *Cancer* 74(6), 1827-1834 (1994).
[172] Negretti L, Bouchireb K, Levy-Piedbois C et al.: Hypofractionated radiotherapy in the treatment of diffuse intrinsic pontine glioma in children: a single institution's experience. *J. Neurooncol.* 104(3), 773-777 (2011).
[173] Walter A, Gajjar A, Ochs J et al.: Carboplatin and etoposide with hyperfractionated radiotherapy in children with newly diagnosed diffuse pontine gliomas: a phase I/II study. *Med. Pediatr. Oncol.* 30(1), 28-33 (1998).
[174] Allen J, Siffert J, Donahue B et al.: A phase I/II study of carboplatin combined with hyperfractionated radiotherapy for brainstem gliomas. *Cancer* 86(6), 1064-1069 (1999).
[175] Bernier-Chastagner V, Grill J, Doz F et al.: Topotecan as a radiosensitizer in the treatment of children with malignant diffuse brainstem gliomas: results of a French Society of Paediatric Oncology Phase II Study. *Cancer* 104(12), 2792-2797 (2005).
[176] Bouffet E, Raquin M, Doz F et al.: Radiotherapy followed by high dose busulfan and thiotepa: a prospective assessment of high dose chemotherapy in children with diffuse pontine gliomas. *Cancer* 88(3), 685-692 (2000).
[177] Kalifa C, Valteau D, Pizer B, Vassal G, Grill J, Hartmann O: High-dose chemotherapy in childhood brain tumours. *Childs Nerv. Syst.* 15(10), 498-505 (1999).
[178] Bradley K, Zhou T, Mcnall-Knapp R et al.: Motexafin-gadolinium and involved field radiation therapy for intrinsic pontine glioma of childhood: a children's oncology group phase 2 study. *Int. J. Radiat. Oncol. Biol. Phys.* 85(1), e55-60 (2013).
[179] Jalali R, Raut N, Arora B et al.: Prospective evaluation of radiotherapy with concurrent and adjuvant temozolomide in children with newly diagnosed diffuse intrinsic pontine glioma. *Int. J. Radiat. Oncol. Biol. Phys.* 77(1), 113-118 (2010).

[180] Bailey S, Howman A, Wheatley K et al.: Diffuse intrinsic pontine glioma treated with prolonged temozolomide and radiotherapy--results of a United Kingdom phase II trial (CNS 2007 04). *Eur. J. Cancer* 49(18), 3856-3862 (2013).

[181] Zaky W, Wellner M, Brown R, Blüml S, Finlay J, Dhall G: Treatment of children with diffuse intrinsic pontine gliomas with chemoradiotherapy followed by a combination of temozolomide, irinotecan, and bevacizumab. *Pediatr. Hematol. Oncol.* 30(7), 623-632 (2013).

[182] Schroeder K, Hoeman C, Becher O: Children are not just little adults: recent advances in understanding of diffuse intrinsic pontine glioma biology. *Pediatr. Res.*, (2013).

[183] Warren K, Killian K, Suuriniemi M, Wang Y, Quezado M, Meltzer P: Genomic aberrations in pediatric diffuse intrinsic pontine gliomas. *Neuro Oncol.* 14(3), 326-332 (2012).

[184] Paugh B, Broniscer A, Qu C et al.: Genome-wide analyses identify recurrent amplifications of receptor tyrosine kinases and cell-cycle regulatory genes in diffuse intrinsic pontine glioma. *J. Clin. Oncol.* 29(30), 3999-4006 (2011).

[185] Zarghooni M, Bartels U, Lee E et al.: Whole-genome profiling of pediatric diffuse intrinsic pontine gliomas highlights platelet-derived growth factor receptor alpha and poly (ADP-ribose) polymerase as potential therapeutic targets. *J. Clin. Oncol.* 28(8), 1337-1344 (2010).

[186] Grill J, Puget S, Andreiuolo F, Philippe C, Macconaill L, Kieran M: Critical oncogenic mutations in newly diagnosed pediatric diffuse intrinsic pontine glioma. *Pediatr. Blood Cancer* 58(4), 489-491 (2012).

[187] Puget S, Philippe C, Bax D et al.: Mesenchymal transition and PDGFRA amplification/mutation are key distinct oncogenic events in pediatric diffuse intrinsic pontine gliomas. *PLoS One* 7(2), e30313 (2012).

[188] Bouffet E, Jakacki R, Goldman S et al.: Phase II study of weekly vinblastine in recurrent or refractory pediatric low-grade glioma. *J. Clin. Oncol.* 30(12), 1358-1363 (2012).

[189] Gururangan S, Fisher M, Allen J et al.: Temozolomide in children with progressive low-grade glioma. *Neuro Oncol.* 9(2), 161-168 (2007).

[190] Gururangan S, Cavazos C, Ashley D et al.: Phase II study of carboplatin in children with progressive low-grade gliomas. *J. Clin. Oncol.* 20(13), 2951-2958 (2002).

[191] Hwang E, Jakacki R, Fisher M et al.: Long-term efficacy and toxicity of bevacizumab-based therapy in children with recurrent low-grade gliomas. *Pediatr. Blood Cancer* 60(5), 776-782 (2013).

[192] Laithier V, Grill J, Le Deley M et al.: Progression-free survival in children with optic pathway tumors: dependence on age and the quality of the response to chemotherapy--results of the first French prospective study for the French Society of Pediatric Oncology. *J. Clin. Oncol.* 21(24), 4572-4578 (2003).

[193] Massimino M, Spreafico F, Riva D et al.: A lower-dose, lower-toxicity cisplatin-etoposide regimen for childhood progressive low-grade glioma. *J. Neurooncol.* 100(1), 65-71 (2010).

[194] Chassot A, Canale S, Varlet P et al.: Radiotherapy with concurrent and adjuvant temozolomide in children with newly diagnosed diffuse intrinsic pontine glioma. *J. Neurooncol.* 106(2), 399-407 (2012).

[195] Warren K, Bent R, Wolters P et al.: A phase 2 study of pegylated interferon α-2b (PEG-Intron(®)) in children with diffuse intrinsic pontine glioma. *Cancer* 118(14), 3607-3613 (2012).

[196] Pollack I, Stewart C, Kocak M et al.: A phase II study of gefitinib and irradiation in children with newly diagnosed brainstem gliomas: a report from the Pediatric Brain Tumor Consortium. *Neuro Oncol.* 13(3), 290-297 (2011).

[197] Haas-Kogan D, Banerjee A, Poussaint T et al.: Phase II trial of tipifarnib and radiation in children with newly diagnosed diffuse intrinsic pontine gliomas. *Neuro Oncol.* 13(3), 298-306 (2011).

[198] Kim C, Kim S, Phi J et al.: A prospective study of temozolomide plus thalidomide during and after radiation therapy for pediatric diffuse pontine gliomas: preliminary results of the Korean Society for Pediatric Neuro-Oncology study. *J. Neurooncol.* 100(2), 193-198 (2010).

[199] Michalski A, Bouffet E, Taylor R et al.: The addition of high-dose tamoxifen to standard radiotherapy does not improve the survival of patients with diffuse intrinsic pontine glioma. *J. Neurooncol.* 100(1), 81-88 (2010).

[200] Sharp J, Bouffet E, Stempak D et al.: A multi-centre Canadian pilot study of metronomic temozolomide combined with radiotherapy for newly diagnosed paediatric brainstem glioma. *Eur. J. Cancer.* 46(18), 3271-3279 (2010).

[201] Wolff J, Driever P, Erdlenbruch B et al.: Intensive chemotherapy improves survival in pediatric high-grade glioma after gross total resection: results of the HIT-GBM-C protocol. *Cancer* 116(3), 705-712 (2010).

[202] Korones D, Fisher P, Kretschmar C et al.: Treatment of children with diffuse intrinsic brain stem glioma with radiotherapy, vincristine and oral VP-16: a Children's Oncology Group phase II study. *Pediatr. Blood Cancer* 50(2), 227-230 (2008).

[203] Sirachainan N, Pakakasama S, Visudithbhan A et al.: Concurrent radiotherapy with temozolomide followed by adjuvant temozolomide and cis-retinoic acid in children with diffuse intrinsic pontine glioma. *Neuro Oncol.* 10(4), 577-582 (2008).

[204] Frappaz D, Schell M, Thiesse P et al.: Preradiation chemotherapy may improve survival in pediatric diffuse intrinsic brainstem gliomas: final results of BSG 98 prospective trial. *Neuro Oncol.* 10(4), 599-607 (2008).

[205] Turner C, Chi S, Marcus K et al.: Phase II study of thalidomide and radiation in children with newly diagnosed brain stem gliomas and glioblastoma multiforme. *J. Neurooncol.* 82(1), 95-101 (2007).

[206] Jennings M, Sposto R, Boyett J et al.: Preradiation chemotherapy in primary high-risk brainstem tumors: phase II study CCG-9941 of the Children's Cancer Group. *J. Clin. Oncol.* 20(16), 3431-3437 (2002).

[207] Jenkin R, Boesel C, Ertel I et al.: Brain-stem tumors in childhood: a prospective randomized trial of irradiation with and without adjuvant CCNU, VCR, and prednisone. A report of the Childrens Cancer Study Group. *J. Neurosurg.* 66(2), 227-233 (1987).

[208] Levin V, Edwards M, Wara W, Allen J, Ortega J, Vestnys P: 5-Fluorouracil and 1-(2-chloroethyl)-3-cyclohexyl-1-nitrosourea (CCNU) followed by hydroxyurea, misonidazole, and irradiation for brain stem gliomas: a pilot study of the Brain Tumor Research Center and the Childrens Cancer Group. *Neurosurgery* 14(6), 679-681 (1984).

[209] Geoerger B, Kieran M, Grupp S et al.: Phase II trial of temsirolimus in children with high-grade glioma, neuroblastoma and rhabdomyosarcoma. *Eur. J. Cancer* 48(2), 253-262 (2012).

[210] Minturn J, Janss A, Fisher P et al.: A phase II study of metronomic oral topotecan for recurrent childhood brain tumors. *Pediatr. Blood Cancer* 56(1), 39-44 (2011).

[211] Nicholson H, Kretschmar C, Krailo M et al.: Phase 2 study of temozolomide in children and adolescents with recurrent central nervous system tumors: a report from the Children's Oncology Group. *Cancer* 110(7), 1542-1550 (2007).

[212] Ruggiero A, Cefalo G, Garré M et al.: Phase II trial of temozolomide in children with recurrent high-grade glioma. *J. Neurooncol.* 77(1), 89-94 (2006).

In: Gliomas: Classification, Symptoms, Treatment and Prognosis ISBN: 978-1-63117-868-9
Editor: David Cory Adamson

Chapter 4

Minimally Invasive Techniques for the Surgical Treatment of Glioma

Heather Kistka, Travis R. Ladner and Lola B. Chambless
Vanderbilt University Department of Neurosurgery,
Nashville, Tennessee, US

Abstract

Gliomas are the second most common primary brain tumor in adults [1]. Their high prevalence and poor prognosis has prompted a significant amount of research into their growth patterns and treatment options. Despite the substantial body of literature on the subject, their infiltrating nature and frequent proximity to eloquent structures continue to present treatment dilemmas to the neurosurgeon. Treatment paradigms differ across the spectrum of low grade glioma (WHO grade 1 and 2) to high grade glioma (WHO grade 3 and 4), but determining the appropriate approach to tumor resection remains a universal challenge.

Surgical Goals

As is the case with any successful treatment plan, the first step in planning glioma resection is establishing goals of care. Patient selection is critical, as some patients who present with very poor performance status may not be appropriate candidates for surgical selection and adjuvant treatment, and it may be appropriate to consider more palliative measures in this group. For patients undergoing surgical treatment, the goals of care generally include: obtaining a maximal safe resection, preserving or improving neurologic status, and expeditious return to independence allowing for early adjuvant therapy when appropriate. These three goals and their relative importance in improving survival have been extensively studied in the literature and must be tailored to a given patient's functional status and tumor grade.

The natural first question facing the neurosurgeon is the extent of planned resection. Although there is no Class 1 evidence available, the general consensus from multiple case series is that a greater extent of resection leads to a survival benefit in all grades of glioma. In WHO grade 4 Glioblastoma Multiforme (GBM), Lacroix et al. reported that resection of >98% of the enhancing tumor was associated with significantly prolonged survival and time to progression and a survival benefit began to be apparent at tumor resection levels >89% [2]. Similar incremental increases in survival were seen with increasing extent of resection in a large series by McGirt et al. [3]. Their results illustrated that extent of resection is independently associated with increased survival when comparing subtotal resection (STR) to near total resection (NTR), as well as comparing NTR to gross total resection (GTR) and these results have been validated by numerous other groups [4–6].

While the bulk of evidence is in favor of maximal possible resection in high grade neoplasms, there has been considerably more debate on the topic in low grade tumors. Still, modern literature has revealed a benefit in terms of overall survival, time to disease progression, and time to malignant transformation with higher degrees of resection. Disparate research results have tended to stem from small sample sizes, retrospective study design and linear rather than volumetric measurement techniques. A recent prospective analysis revealed increased recurrence-free survival and time to malignant progression in patients with greater extent of resection [7]. However, a review of earlier literature found that prospective trials tended to favor extent of resection as an important clinical variable while retrospective series did not have similar findings [4]. The authors suggested this may be due to selection bias. More recently, Ius et al. reported that all studies using volumetric measurements found a survival advantage in patients with greater extent of resection and lower residual tumor burden [5]. There was also an advantage in terms of time to tumor progression and time to malignant degeneration. Therefore, despite some variability, the available body of literature supports maximal resection of low grade gliomas when possible.

In balance with the goal of an image-complete tumor resection is the desire to preserve or improve neurologic function. In addition to being potentially devastating for the patient, creating a new permanent neurologic deficit has been shown to decrease survival in patients with GBM, therefore negating any benefit of increased extent of resection [8]. In low grade gliomas, most patients have minimal if any preoperative neurologic deficit [9]. It is, therefore, difficult to weigh the risks of significant neurologic deficit in a patient with years of expected survival against the potential longer term survival benefit of a GTR. However, the more favorable prognosis in patients with low grade gliomas is advantageous in that they have more time to recover from a deficit. Patients with high grade tumors do not have the same luxury of time for rehabilitation and frequently do not recover significantly when left with a serious neurologic deficit after resection [8, 10].

The literature suggests that the goal in glioma surgery should be a balancing act between resecting the maximal amount of tumor possible and maintaining neurologic function. This is increasingly facilitated by technological developments as well as new operative techniques. The minimally invasive approach to surgery takes advantage of these advancements in the field to minimize the damage to surrounding tissues, while achieving equal if not improved extent of resection compared to traditional approaches. The minimally invasive approach is particularly appealing in gliomas which are frequently located deep within the brain, often involving the periventricular zone [11]. Resection therefore frequently requires disruption of normal parenchyma. With a minimally invasive approach, one hopes to limit approach-related damage to adjacent cortex.

Furthermore, minimally invasive techniques address the third goal of rapid recovery by decreasing many causes of perioperative morbidity. This has been borne out well in the field of general surgery, which has migrated to laparoscopic procedures in many cases, including appendectomy, cholecystectomy, anti-reflux surgery, and Roux-en-Y gastric bypass [12]. Shorter, less invasive surgical procedures lead to early mobilization and shorter lengths of stay [12, 13]. This corresponds to lower rates of deep venous thrombosis [14], the most common complication of craniotomy for brain tumor, and catheter related urinary tract infections [15]. In addition, a smaller incision improves the ease of wound care which is believed to decrease the incidence of surgical site infections. Optimal wound healing is paramount in the high grade glioma population as the standard of care involves adjunctive radiation soon after resection [16].

Pre-Operative Planning

The minimally invasive surgeon must rely more heavily on preoperative planning to achieve the aforementioned goals. In addition to the standard high quality preoperative MRI, recent imaging advances have provided new ways to explore the functional circuitry unique to each individual. These modalities have emerged as useful adjuncts to the traditional guidance systems.

Functional MRI (fMRI)

The major challenge to achieving a maximal safe tumor resection is the preservation of eloquent tissue. The term "eloquent" is used by glioma surgeons to describe cortical or subcortical structures which are crucial to the normal neurologic function of the patient and which must be preserved to maintain good quality of life postoperatively. For example, the primary motor and language cortices are classic eloquent structures carefully avoided during tumor resections. These areas, particularly language cortex, can have significant anatomic variability especially when displaced by an invasive tumor. Traditionally, the location of these areas has been mapped in real time via a large exposure in an awake craniotomy. However, the advent of fMRI has provided a less invasive method for the surgeon to localize delicate structures. This imaging technique is based on the principle assumption that there is an increased flow of oxygenated blood to the cortex when completing a task which requires activation of that area. The blood oxygen level dependent (BOLD) signal is measured during specific tasks and overlaid on a structural MRI obtained during the same sitting as demonstrated in Figure 1. Knowing the relative location of eloquent areas in relation to the tumor can greatly assist the surgeon in planning the safest, most direct and therefore least invasive approach to a given tumor. However, these images still lack structural precision and may indicate as functionally relevant areas which could in fact be resected without postoperative deficit. When combined with other minimally invasive imaging techniques such as DTI (described below) fMRI studies are over 90% accurate in determining the precise location of eloquent structures and preserving function in patients without the need for an awake craniotomy [17, 18].

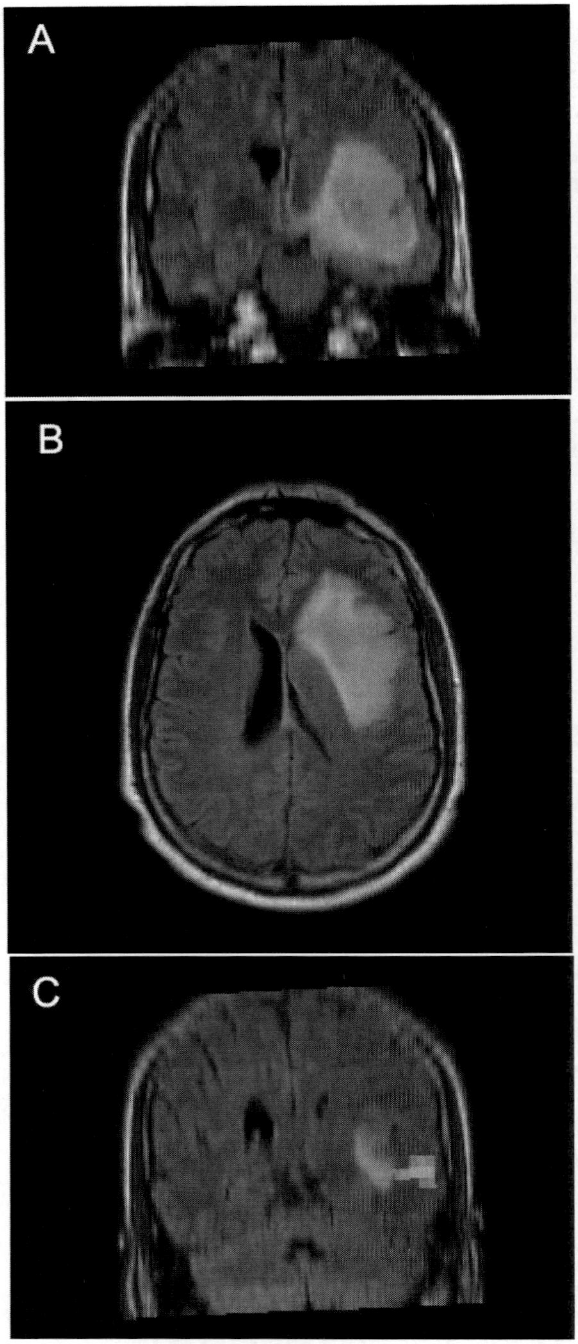

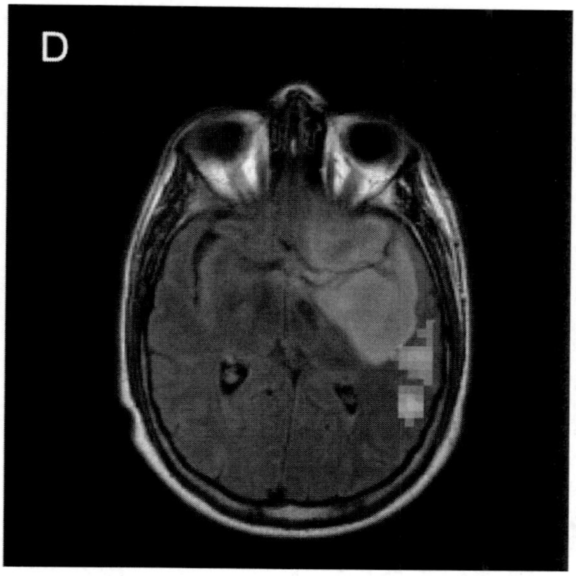

Figure 1. Understanding the relative location of eloquent areas in relation to the tumor using functional MRI (fMRI) can greatly assist the surgeon in planning the least invasive approach to a given tumor. Preoperative fMRI with word generation task in (A) coronal and (B) axial planes demonstrates activation of Broca's area adjacent to tumor (larger red region.) Preoperative fMRI with word reading task in (C) coronal and (D) axial planes demonstrates activation of Wernicke's area adjacent to tumor (blue). This patient subsequently underwent microsurgical resection of this 8 x 5 cm left insular Grade II astrocytoma using neuronavigation via frontotemporal approach.

Traditional awake craniotomy, while effective, is maximally rather than minimally invasive. It is significantly more anxiety provoking for the patient and involves additional time for preparation and special anesthetic considerations [19]. It often involves a large craniotomy and exposure of a wider area of cortex than that necessary for tumor resection in order to facilitate mapping. Even so, this technique is not 100% sensitive in identifying eloquent areas particularly at tumor margins [20]. Many patients with gliomas simply cannot tolerate awake craniotomy, even under ideal conditions. In a qualitative study of the experience of 21 patients undergoing awake craniotomy, greater than 50% of patients reported discomfort during the craniotomy because of noise and vibrations from the drill, pain, and uncomfortable positioning [21]. In addition to subjective patient complaints, awake craniotomy has a reported greater incidence of hypertension, hypotension, and tachycardia than surgery with general anesthesia [22]. However, awake craniotomy remains the gold standard for functional mapping particularly in challenging cases involving the language cortex. To address these limitations and move towards a less invasive approach, many advocates for this technique have moved towards "negative mapping" where a smaller exposure is made and the absence of functional inhibition is used as indication that a particular region can be safely resected. In a subset of patients, this technique may be critical for obtaining maximal safe tumor resection, and the glioma surgeon should be prepared to utilize it in conjunction with preoperative imaging modalities when necessary.

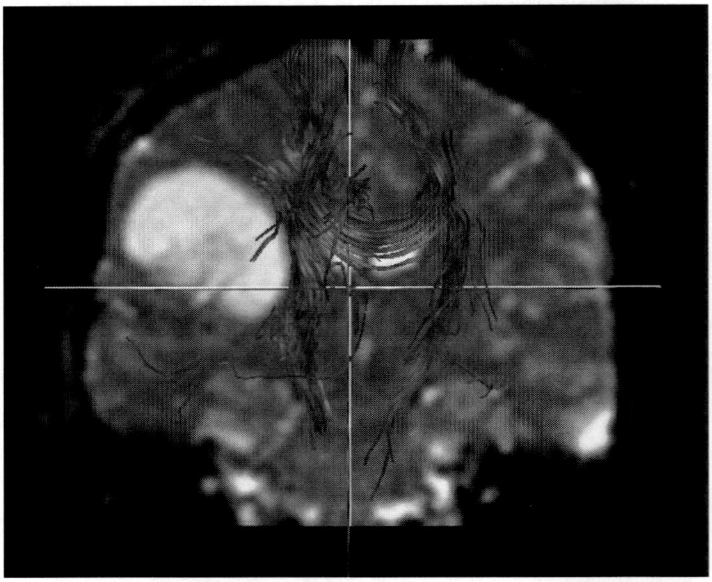

Figure 2. Diffusion Tensor Imaging (DTI) is used to visualize critical structures between functionally eloquent areas. This modality enables assessment of neuronal connectivity through visualization of the brain's major white matter tracts. DTI therefore allows better guidance of surgical approach and resection. DTI in this patient shows bilateral corticospinal tract fibers in coronal section in relationship to right-sided tumor. This patient underwent microsurgical resection of this 5 x 3 cm right frontal Grade II oligodendroglioma using neuronavigation via right-sided craniotomy.

Diffusion Tensor Imaging (DTI)

The advent of diffusion tensor imaging (DTI) is an additional tool for the neurosurgeon to visualize critical structures between functionally eloquent areas. This technology is founded upon the assumption that water molecules will travel more freely down axon fibers than through membranes. Calculating these molecules' fractional anisotropy, or ability to diffuse along various axes, can lead to well defined visualization of long fiber tracts. This information is being applied with increasing accuracy and success in the resection of tumors near the pyramidal tracts and language cortices as demonstrated in the example depicted in figure 2. The current evidence supports an increase in extent of resection and reduction of postoperative deficits when using DTI imaging as an adjunct to traditional techniques of direct subcortical stimulation and awake craniotomy [6, 23, 24]. Zhu et al. found that DTI was 92.6% sensitive and 93.2% specific when compared to direct subcortical stimulation of the pyramidal tracts during glioma resection [24]. The technique is most reliable when applied to the more anatomically homogeneous pyramidal tracts, but it is being used with increasing success in language areas as well [25, 26].

The current limitations of DTI involve the inability to image small crossing fibers tracts as well as limitations related to intraoperative brain shift. The margin of error due to brain shift has been studied by many groups and found to average between 5 and 10mm [27]. In a quantitative study by Roberts et al., craniotomy area was not associated with degree of brain shift; however, gravity played a dominant role in brain shift, attributed to displacement of

CSF and loss of buoyancy [27]. The direction of this shift is affected by both tumor location and patient position. Patients with tumors adjacent to the ventricle tend to have inward shift with loss of CSF during resection and more peripherally located tumors tend to exhibit outward shift as pressure is relieved from the white matter tracts during tumor resection [28, 29]. Although one would expect this phenomenon to be less important in a minimally invasive approach with less bony removal, there is currently no evidence to support this belief. In fact, shift has been documented in burr hole procedures as well as large craniotomies [28]. This is likely due to the multifactorial nature of the process which is dependent on the relative mass effect caused by tumor, CSF and the skull. Minimally invasive procedures rely on CSF egress and tumor resection to provide a working corridor and are therefore still susceptible to brain shift. Given this variability, DTI is currently recommended as an adjunct to a multimodal approach to surgical planning and the surgeon must recognize that these variables require assessment throughout the case.

Surgical Approach

With all of this advanced imaging data at his or her disposal, the neurosurgeon's task is to integrate the available information into a minimally invasive surgical plan. This involves reducing bony exposure and cosmetic deformity, and most importantly, minimizing disruption of normal tissue. Although the idea of exposure through a small craniotomy has been around for many years, it was only after the development of the lighted operating microscope and eventually the endoscope that surgeons have been able to practically realize this vision. According to the two-point technique, the optimal trajectory to approach a lesion in an eloquent area is the shortest distance from the center of the lesion to the surface, while avoiding critical structures [30].

The keyhole concept was first described by Wilson in 1971 [31] but was not widely popularized until van Lindert et al. [32] published details of their experience with the supraorbital approach in 1998. The authors described a minimally invasive, cosmetically appealing alternative to a traditional large craniotomy for aneurysm clipping. Precise pre-surgical imaging, planning and patient positioning can allow the surgeon to access a wide variety of structures with slight variations on a standard approach. After carefully marking out key landmarks and ideal craniotomy placement, an incision is made in the eyebrow lateral to the supraorbital nerve. The frontal fascia is cut at the temporal line and the temporalis muscle is retracted posteriorly. A single burr hole is placed in the temporal bone and used to turn a small craniotomy flap tailored to the area of interest. Remaining bony prominences (orbital rim, anterior clinoid process, sphenoid wing, etc.) obscuring the surgeon's view are then drilled extradurally to maximize the working corridor while minimizing retraction. Cadaveric [33] and morphometric [34] studies have validated the concept that the view of the skull base afforded to the surgeon via a minimally invasive approach is similar to that of a traditional pterional craniotomy.

Although this approach was initially employed for aneurysm clipping and treatment of skull base lesions it has since been expanded upon and validated for intra-axial tumor resection in the orbitofrontal, frontal, medial temporal lobe as well [35]. An ideal case for this approach is depicted in figure 3. Not only are the craniotomy and length of incision minimized via the eyebrow approach, it frequently also provides the most direct route to a lesion with minimal cortical disruption [36]. As this is a fairly new technique, there are not currently any large series illustrating its efficacy [36]. Reisch and Pernecezky report excision of 18 frontal and temporal astrocytomas [37] and Ditzel FIlho et al. describe a mean corticectomy diameter of 15 mm to achieve resection of tumors with mean size of 37 mm [38]. Adjunctive use of the ultrasound and endoscope may be necessary in these cases to avoid leaving residual tumor that may not be well visualized at the borders of the resection cavity [35, 36, 38].

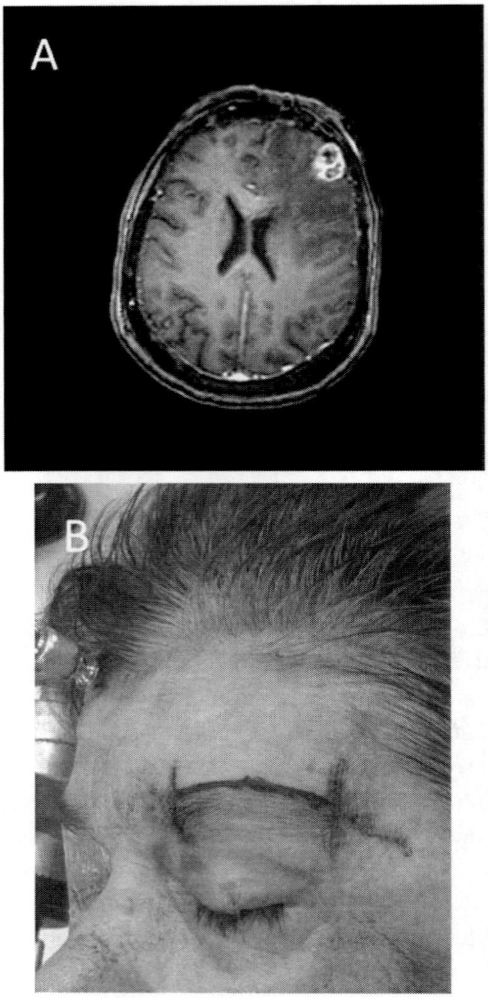

Figure 3. The "eyebrow incision" may be suitable for a minimally invasive approach to some intrinsic tumors of the frontal lobe. In some cases, this may allow the surgeon to avoid a much larger and more morbid bicoronal craniotomy. (A) T1-post-contrast MRI of a patient with a GBM located in the left frontal pole. (B) Planned incision (between hatchmarks) for approach to this lesion. If additional lateral exposure is needed, the incision could be extended beyond the brow as indicated. Planning a method to expand exposure in the setting of intraoperative challenges is a key component to successfully executing minimally invasive tumor resections. This patient underwent microsurgical resection of this Grade IV GBM.

Although the cosmetic results of this approach are favored by patients and plastic surgeons [39] it is not without morbidity. Frontalis palsy has been reported to occur at a higher rate in this approach; however, if attention is paid to the lateral extent of the incision, this can occur at a rate of less than one percent [35]. Additionally, some have been concerned that the orbital trauma of the supraorbital keyhole approach may lead to cosmetic deformities; however, the complication profile including CSF leak, infection and cosmetic deformity in retrospective series is comparable to that in pterional or orbitozygomatic approaches [39].

The keyhole concept in neurosurgery is widely associated with the supraorbital approach. However, its usefulness is broadened when one remembers that it applies to a geometric concept rather than a single approach. In this way, the concept has been used to address lesions adjacent to the tentorium and falx as well as via a retrosigmoid approach [36]. Additional studies have been performed which validate the feasibility of the occipital transtentorial keyhole approach to the inferior and medial temporal lobe and pineal region. Cadaveric studies have illustrated that although the working angles are narrow, the exposure via this approach is similar to that of traditional supracerebellar infratentorial and transtentorial approaches [40].

Although a small craniotomy may be appealing to both patient and surgeon, the surgeon must be aware that this may not be appropriate in every patient. At the forefront of surgical decision making should be the principal tenant of the keyhole concept: the further away the area of interest, the larger the field of view granted by a small incision. For this reason, deep-seated lesions are most amenable to a keyhole approach whereas a lesion close at the convexity of the cortical surface will still require a craniotomy as large as the tumor to achieve complete resection. As we refer to the term "minimally invasive" to mean minimal disruption of normal tissue, this is still a minimally invasive approach, albeit with a larger incision. Additionally, the neurosurgeon must take into account anatomical variations such as a large frontal sinus or prominent skull base anatomy that may prevent him or her from obtaining the necessary trajectory in surgery [35]. In addition, the surgeon utilizing a keyhole approach must be prepared to make several adjustments to traditional technique. For example, it may be critical to adjust the patient or the microscope significantly throughout the case to allow for optimal visualization of the entire tumor bed. The organization of the room and operative equipment must be planned with this in mind. Close attention to patient positioning is key – the patient must be secure enough to tolerate changes in orientation with close attention to padding of potential pressure points which must be anticipated at the outset of the case. In addition, the surgeon must be prepared to use angled instruments such as bipolars and suction and should have ready access to angled endoscopes to optimize the view if necessary. Finally, as with any craniotomy, the surgeon and anesthesiologist must carefully plan the use of steroids, anti-epileptics, diuretics, and anesthetic agents to maintain adequate cerebral perfusion pressures while minimizing intracranial edema and avoiding early postoperative complications such as seizure. Conscientious attention to these details before incision is critical to the ultimate success of the operation.

Intraoperative Tools

Stereotactic Neuronavigation

After careful planning of a minimally invasive approach, many tools exist to assist the surgeon in achieving a maximum safe resection. Accurate navigation systems are invaluable in planning a minimally invasive craniotomy. Prior to the advent of this technology, anatomic landmarks provided guidelines for the surgeon, but without knowing the exact location of a given lesion, craniotomies were naturally larger to expand the surgeon's field of view.

After induction of anesthesia and proper positioning of the patient in a Mayfield head holder, the patient's head position is linked to a detailed structural MRI. The accuracy of registration is verified using known anatomic landmarks. The surgeon may then use the probe to explore the borders of the tumor and their relationship to critical structures as they relate to precise intraoperative positioning. The nuances of the exact positioning of the incision and trajectory for surgery are planned prior to the beginning of surgery. The patient positioning can also be altered at this stage to allow for better visualization during surgery.

Although neuronavigation is a critical starting point for a minimally invasive operation, the technology has limitations and therefore cannot be used in isolation. First of all, the accuracy of registration is not exact [27, 28, 41]. There are a number of reasons for these discrepancies. For example, the patient's head is frequently in a different position than that used to obtain the MRI. This simple change of position is believed to result in some amount of brain shift. Additionally, the position of the tumor and surrounding brain will invariably change after the craniotomy and dural opening. One may expect this phenomenon to be negligent with a smaller craniotomy, but shifts have been demonstrated even after burr hole placement only [27, 28]. Additionally, a guiding principle of minimally invasive craniotomy involves promoting CSF egress from the ventricular system and cisterns early on in an operation to expand a working corridor with minimal retraction. This process results in inward shift which counteracts the predicted outward shift expected from increased intracranial pressure. Furthermore, the surgical cavity naturally collapses during resection further altering the relationship of the brain-tumor interface as it was represented on a preoperative image. As the degree to which these forces counteract each other cannot be accurately predicted, the surgeon may opt to employ intraoperative imaging techniques.

Endoscopy

The advent of the endoscope is arguably the most important innovation in minimally invasive surgery to date. Endoscopy provides a deep source of direct illumination within the operative field and allows visualization of structures that are typically hidden from view [35, 42]. Although some minimally invasive surgery may be done exclusively with a microscope or endoscope, using these tools in combination is a common approach in the management of glioma. In this technique, the microscope is often used for the majority of the initial dissection [35, 36, 42]. The endoscope is then introduced towards the end of the case to inspect for residual tumor in a deep resection cavity, as in the case depicted in figure 4. Use of the endoscope in this manner is particularly useful in increasing visualization of areas where the tumor may be intimately related to cranial nerves or critical vascular structures. Angled endoscopes and instruments may also be used to work around corners to inspect for any residual tumor that may not be visualized by a direct microscopic view. Tumor resection may then continue under endoscopic guidance. This may be performed by a single surgeon holding the endoscope in the nondominant hand with a dissector in another or, preferably, via a three-hand approach wherein one surgeon guides the endoscope while another performs two-handed careful microsurgical dissection. If an assistant is not available, the endoscope may also be secured in a holder.

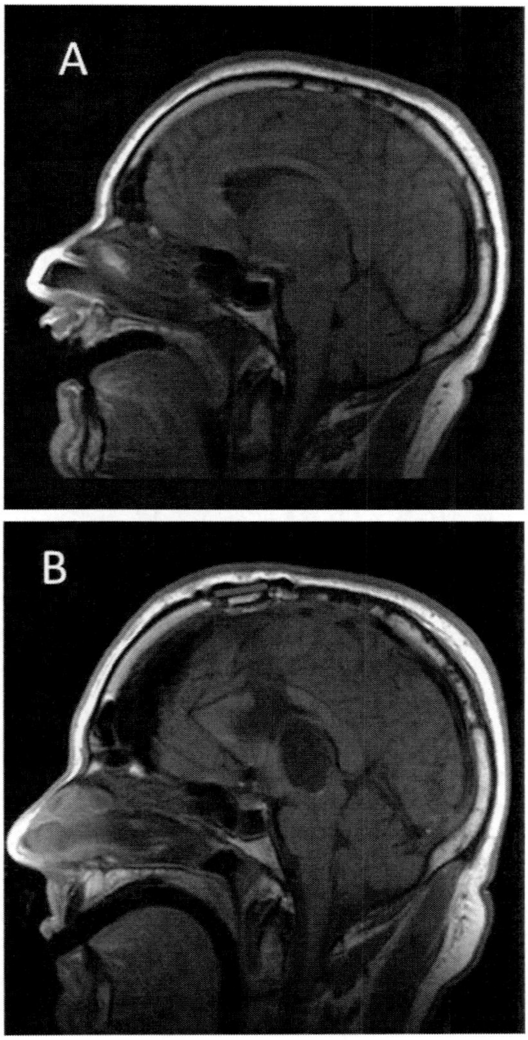

Figure 4. Deep-seated intrinsic tumors are well-suited to keyhole approaches. (A) Preoperative T1 MRI demonstrating a large thalamic GBM. (B) Postoperative T1 MRI demonstrating resection of the GBM via a 2.4cm craniotomy for an interhemispheric transcallosal approach (craniotomy extent in red.) This resection could not be performed through a minimally invasive approach without the judicious use of the neuroendoscope to provide deep illumination of the resection cavity.

A critical facet of performing a successful endoscopic surgery involves the use of proper narrow and angled instruments to operate in small corridors and around corners in addition to a well-controlled angled suction device [36, 43]. Beyond choosing the length and angle of the scope, the surgeon may also use a rigid or flexible endoscope. The flexible scopes have the advantage of extra maneuverability and possibly less damage to adjacent tissue, but the optical resolution is not as clear.

A frequently cited difficulty with the endoscope is that it only provides a two dimensional view of the surgical field [44]. More recently, stereoscopic endoscopes have been developed to allow the surgeon to view the images in three dimensions with the aid of special glasses thereby circumventing the need to perform surgery in three dimensions based on a two dimensional image. Although there is a learning curve associated with any new technology, in the largest single series, Fries and Perneczky reported that their operative times were reduced by 10-120 minutes when performing 380 endoscopically assisted intracranial procedures, 205 of which were tumors [42].

Retraction

Most disruption of normal tissue in neurosurgery is related to retraction injury rather than direct cortical destruction. Minimizing retraction is a central tenet of the minimally invasive approach. Tubular retractor systems may be utilized with or without endoscopy to limit the damage to surrounding tissue when accessing a deep lesion [36]. This concept was first introduced by Kelly et al. in 1988 [45]. Subsequently, Otsuki et al. reported operating on fifteen deep-seated intra-axial lesions through a burr hole and rigid eight millimeter tube [46]. The guiding tube was stereotactically introduced into the brain according to a pre-planned trajectory and secured to rigid fixation. In this fashion, they were able to achieve gross total resection of seven of the lesions, the largest of which was 2.6 cm. Moshel, Link and Kelly reported their experience with 72 thalamic pilocytic astrocytomas achieving gross total resection in 58 patients with a low morbidity and mortality [47]. Since then, the technique has slowly gained popularity. Kassam et al. resected 21 intraparenchymal lesion using a tubular retraction system and endoscopic guidance only [48]. Raza et al. described the first use of a retractor system designed particularly for intracranial use in 2010 [49]. These dilating retractors are designed to split apart white matter tracts rather than sever them, thereby doing less damage to functional tracts during resection of deep tumors [50]. They are made of transparent material allowing the surgeon to visualize any tissue damage that may be caused by their insertion. This is a great improvement over opaque systems which can lead to occult hemorrhage. In addition to limiting the need to cut white matter tracts, the use of a constant, equally distributed force to retract surrounding brain is purported to cause less damage than repetitive, unequal, intermittent retraction in conventional surgery [50] which can lead to contusions and venous infarction [51].

Comparisons of this new technology with existing techniques are forthcoming, but once again, patient and tumor selection are key factors in determining success. For example, tubular retraction systems may not be suitable for resection of highly vascular tumors due to the difficulty of achieving hemostasis through a small operative corridor. Some of these limitations were studied by Jo et al. who were able to perform GTR of tumor in two thirds of patients via an 11 mm tube [52]. They found that tumor size > 3 cm and a calcified component were negative prognostic factors for their ability to completely resect tumors using this system. This finding is due to the natural need for piecemeal resection when operating through a small corridor. Similarly, Almenawer et al. achieved GTRof 70% of tumors in their series using a serial dilation technique adapted from spinal surgery to achieve a larger working corridor [53] and Greenfield et al. report GTR of 10/10 tumors with a similar technique [50].

Despite these examples of success, some surgeons prefer to perform resection of intraaxial tumors without the use of any fixed retractors at all. With judicious surgical planning and patient positioning, it is possible to work through a narrow cortical channel which is kept open through gentle retraction by the surgeon's suction and other instruments. Close attention to positioning and movement of the patient during the operation may allow gravity to help keep the surgical corridor open. Targeted intermittent light retraction of this type may facilitate work around larger lesions and may also limit damage to white matter tracks. Some have gone so far as to eliminate the use of retraction completely. Spetzler and Sanai recently described a series of 223 patients with complex vascular and skull base lesions selected for retractorless resection, of which 97% were successfully treated without the use of a self-retaining retractor system [54].

Intraoperative Fluorescence

Direct visualization of residual tumor can be further improved in GBM resection with the addition of 5-aminolevulinic acid (5-ALA). This orally administered compound is ingested prior to surgery. The prodrug undergoes intracellular metabolism into a fluorescent molecule, protophorphyrin IX [55–57] which accumulates preferentially in tumor cells and epithelial tissues. When illuminated with blue light, the compound emits a red-violet light allowing the location of residual tumor cells to be visualized with the naked eye. The use of this compound was found to be associated with a significant increase in the extent of resection as well as progression free survival in a randomized controlled European trial [56]. However, neither neuronavigation nor the Stupp protocol [16] were routinely used at the time of the trial. Single center experiences report a >98% resection in all cases [58], but the exact degree of benefit of 5-ALA in modern neurooncologic practice remains unknown. Three separate clinical trials are underway in the United States to answer this question (NCT01575275, NCT01128218, and NCT01445691). However, the utility of this technique in minimally invasive surgery is intuitively high. It promotes easy identification of tumor in a small operative field and initial reports have encouraging high rates of GTR [59]. Moreover, the florescence has been very reliable when compared to histologic samples. One study revealed that one hundred percent of pathologic samples that appeared bright red intraoperatively were consistent with GBM. A vague pink hue was associated with tumor involvement in 97% and the absence of fluorescence had a 66% negative predictive value for tumor [60]. The persistence of cellular atypia in areas without 5-ALA detection is similar to what is seen in low grade gliomas. For this reason, 5-ALA is not usually employed in low grade glioma resection; however, preliminary data have revealed that the use of confocal microscopy may aid in visualization of 5–ALA fluorescence in low grade gliomas. Although the sample sizes are small, the presence or absence of fluorescence correlated with histopathologic diagnosis in all cases. This included 3 cases in which neuronavigation indicated that no further tumor was present, but 5-ALA fluorescence and histopathologic analyses were positive for tumor cells [61]. These data highlight the imperfections in neuronavigation that may be improved upon with adjunctive techniques.

Functional Mapping

Although several intraoperative technologies are aimed at increasing extent of resection, it is not recommended that they be used in isolation. Initial reports of resection with 5-ALA guidance revealed a greater incidence of post-operative deficits [56, 62]. Adjunctive functional monitoring is therefore recommended in cases involving eloquent tissue to ensure that an aggressive resection does not lead to a devastating neurologic deficit [63, 64]. For patients under general anesthesia, motor mapping can be performed by direct electrical stimulation of cortical and subcortical sites while observing motor evoked potentials as well as motor movements [65]. A recent meta-analysis demonstrated decreased neurological deficits and greater extent of resection with the use of intraoperative stimulation brain mapping in glioma resection [66]. Traditionally, cortical mapping has been the gold standard to map out functionally relevant anatomy with the use of a large craniotomy and surface grids. This "positive" monitoring provided a map of areas which would lead to a deficit if disturbed. However, with the advent of more sophisticated neuromonitoring and the understanding that traditional anatomy is often disrupted by tumor infiltration, most neurosurgeons have turned to "negative" monitoring. In this technique, the surgeon takes a limited approach to the tumor and tests the area of planned resection for any response throughout the case. This approach results in similar functional outcomes with less invasive surgery [67, 68].

Robotics

The combination of a small opening, long surgical corridor and incorporation of several different technologies render keyhole surgery an ideal area for robotic assistance. Several systems have been developed to date without overwhelming success; however, with each trial, the necessary facets of neurosurgical robotic technology continue to be elucidated [69]. To date, the system most applicable to keyhole neurosurgery is the da Vinci Surgical System® (Intuitive Surgical®), which was developed to work under endoscopic guidance in small corridors. Successful supraorbital keyhole craniotomies were recently performed on cadavers using this system [70]. Hong et al. note that the robot had the advantages of superior instrumentation which provides seven degrees of freedom and ninety degrees of articulation compared to four degrees of freedom and zero degrees of articulation with traditional endoscopic instruments. They also reported good stereoscopic visualization of deep critical structures and a useful tremor reduction technology. The current drawbacks include the inability to perform a craniotomy with the current available instrumentation as well as the three arm design which can lead to collisions and interfere with surgery if not positioned properly at the start of the case. Additional work is being performed to provide surgeons with haptic feedback to increase their comfort with this new technology [69]. Although the learning curve is steep for any new surgical technique, robotic assisted surgery holds the promise of eliminating current downsides of minimally invasive surgery (decreased surgical maneuverability, poor visualization, and need for surgical assistant to guide the endoscope) while maintaining the benefits.

Intraoperative Imaging

One way to improve accurate understanding of tumor borders is intraoperative imaging. These techniques provide real-time assessment of the anatomical features of the tumor and adjacent structures which can be very useful in adjusting surgical plans. However, these obvious benefits must be balanced against the difficulty of employing these technologies in the operating room, as well as the time and cost added to the case. Current technological advances in this arena are primarily focused on reducing these challenges while making this technology more readily accessible and more facile in a variety of situations.

Intraoperative MRI

The use of intraoperative MRI (iMRI) has grown in popularity as a way to identify residual tumor that may be amenable to resection before leaving the operating room. Most groups utilize the iMRI scan to assess their initial extent of resection and guide further resection if necessary. Others even obtain their preoperative imaging immediately before surgery to limit the effect of brain shift and obtain the most accurate intraoperative stereotactic guidance possible. To further increase accuracy, three-dimensional ultrasound can then be performed at several points throughout a case and used to update the stereotactic imaging [29, 71]. Several observational series have concluded that iMRI both improves extent of resection and survival in patients with glioma. These studies also report a significant survival benefit associated with a greater extent of resection. The only prospective randomized controlled trial to date revealed that the use of iMRI increased the rate of GTR and that extent of resection was a significant predictor of prolonged progression free survival in multivariate analysis [72]. A large study of low grade glioma resection using iMRI revealed a trend toward increased survival in the GTRsubgroup but this was not statistically significant [73]. In general, the low grade literature has been less conclusive as to the benefit of iMRI, likely related to a number of factors including heterogeneity of tumor histology and management, smaller patient populations, and the necessity of longer follow up. Additionally, vague tumor borders based on T2 hyperintensity lead to difficulty when determining the extent of resection. This is a problem that may be overcome by utilizing additional intraoperative MRI sequences. Pamir et al. demonstrated that magnetic resonance spectroscopy was 87.5% sensitive and 100% specific for residual tumor when compared to histologic analysis in their small series [74]. Furthermore, evidence of restricted diffusion on diffusion weighted imaging sequences was 60% sensitive and 100% specific for post-operative changes. Although both lack sensitivity, the specificity is encouraging and implies that an algorithm may eventually be developed which takes into account the appearance of questionable residual tumor on multiple sequences to decrease false negatives and improve extent of resection.

The challenges of iMRI relate primarily to the machine itself as well as the cost. Fundamentally, these are machines which require a large amount of space and the absolute avoidance of diamagnetic materials which are ubiquitous in the typical operating room. This requires either retrofitting the operating room with specific materials and instruments or moving the patient to the scanner in an adjacent room intraoperatively. A variety of systems are commercially available which seek to minimize these issues in a number of ways. However, the cost of installation of these systems remains quite high, with estimates ranging from $1 million to $7 million, necessitating frequent use for justification of capital expenditures [75, 76].

Ultrasound

Comparatively, intraoperative ultrasound is a relatively easy and cost effective technique to visualize the anatomy of a tumor as it changes throughout resection. It requires relatively little special equipment and provides excellent temporal resolution of the resection process. Some groups advocate the use of a sophisticated three dimensional ultrasound which can update stereotactic navigation during surgery [29, 71]. Even a two dimensional view at the outset of a case is frequently helpful in assessing the adequacy and accuracy of the craniotomy placement as well as planning the precise trajectory for optimal tumor resection. Unfortunately, the resolution on most equipment is not precise enough to delineate definite borders between tumor and normal tissue, particularly in infiltrating lesions like gliomas. This border is further obscured intraoperatively by edema and debris that may alter the ultrasonic appearance of normal brain during resection. Furthermore, its utility is limited in very small craniotomies that may not allow an adequate bone window for visualization. Three probes are commonly used: spinal (14 × 3 mm), burr hole (8 × 8 mm) and cranial (30 × 12 mm). However, sizes can vary among manufacturers [77]. Ultrasound is therefore most often used as an adjunct in the debulking stage of an operation to optimize angles and identify large sections of residual tumor but is not thought to be a reliable method for identifying small tumor remnants at the end of a glioma resection.

Complication Avoidance

Despite the cosmetic and functional benefit of the minimally invasive approach to glioma resection, many surgeons still worry that a small field does not allow for adequate maneuverability in the face of complications such as significant hemorrhage. Advocates of minimally invasive techniques maintain that many potential injuries can be avoided with increased experience and meticulous technique. There are several central tenets of the minimally invasive approach that must be understood to carry out these procedures safely.

Surgeons inexperienced with this type of approach should develop their minimally invasive skills in a steady fashion over many cases. The "typical" craniotomy and approach can slowly be dialed down in size over time. At the completion of each case, the surgeon should turn a critical eye to his or her approach, and ask what portions of the exposure may not have been necessary. Simple steps such as maximizing the size of the craniotomy within a small incision may lead to significant reductions in the size and morbidity of the exposure.

Surgeons experienced with endoscopic, minimally invasive approaches emphasize the importance of preoperative planning in minimizing complications and frustration with these approaches. Particularly during the learning curve of a surgeon and an institution, it is important to verify that all of the necessary equipment is present and in working order prior to beginning a case. Additionally, planning the appropriate trajectory to address a given tumor is of paramount importance when working through a smaller opening [78]. Accurate neuronavigation and the availability of intraoperative ultrasound are critical in this regard.

As surgeons begin to gain experience with this type of technique, it is important to consider a surgical fall-back plan. If the surgeon finds that he or she is unable to obtain adequate visualization or maneuverability through a minimally invasive approach, the case should be set up in such a way that the surgeon can expand the exposure easily to ensure that the operation can be completed safely. Careful attention to positioning, prepping and draping can make intraoperative adjustments straightforward and can reduce the risk of serious complications.

When using a minimally invasive approach, the surgeon will be wise to take special care on the handling of instruments passing through the narrow surgical corridor. Instruments should always be inserted and removed from the field under direct vision to avoid injury to neurovascular structures outside the field of view. Additionally, the endoscope should be inserted and removed in one trajectory only and rotated about its long axis to improve vision rather than be swung back and forth through the brain. The addition of a rigid retractor system or an assistant whose main focus is avoiding potentially dangerous movements of the endoscope is helpful in this regard [36, 78]. Finally, dural closure is naturally more of a challenge in a small field. Therefore, meticulous attention to detail and consideration of adjunctive products to decrease the risk of CSF leak are advised [35, 36].

Conclusion

The surgical management of glioma remains a serious challenge. Patients with glioma face a very difficult diagnosis, and good surgical treatment can make a tremendous difference in terms of overall survival and quality of life. The surgeon's goals are increasingly clear: obtain a maximal resection while minimizing the risk of neurologic injury and reducing overall morbidity to improve quality of life and promote early access to adjuvant treatment. With these goals in mind, minimally invasive approaches to glioma resection are becoming increasingly attractive to both the surgeon and the patient. With experience, these approaches, which involve less damage to scalp, skull and surrounding brain tissue, can provide results equal to or better than traditional large craniotomies in less time. Although there is a learning curve with any new technique, the benefit of minimal injury to eloquent structures, shorter recovery periods, earlier access to adjuvant therapy, and excellent cosmetic results outweigh the increased costs of acquiring a new skill set. Ongoing technological advances in intraoperative imaging, functional mapping, and instrumentation such as robotics promise to make these approaches even more attractive over time, and it is increasingly clear that this approach will be critically important to the future of glioma surgery.

Acknowledgments

The authors would like to thank Victoria Morgan, Matthew Day, and Megan Strother for their expertise and technical assistance in producing the included fMRI and DTI images.

References

[1] Ostrom QT, Gittleman H, Farah P, Ondracek A, Chen Y, Wolinsky Y, et al. CBTRUS Statistical Report: Primary Brain and Central Nervous System Tumors Diagnosed in the United States in 2006-2010. *Neuro Oncol.* 2013 Nov 1;15(suppl 2):ii1–ii56.

[2] A multivariate Analysis of 416 patients with GBM: prognosis, EOR and survival_Lacroix.pdf [Internet]. [cited 2013 Aug 27]. Available from: http://thejns.org.proxy.library.vanderbilt.edu/doi/pdf/10.3171/jns.2001.95.2.0190

[3] McGirt MJ, Chaichana KL, Gathinji M, Attenello FJ, Than K, Olivi A, et al. Independent association of extent of resection with survival in patients with malignant brain astrocytoma. *J. Neurosurg.* 2009 Jan;110(1):156–62.

[4] Keles GE, Lamborn KR, Berger MS. Low-grade hemispheric gliomas in adults: a critical review of extent of resection as a factor influencing outcome. *J. Neurosurg.* 2001 Nov;95(5):735–45.

[5] Ius T, Isola M, Budai R, Pauletto G, Tomasino B, Fadiga L, et al. Low-grade glioma surgery in eloquent areas: volumetric analysis of extent of resection and its impact on overall survival. A single-institution experience in 190 patients: clinical article. *J. Neurosurg.* 2012 Dec;117(6):1039–52.

[6] Kuhnt D, Becker A, Ganslandt O, Bauer M, Buchfelder M, Nimsky C. Correlation of the extent of tumor volume resection and patient survival in surgery of glioblastoma multiforme with high-field intraoperative MRI guidance. *Neuro-oncology.* 2011 Dec;13(12):1339–48.

[7] Majchrzak K, Kaspera W, Bobek-Billewicz B, Hebda A, Stasik-Pres G, Majchrzak H, et al. The assessment of prognostic factors in surgical treatment of low-grade gliomas: a prospective study. *Clin. Neurol. Neurosurg.* 2012 Oct;114(8):1135–44.

[8] McGirt MJ, Mukherjee D, Chaichana KL, Than KD, Weingart JD, Quinones-Hinojosa A. Association of surgically acquired motor and language deficits on overall survival after resection of glioblastoma multiforme. *Neurosurgery.* 2009 Sep;65(3):463–469; discussion 469–470.

[9] Pignatti F, Bent M van den, Curran D, Debruyne C, Sylvester R, Therasse P, et al. Prognostic Factors for Survival in Adult Patients With Cerebral Low-Grade Glioma. *JCO.* 2002 Apr 15;20(8):2076–84.

[10] Lote K, Egeland T, Hager B, Stenwig B, Skullerud K, Berg-Johnsen J, et al. Survival, prognostic factors, and therapeutic efficacy in low-grade glioma: a retrospective study in 379 patients. *JCO.* 1997 Sep 1;15(9):3129–40.

[11] Ellingson BM, Lai A, Harris RJ, Selfridge JM, Yong WH, Das K, et al. Probabilistic Radiographic Atlas of Glioblastoma Phenotypes. *AJNR Am. J. Neuroradiol.* 2013 Mar 1;34(3):533–40.

[12] Nguyen NT, Hinojosa MW, Fayad C, Varela E, Konyalian V, Stamos MJ, et al. Laparoscopic Surgery Is Associated With a Lower Incidence of Venous Thromboembolism Compared With Open Surgery. *Annals of Surgery December* 2007. 2007;246(6):1021–7.

[13] Kumar S, Al-Wahab Z, Sarangi S, Woelk J, Morris R, Munkarah A, et al. Risk of postoperative venous thromboembolism after minimally invasive surgery for endometrial and cervical cancer is low: A multi-institutional study. *Gynecologic Oncology*. 2013 Jul;130(1):207–12.

[14] Khaldi A, Helo N, Schneck MJ, Origitano TC. Venous thromboembolism: deep venous thrombosis and pulmonary embolism in a neurosurgical population: Clinical article. *Journal of Neurosurgery*. 2011 Jan;114(1):40–6.

[15] Nosova K, Nuño M, Mukherjee D, Lad SP, Boakye M, Black KL, et al. Urinary tract infections in meningioma patients: analysis of risk factors and outcomes. *Journal of Hospital Infection*. 2013 Feb;83(2):132–9.

[16] Stupp R, Mason WP, Van den Bent MJ, Weller M, Fisher B, Taphoorn MJB, et al. Radiotherapy plus Concomitant and Adjuvant Temozolomide for Glioblastoma. *New England Journal of Medicine*. 2005;352(10):987–96.

[17] Berntsen EM, Gulati S, Solheim O, Kvistad KA, Torp SH, Selbekk T, et al. Functional magnetic resonance imaging and diffusion tensor tractography incorporated into an intraoperative 3-dimensional ultrasound-based neuronavigation system: impact on therapeutic strategies, extent of resection, and clinical outcome. *Neurosurgery*. 2010 Aug;67(2):251–64.

[18] Gulati S, Berntsen EM, Solheim O, Kvistad KA, Håberg A, Selbekk T, et al. Surgical resection of high-grade gliomas in eloquent regions guided by blood oxygenation level dependent functional magnetic resonance imaging, diffusion tensor tractography, and intraoperative navigated 3D ultrasound. *Minim. Invasive Neurosurg*. 2009 Feb;52(1):17–24.

[19] Gupta DK, Chandra PS, Ojha BK, Sharma BS, Mahapatra AK, Mehta VS. Awake craniotomy versus surgery under general anesthesia for resection of intrinsic lesions of eloquent cortex—A prospective randomised study. *Clinical Neurology and Neurosurgery*. 2007 May;109(4):335–43.

[20] Kim SS, McCutcheon IE, Suki D, Weinberg JS, Sawaya R, Lang FF, et al. Awake craniotomy for brain tumors near eloquent cortex: correlation of intraoperative cortical mapping with neurological outcomes in 309 consecutive patients. *Neurosurgery*. 2009 May;64(5):836–845; discussion 345–346.

[21] Palese AD, Skrap M, Fachin MB, Visioli S, Zannini L. The Experience of Patients Undergoing Awake Craniotomy: In the Patients' Own Words. A Qualitative Study. *Cancer Nursing* March/April 2008. 2008;31(2):166–72.

[22] Skucas AP, Artru AA. Anesthetic Complications of Awake Craniotomies for Epilepsy Surgery. *Anesthesia & Analgesia* March 2006. 2006;102(3):882–7.

[23] Wu J-S, Zhou L-F, Tang W-J, Mao Y, Hu J, Song Y-Y, et al. Clinical evaluation and follow-up outcome of diffusion tensor imaging-based functional neuronavigation: a prospective, controlled study in patients with gliomas involving pyramidal tracts. *Neurosurgery*. 2007 Nov;61(5):935–948; discussion 948–949.

[24] Zhu F-P, Wu J-S, Song Y-Y, Yao C-J, Zhuang D-X, Xu G, et al. Clinical application of motor pathway mapping using diffusion tensor imaging tractography and intraoperative

direct subcortical stimulation in cerebral glioma surgery: a prospective cohort study. *Neurosurgery*. 2012 Dec;71(6):1170–1183; discussion 1183–1184.

[25] Bello L, Castellano A, Fava E, Casaceli G, Riva M, Scotti G, et al. Intraoperative use of diffusion tensor imaging fiber tractography and subcortical mapping for resection of gliomas: technical considerations. *Neurosurg. Focus*. 2010 Feb;28(2):E6.

[26] Bertani G, Fava E, Casaceli G, Carrabba G, Casarotti A, Papagno C, et al. Intraoperative mapping and monitoring of brain functions for the resection of low-grade gliomas: technical considerations. *Neurosurg. Focus*. 2009 Oct;27(4):E4.

[27] Roberts DW, Hartov A, Kennedy FE, Miga MI, Paulsen KD. Intraoperative Brain Shift and Deformation: A Quantitative Analysis of Cortical Displacement in 28 Cases. *Neurosurgery* October 1998. 1998;43(4):749–58.

[28] Nimsky C, Ganslandt O, Hastreiter P, Wang R, Benner T, Sorensen AG, et al. Intraoperative Diffusion-Tensor MR Imaging: Shifting of White Matter Tracts during Neurosurgical Procedures—Initial Experience1. *Radiology*. 2005 Jan 1;234(1):218–25.

[29] Ohue S, Kohno S, Inoue A, Yamashita D, Harada H, Kumon Y, et al. Accuracy of diffusion tensor magnetic resonance imaging-based tractography for surgery of gliomas near the pyramidal tract: a significant correlation between subcortical electrical stimulation and postoperative tractography. *Neurosurgery*. 2012 Feb;70(2):283–293; discussion 294.

[30] Adam P. Brown, B. Gregory Thompson, Robert F. Spetzler. The Two-Point Method: Evaluating Brain Stem Lesions. *BNI Quarterly*. 1996;12(1).

[31] Wilson DH. Limited exposure in cerebral surgery. Technical note. *J. Neurosurg*. 1971 Jan;34(1):102–6.

[32] Van Lindert E, Perneczky A, Fries G, Pierangeli E. The supraorbital keyhole approach to supratentorial aneurysms: concept and technique. *Surg. Neurol*. 1998 May; 49(5):481–489; discussion 489–490.

[33] Cheng C-M, Noguchi A, Dogan A, Anderson GJ, Hsu FPK, McMenomey SO, et al. Quantitative verification of the keyhole concept: a comparison of area of exposure in the parasellar region via supraorbital keyhole, frontotemporal pterional, and supraorbital approaches. *J. Neurosurg*. 2013 Feb;118(2):264–9.

[34] Beretta F, Andaluz N, Chalaala C, Bernucci C, Salud L, Zuccarello M. Image-guided anatomical and morphometric study of supraorbital and transorbital minicraniotomies to the sellar and perisellar regions: comparison with standard techniques. *J. Neurosurg*. 2010 Nov;113(5):975–81.

[35] Wilson DA, Duong H, Teo C, Kelly DF. The Supraorbital Endoscopic Approach for Tumors. *World Neurosurg*. 2013 Feb 5;

[36] Garrett M, Consiglieri G, Nakaji P. Transcranial minimally invasive neurosurgery for tumors. *Neurosurg. Clin. N. Am*. 2010 Oct;21(4):595–605, v.

[37] Reisch R, Perneczky A. Ten-year experience with the supraorbital subfrontal approach through an eyebrow skin incision. *Neurosurgery*. 2005 Oct;57(4 Suppl):242–255; discussion 242–255.

[38] Ditzel Filho LFS, McLaughlin N, Bresson D, Solari D, Kassam AB, Kelly DF. Supraorbital Eyebrow Craniotomy for Removal of Intraaxial Frontal Brain Tumors: A Technical Note. *World Neurosurgery* [Internet]. [cited 2013 Jul 11]; Available from: http://www.sciencedirect.com/science/article/pii/S187887501201340X

[39] Beseoglu K, Lodes S, Stummer W, Steiger H-J, Hänggi D. The transorbital keyhole approach: early and long-term outcome analysis of approach-related morbidity and cosmetic results. Technical note. *J. Neurosurg.* 2011 Mar;114(3):852–6.

[40] Ma Y, Lan Q. An Anatomic Study of the Occipital Transtentorial Keyhole Approach. *World Neurosurgery* [Internet]. [cited 2013 Jul 11]; Available from: http://www.sciencedirect.com/science/article/pii/S187887501200410X

[41] Kuhnt D, Bauer MHA, Nimsky C. Brain shift compensation and neurosurgical image fusion using intraoperative MRI: current status and future challenges. *Crit. Rev. Biomed. Eng.* 2012;40(3):175–85.

[42] Fries G, Perneczky A. Endoscope-assisted Brain Surgery: Part 2-Analysis of 380 Procedures. *Neurosurgery* February 1998. 1998;42(2):226–31.

[43] Ishii M, Gallia GL. Application of Technology for Minimally Invasive Neurosurgery. *Neurosurgery Clinics of North America.* 2010 Oct;21(4):585–94.

[44] Dehdashti AR, Ganna A, Witterick I, Gentili F. Expanded endoscopic endonasal approach for anterior cranial base and suprasellar lesions: indications and limitations. *Neurosurgery.* 2009 Apr;64(4):677–687; discussion 687–689.

[45] Kelly PJ, Goerss SJ, Kall BA. The stereotaxic retractor in computer-assisted stereotaxic microsurgery. Technical note. *J. Neurosurg.* 1988 Aug;69(2):301–6.

[46] Otsuki T, Jokura H, Yoshimoto T. Stereotactic guiding tube for open-system endoscopy: a new approach for the stereotactic endoscopic resection of intra-axial brain tumors. *Neurosurgery.* 1990 Aug;27(2):326–30.

[47] Moshel YAMD, Link MJ, Kelly PJ. Stereotactic Volumetric Resection of Thalamic Pilocytic Astrocytomas. *Neurosurgery* July 2007. 2007;61(1):66–75.

[48] Kassam AB, Engh JA, Mintz AH, Prevedello DM. Completely endoscopic resection of intraparenchymal brain tumors. *J. Neurosurg.* 2009 Jan;110(1):116–23.

[49] Raza SM, Recinos PF, Avendano J, Adams H, Jallo GI, Quinones-Hinojosa A. Minimally Invasive Trans-Portal Resection of Deep Intracranial Lesions. min - *Minimally Invasive Neurosurgery.* 2011 Apr 20;54(01):5–11.

[50] Greenfield JP, Cobb WS, Tsouris AJ, Schwartz TH. Stereotactic minimally invasive tubular retractor system for deep brain lesions. *Neurosurgery.* 2008 Oct;63(4 Suppl 2):334–339; discussion 339–340.

[51] Zhong J, Dujovny M, Perlin AR, Perez-Arjona E, Park HK, Diaz FG. Brain retraction injury. *Neurol. Res.* 2003 Dec;25(8):831–8.

[52] Jo K-I, Chung SB, Jo K-W, Kong D-S, Seol H-J, Shin H-J. Microsurgical resection of deep-seated lesions using transparent tubular retractor: pediatric case series. *Childs Nerv. Syst.* 2011 Nov;27(11):1989–94.

[53] Almenawer SA, Crevier L, Murty N, Kassam A, Reddy K. Minimal access to deep intracranial lesions using a serial dilatation technique: case-series and review of brain tubular retractor systems. *Neurosurg. Rev.* 2013 Apr;36(2):321–329; discussion 329–330.

[54] Spetzler RF, Sanai N. The quiet revolution: retractorless surgery for complex vascular and skull base lesions. *J. Neurosurg.* 2012 Feb;116(2):291–300.

[55] Stummer W, Stocker S, Wagner S, Stepp H, Fritsch C, Goetz C, et al. Intraoperative detection of malignant gliomas by 5-aminolevulinic acid-induced porphyrin fluorescence. *Neurosurgery.* 1998 Mar;42(3):518–525; discussion 525–526.

[56] Stummer W, Pichlmeier U, Meinel T, Wiestler OD, Zanella F, Reulen H-J, et al. Fluorescence-guided surgery with 5-aminolevulinic acid for resection of malignant glioma: a randomised controlled multicentre phase III trial. *Lancet Oncol.* 2006 May;7(5):392–401.

[57] Duffner F, Ritz R, Freudenstein D, Weller M, Dietz K, Wessels J. Specific intensity imaging for glioblastoma and neural cell cultures with 5-aminolevulinic acid-derived protoporphyrin IX. *J. Neurooncol.* 2005 Jan;71(2):107–11.

[58] Díez Valle R, Tejada Solis S, Idoate Gastearena MA, García de Eulate R, Domínguez Echávarri P, Aristu Mendiroz J. Surgery guided by 5-aminolevulinic fluorescence in glioblastoma: volumetric analysis of extent of resection in single-center experience. J. *Neurooncol.* 2011 Mar;102(1):105–13.

[59] Prat-Acín R, Galeano-Senabre I, Pancucci G, Evangelista R, Ayuso-Sacido A, Botella C. Supraorbital trans-eyebrow craniotomy and fluorescence-guided resection of fronto-basal high grade gliomas. *Clinical Neurology and Neurosurgery.* 2013 Sep;115(9):1586–90.

[60] Idoate MA, Díez Valle R, Echeveste J, Tejada S. Pathological characterization of the glioblastoma border as shown during surgery using 5-aminolevulinic acid-induced fluorescence. *Neuropathology.* 2011;31(6):575–82.

[61] Sanai N, Snyder LA, Honea NJ, Coons SW, Eschbacher JM, Smith KA, et al. Intraoperative confocal microscopy in the visualization of 5-aminolevulinic acid fluorescence in low-grade gliomas. J. Neurosurg. 2011 Oct;115(4):740–8.

[62] Aldave G, Tejada S, Pay E, Marigil M, Bejarano B, Idoate MA, et al. Prognostic Value of Residual Fluorescent Tissue in Glioblastoma Patients After Gross Total Resection in 5-Aminolevulinic Acid-Guided Surgery. [Miscellaneous Article]. *Neurosurgery* June 2013. 2013;72(6):915–21.

[63] Schucht P, Beck J, Abu-Isa J, Andereggen L, Murek M, Seidel K, et al. Gross total resection rates in contemporary glioblastoma surgery: results of an institutional protocol combining 5-aminolevulinic acid intraoperative fluorescence imaging and brain mapping. *Neurosurgery.* 2012 Nov;71(5):927–935; discussion 935–936.

[64] Senft C, Forster M-T, Bink A, Mittelbronn M, Franz K, Seifert V, et al. Optimizing the extent of resection in eloquently located gliomas by combining intraoperative MRI guidance with intraoperative neurophysiological monitoring. *J. Neurooncol.* 2012 Aug;109(1):81–90.

[65] Duffau H, Capelle L, Denvil D, Sichez N, Gatignol P, Taillandier L, et al. Usefulness of intraoperative electrical subcortical mapping during surgery for low-grade gliomas located within eloquent brain regions: functional results in a consecutive series of 103 patients. *J. Neurosurg.* 2003 Apr;98(4):764–78.

[66] Hamer PCDW, Robles SG, Zwinderman AH, Duffau H, Berger MS. Impact of Intraoperative Stimulation Brain Mapping on Glioma Surgery Outcome: A Meta-Analysis. *JCO.* 2012 Jul 10;30(20):2559–65.

[67] Sanai N, Berger MS. Intraoperative stimulation techniques for functional pathway preservation and glioma resection. *Neurosurg. Focus.* 2010 Feb;28(2):E1.

[68] Bodily L, Mintz AH, Engh J. Combined Awake Craniotomy with Endoscopic Port Surgery for Resection of a Deep-Seated Temporal Lobe Glioma: A Case Report. *Case Reports in Medicine.* 2013;2013:1–3.

[69] Marcus HJ, Seneci CA, Payne CJ, Nandi D, Darzi A, Yang G-Z. Robotics in Keyhole Transcranial Endoscope-assisted Microsurgery: A Critical Review of Existing Systems and Proposed Specifications for New Robotic Platforms. *Neurosurgery*. 2013 Aug 5;

[70] Hong W-C, Tsai J-C, Chang SD, Sorger JM. Robotic skull base surgery via supraorbital keyhole approach: a cadaveric study. *Neurosurgery*. 2013 Jan;72 Suppl 1:33–8.

[71] Nossek E, Korn A, Shahar T, Kanner AA, Yaffe H, Marcovici D, et al. Intraoperative mapping and monitoring of the corticospinal tracts with neurophysiological assessment and 3-dimensional ultrasonography-based navigation: Clinical article. *Journal of Neurosurgery*. 2011 Mar;114(3):738–46.

[72] Senft C, Bink A, Franz K, Vatter H, Gasser T, Seifert V. Intraoperative MRI guidance and extent of resection in glioma surgery: a randomised, controlled trial. *Lancet Oncol.* 2011 Oct;12(11):997–1003.

[73] Claus EB, Horlacher A, Hsu L, Schwartz RB, Dello-Iacono D, Talos F, et al. Survival rates in patients with low-grade glioma after intraoperative magnetic resonance image guidance. *Cancer*. 2005;103(6):1227–33.

[74] Pamir MN, Özduman K, Yıldız E, Sav A, Dinçer A. Intraoperative magnetic resonance spectroscopy for identification of residual tumor during low-grade glioma surgery: clinical article. *J. Neurosurg*. 2013 Jun;118(6):1191–8.

[75] Makary M, Chiocca EA, Erminy N, Antor M, Bergese SD, Abdel-Rasoul M, et al. Clinical and economic outcomes of low-field intraoperative MRI-guided tumor resection neurosurgery. *Journal of Magnetic Resonance Imaging*. 2011;34(5):1022–30.

[76] Ntoukas V, Krishnan R, Seifert VM. The New Generation Polestar N20 For Conventional Neurosurgical Operating Rooms: A Preliminary Report. *Neurosurgery* March 2008. 2008;62(3):82–90.

[77] Ivanov M, Wilkins S, Poeata I, Brodbelt A. Intraoperative ultrasound in neurosurgery – a practical guide. *British Journal of Neurosurgery*. 2010 Oct;24(5):510–7.

[78] Sughrue ME, Mills SA, Young RL. Complication Avoidance in Minimally Invasive Neurosurgery. *Neurosurgery Clinics of North America*. 2010 Oct;21(4):699–702.

In: Gliomas: Classification, Symptoms, Treatment and Prognosis ISBN: 978-1-63117-868-9
Editor: David Cory Adamson

Chapter 5

Advances in Targeted Radiation Therapy for High-Grade Gliomas

Michael F. Gensheimer, Lia M. Halasz and Shilpen Patel*
University of Washington Medical Center, WA, US

Abstract

Radiation therapy plays an important role in the treatment of high-grade gliomas; it improves survival and can relieve neurologic symptoms. However, the diffuse growth pattern and radioresistance of high-grade gliomas make radiation treatment of these tumors challenging. New techniques in MRI and molecular imaging provide an *in vivo* view of the biology of gliomas. Cellular proliferation, oxygenation, perfusion, and water diffusion can be measured in tumor regions with high resolution. In parallel with these advances in imaging, technical progress in radiation therapy delivery has made it possible to precisely target tumor subvolumes while maximally sparing surrounding healthy brain structures. Particle beam radiation using protons or carbon ions is one promising approach to improving therapeutic index. In this chapter we review recent work on functional glioma imaging and physical targeting of radiation dose. We also explore topics at the intersection of these research areas such as radiation dose painting. The eventual goal is to improve the therapeutic index of radiation therapy for gliomas by increasing tumor cell kill and reducing normal tissue toxicity.

Introduction

Gliomas are neoplasms that arise from glial cells--the supporting cells of the central nervous system. High-grade gliomas (HGG) are defined as the subset of gliomas with a more aggressive growth and recurrence pattern. HGG is divided into anaplastic astrocytoma, anaplastic oligodendroglioma, anaplastic oligoastrocytoma (all WHO grade III), and

* Corresponding author: Shilpen Patel, University of Washington Medical Center, 1959 NE Pacific St, Box 356043, Phone: 206-598-4100. Fax: 206-598-3786. Email: shilpenp@uw.edu.

glioblastoma (GBM, WHO grade IV). HGGs are aggressive neoplasms which are rarely curable.

Radiation therapy is an important component of treatment for HGG. After maximal safe resection, external beam radiation has been shown in randomized trials to extend survival for HGG patients (Walker). However, even with modern trimodality treatment (surgery followed by radiation therapy with concurrent and adjuvant temozolomide), median survival for GBM is only 15 months and 5-year survival is 10% (Stupp 2009). Survival after treatment of WHO grade III gliomas is better than for GBM, but long-term survival is still rare.

Radiation therapy for HGG is challenging because not only are these tumors radioresistant, but they also exhibit a diffuse growth pattern with microscopic spread into surrounding healthy brain. Whereas external beam radiation therapy to 60 Gy is sufficient to control microscopic disease in most tumor types, the growth of HGG is delayed but not prevented with this dose of radiation. A classic study from Wallner and colleagues at Memorial Sloan-Kettering Cancer Center showed that whole brain radiation therapy to 40 Gy with a further boost to the site of the resected tumor, 78% of tumors recurred within 2 cm of the of the initial enhancing mass--in other words, at the site that received the highest radiation dose (Wallner). This propensity for central recurrence within the radiation field has also been documented with modern partial brain radiation therapy with concurrent temozolomide (Sherriff). Radiation dose escalation has been disappointing; in a study from the University of Michigan, most failures occurred centrally even when dose was escalated to 90 Gy (Chan).

While HGGs tend to recur centrally, their diffuse growth pattern was illustrated vividly when surgeons performed hemispherectomy for GBM, only to see the tumors recur in the contralateral hemisphere (Claes). This striking finding illustrates that no matter how precise the targeting of surgery and radiation therapy, GBM and most WHO grade III gliomas will not be curable except with novel treatments such as targeted systemic agents.

Why, then, should we devote resources to improving targeting of radiation dose for HGG? There are multiple reasons:

- HGGs, especially GBM, are usually spatially heterogeneous in terms of perfusion, proliferation, hypoxia, and function of the surrounding brain parenchyma. Radiation therapy clearly has activity against HGG, as demonstrated by delay of recurrence and improved survival. Therefore, there is a strong theoretical justification for optimizing radiation dose delivery to focus on areas of increased tumor cell density, radioresistance, or recurrence risk.
- While past trials have not shown a benefit from radiation dose escalation or boosting dose to part of the tumor, we may not have had the tools to target the right areas. Emerging imaging technologies such as FET (O-(2-[18F]fluoroethyl)-L-tyrosine) PET may have a complementary role to MRI in identifying areas of highest glioma cell density (Pauleit).
- There has been a gradual trend toward treating with a reduced volume in HGG, with equivalent or improved survival outcomes. Using advanced imaging or physical targeting methods such as particle beam therapy, further volume reduction may be possible, which could theoretically reduce neurotoxicity.
- New molecularly targeted agents are being introduced at a rapid rate. In other disease sites, the efficacy of radiation therapy has been dramatically improved with the

addition of concurrent systemic therapy (transitional cell carcinoma of the bladder, esophageal cancer). If more effective systemic therapies for HGG are developed which synergize with radiation therapy, precise targeting of various tumor areas may become more effective and important.

Identifying the Target

In current practice, post-operative contrast-enhanced MRI is the main imaging modality used for radiation target delineation. T1-weighted gadolinium-enhanced and T2-weighted sequences are acquired. The enhancing region on the T1-weighted sequence is thought to represent the mass-like part of the tumor; the larger hyperintense region on T2-weighted sequence is thought to represent infiltration of glioma cells into surrounding brain. Figure 1 shows representative MRI images for a patient with glioblastoma multiforme. The Radiation Therapy Oncology Group trials generally specify that the larger T2-hyperintense region plus a margin should be treated to a dose of around 46 Gy in five weeks, followed by a boost to the enhancing mass to a total dose of 60 Gy. However, there are varying practice patterns across the United States and EORTC trials generally specify treating the T2-hyperintesnse region to the prescribed dose with a smaller margin.

It has been known for some time that CT and MRI underestimate the extent of HGG. Investigators at the Mayo Clinic performed CT, MRI, and stereotactic biopsies in 40 patients with gliomas (Kelly). Of specimens obtained just outside of the area of T2 prolongation, around half had isolated tumor cells on pathologic examination.

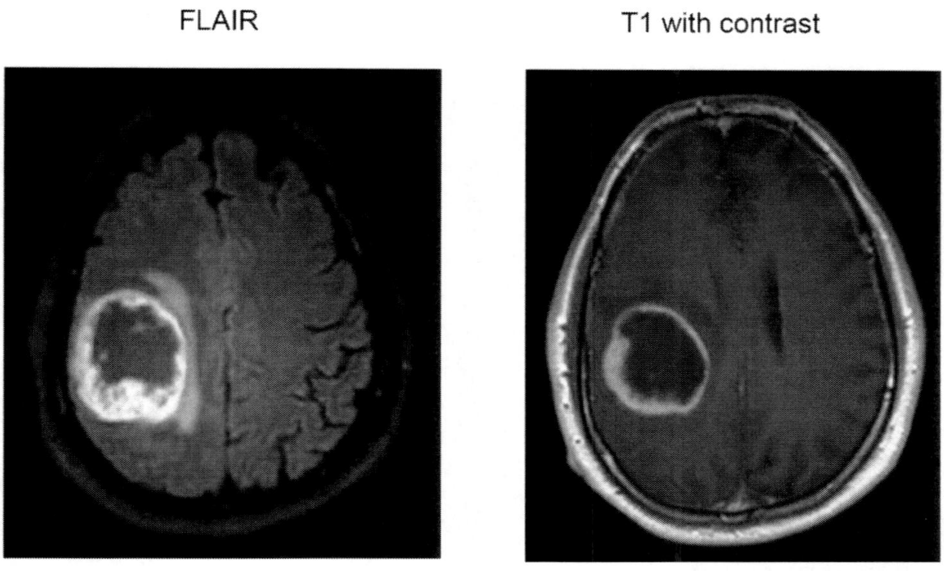

Figure 1. MRI in a 60 year old patient with glioblastoma multiforme. Left: T2-weighted FLAIR sequence shows surrounding edema. Right: T1-weighted contrast-enhanced sequence shows rim-enhancing mass.

At the same time, HGG and especially GBMs are spatially heterogeneous, with varying cellularity, oxygenation, and proliferation within the main bulk of the tumor. This can be seen on traditional imaging, as on contrast-enhanced MRI, GBM often demonstrates a ring-enhancing appearance indicating central necrosis. However, anatomical imaging with CT or MR does not provide a direct window into molecular heterogeneity in tumors. There is emerging evidence that some GBMs are composed of genetically distinct subpopulations, all derived from a single precursor cell. Amplification of tyrosine kinases drives growth of GBMs and is an important step in tumorigenesis. Snuderl and colleagues performed fluorescence in situ hybridization for multiple tyrosine kinases in 350 GBM samples (Snuderl). They unexpectedly found that several tumors were composed of subpopulations with amplification of mutually exclusive tyrosine kinases. These subpopulations would be expected to have varied radiobiological properties such as sensitivity to radiation.

Clearly, anatomical imaging is inadequate for determining the extent of HGG or fully examining heterogeneity within the tumor. Much current research focuses on the goal of biological or functional imaging, which holds great promise for improving prognostication and treatment for gliomas.

Nuclear Medicine Techniques

PET and SPECT imaging can provide a window into molecular activity in and around cancer cells. The most common PET tracer used in clinical use, fluorodeoxyglucose (FDG), is less useful in the brain than for other sites because signal from tumor can be drowned out by high uptake in normal brain (Chen). However, some groups have found delayed imaging to improve distinction between gliomas and normal gray matter; see figure 2 (Spence).

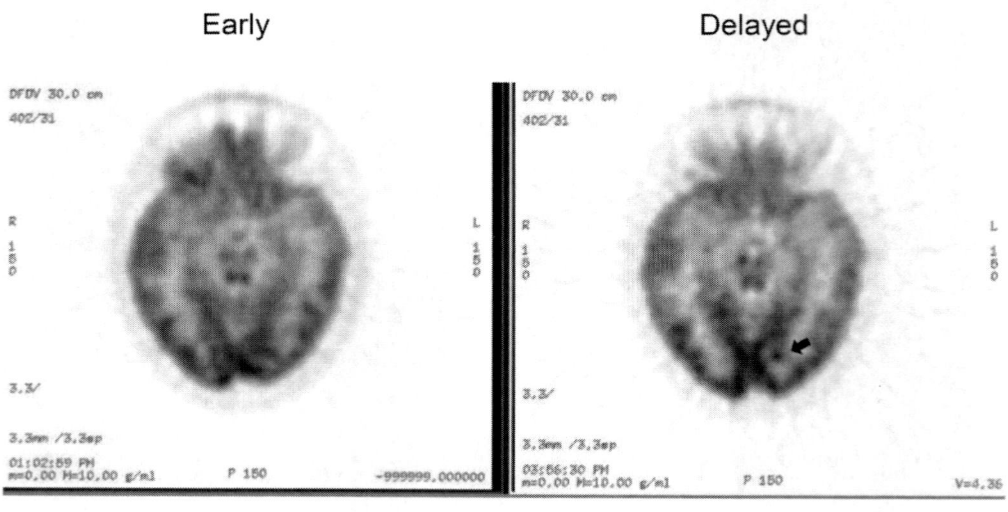

Figure 2. Early and delayed FDG PET images in a patient with a left occipital brain metastasis. High uptake in healthy brain obscures the mass when imaged 55 minutes after tracer injection (left), but the mass is clearly visible 229 minutes after injection (right, with arrow).

Newer tracers have been shown to improve tumor-to-normal signal ratio and can image specific cellular activities. These tracers could help move biologically targeted radiation therapy closer to clinical practice.

18F-FLT is a tracer which, as a thymidine analogue, is taken up in rapidly dividing cells through the activity of thymidine kinase. Chen and colleagues at UCLA performed FLT PET and standard FDG PET imaging in twenty-five patients with WHO grade II-IV gliomas, mostly GBMs (Chen). FLT PET uptake above background was 100% sensitive and specific for distinguishing high-grade versus low-grade gliomas. Five patients with treated gliomas which were stable on MRI had positive FLT PET but negative FDG PET. Strikingly, all five patients had tumor progression within 3 months of the PET scans. Fourteen tumors were resected and Ki-67 score, a marker for cellular proliferation, was obtained on the pathology specimens. Maximum FLT uptake correlated well with Ki-67 ($r = 0.84$, $p < 0.0001$), whereas maximum FDG uptake had only a moderate correlation ($r = 0.51$). More recently, the same group showed that FLT PET is useful for early response assessment to therapy (Schwarzenberg). Thirty patients treated with bevacizumab for recurrent HGG received MRI and FLT PET before and 6 weeks after initiation of therapy. Relative decrease in FLT uptake was more predictive of overall survival and progression-free survival than standard MRI response criteria (for overall survival, $p < 0.001$ and 0.01, respectively).

Another promising tracer is O-(2-[18F]fluoroethyl)-L-tyrosine, abbreviated as FET. FET is a labeled amino acid that is preferentially taken up by tumor cells compared to normal brain. Pauleit and colleagues performed an intriguing study in which thirty-one patients with suspected gliomas underwent stereotactic biopsy, guided by a combination of MRI and FET PET imaging (Pauleit). Biopsies guided by MRI had good sensitivity for tumor of 96%, but specificity was only 53%. By contrast, FET PET had sensitivity of 92% and improved specificity of 81%. This indicates that some areas of peritumoral inflammation and edema can be mistaken for active tumor on MRI, but this problem can be corrected by the addition of functional imaging.

A related study has more direct relevance to radiation therapy planning (Piroth, 2011). Piroth and colleagues at the RWTH Aachen University Hospital in Aachen, Germany performed postoperative, pre-radiation therapy FET PET and standard MRI. The volume of residual active tumor was defined by tumor to blood ratio of FET uptake of greater than 1.6. When tumor volume on FET PET was >25 ml, overall survival was 6.9 months, compared to 20.0 months when volume was < 25 ml ($p < 0.001$). On multivariate analysis with Cox regression, active tumor volume on FET PET strongly predicted survival duration, but enhancing volume on MRI was not an independent predictor of survival.

The same group performed a follow-up study with the hypothesis that radiation dose escalation to the area of greatest activity on FET PET could improve disease control and survival for GBM (Piroth, 2012). Twenty-two patients were treated with intensity-modulated radiation therapy. They received a dose of 60 Gy to a larger, MRI-defined volume and then an additional 12 Gy boost to a smaller area with tumor-to-brain ratio of FET uptake of at least 1.6. Concurrent and adjuvant temozolomide chemotherapy was used in a standard fashion. Unfortunately, median overall survival of 14.8 months was not improved compared to standard treatment. This may be due not to deficiencies in targeting, but to the resistance of GBM to even high-dose radiation as shown in multiple dose-escalation studies using conventional imaging.

MR-based Techniques

Contrast-enhanced MRI has been the cornerstone of radiation target delineation for HGG for around twenty years. MR techniques have advantages of high spatial resolution compared to PET/SPECT, and high temporal resolution when using techniques such as dynamic contrast-enhanced MRI. They are also generally less expensive than PET, and because there is no radiation dose to the patient, MRI can be repeated frequently. Research at the intersection of MR and radiation therapy falls into two groups: 1) more clever use of standard anatomic imaging to delineate targets and assess response to treatment, and 2) use of advanced MRI methods to accomplish biological imaging.

The first group is epitomized by the mathematical modeling work of Kristin Swanson and colleagues at the University of Washington. They developed a model of glioma tumor growth that uses pretreatment standard MRI to predict tumor growth rate and directions of expansion (Swanson 2003). The model starts with the assumption that the rate of change of tumor cell population at any location can be expressed as the sum of diffusion of tumor cells into the location and the net proliferation of cells at the location. They hypothesized that each patient's tumor has varying predilection for proliferation and diffusion/invasion. Tumors with a large ratio of contrast-enhancing volume to T2-hyperintense volume are thought to progress more through proliferation, and those with a small enhancing volume but large T2-hyperintense volume progress more through diffusion. The model has been shown to correlate well with clinical outcomes. For instance, it is able to predict survival time accurately (Swanson 2008). The model has obvious applications to radiation therapy. In a preclinical computer simulation, an optimized radiation plan was created to deliver the highest dose to areas of highest cell density as predicted by the mathematical model (Holdsworth). Tumor control probability and normal tissue complication probability were predicted to be improved compared to a standard radiation plan.

Advanced MR techniques with potential applications to HGG radiotherapy include perfusion methods to measure blood flow, diffusion imaging to measure diffusion rate of water in tissues, and spectroscopic methods to measure concentrations of molecules in cells.

Dynamic contrast-enhanced MRI takes advantage of the high spatial and temporal resolution of MRI to image at multiple time points before and immediately after the injection of contrast material. For each voxel, a curve representing the time course of contrast uptake can be generated. The rate and quantity of contrast uptake and release by tissues can be studied. Researchers at the University of Michigan hypothesized that GBMs with large areas of high vascular permeability ("leaky blood vessels" due to blood-brain barrier disruption from tumor) would prove to be more aggressive (Cao). In twenty HGG patients, tumor vascular leakage volume as measured on dynamic contrast-enhanced MRI was more predictive of survival than parameters from standard MRI or tumor grade (III vs. IV). Though not mentioned by the authors, this work has natural application to radiation target delineation.

Diffusion-weighted MRI measures the random motion of water as it diffuses between cells. In multiple disease sites, lower rates of diffusion are correlated with increased tumor cell density, histologic grade, and aggressive biology (Galban). Diffusion-weighted MRI is emerging as a valuable method for early response assessment to treatment. Galban and colleagues performed pre-treatment and mid-radiation therapy diffusion-weighted MRI and dynamic susceptibility contrast-MRI in 45 HGG patients. When water diffusion rate increased and blood uptake decreased during treatment, patients had improved 1-year survival (p <

0.0001). This work raises the tantalizing possibility of imaging changes in tumor biology mid-treatment, then adjusting the remainder of the radiation treatment based on these findings. Total radiation dose, spatial dose distribution, or duration of adjuvant chemotherapy could be modulated.

A common clinical problem involves distinguishing radiation injury from tumor progression on follow-up MRIs. A growing tumor causes an increase in the size of the contrast-enhancing volume and surrounding edema. However, radiation effects can cause a similar MRI appearance even in the absence of tumor progression. Radiation injury can be seen months to years after treatment, and may be due to disruption of the blood-brain barrier from endothelial cell death (Brandsma). Patients sometimes undergo resection of the recurrent contrast-enhancing area, only for pathology to demonstrate inflammatory reaction and no viable tumor. Advanced MR techniques hold promise in distinguishing tumor progression from radiation injury. ^{1}H magnetic resonance spectroscopy (MRS) allows the concentration of various metabolites to be measured *in vivo.* Some of the most impressive results were reported from China (Zeng). Twenty-eight patients with new contrast-enhancing lesions at the location of a previously irradiated HGG underwent MRS. The ratios of choline, creatine, and *N*-acetylaspartate concentration were significantly different in the nine patients with radiation injury compared to the nineteen with progression. Diagnostic accuracy was 96.2%. At our institution, a combination of standard MRI, MRS, and/or FDG PET is used in this situation, but there is room for improvement and some patients still undergo resection which in retrospect was not necessary.

More radical MR techniques are coming over the horizon, but their specific applications and eventual impact on clinical practice still need to be determined. In the last few years, there has been intense interest in hyperpolarized ^{13}C MR spectroscopic imaging (MRSI). The low signal-to-noise ratio of standard ^{1}H MRS means that in practice, only one location or a few locations in the tumor can be interrogated. In contrast, in hyperpolarized ^{13}C MRSI, ^{13}C labeled compounds are hyperpolarized outside of the body, then injected intravenously and imaged. The hyperpolarization process increases signal-to-noise ratio by a factor of 10,000, putting high-resolution spectroscopic imaging into reach (Chaumeil). Though the technique is still in its infancy, the first human trial is ongoing in prostate cancer patients. Hyperpolarized ^{13}C MRSI also holds promise in HGG. At the University of California San Francisco, the technique was applied to a rat model of GBM. Rats treated with the mTOR inhibitor everolimus and a control group were imaged before and two days and seven days after initiation of treatment. At day 7, there was a significant drop in lactate-to-pyruvate ratio in the treated animals only. Conventional MRI did not show a decrease in tumor size until day 15. This study is impressive because it was performed using a clinical MRI scanner and demonstrated *in vivo* MRSI in a clinically relevant model system. However, before hyperpolarized ^{13}C imaging is ready for the mainstream, spatial resolution will need to be improved (4mm x 4mm in this study) and safety in humans needs to be demonstrated. There could be myriad applications to radiation therapy, such as identifying tumor regions with increased proliferation or hypoxia, or performing mid-treatment imaging to identify regions with early response or resistance to treatment.

Delivering Dose to the Target

While recent research in HGG imaging has not yet had much influence on everyday clinical practice, technical advances in radiation treatment delivery have already made their mark in the clinic. These can be divided into improvements in the precision and shaping of standard photon/X-ray therapy, and use of particle beam therapy such as carbon ion or proton radiotherapy.

The last few decades have seen relentless improvements in the precision of radiation therapy delivery. X-ray therapy is typically delivered using a linear accelerator. Many linear accelerators are now fitted with on-board imaging devices such as cone beam CT. Use of cone beam CT protocols during HGG treatment allows use of tighter target volume margins and consequent reduction in doses to surrounding normal structures like healthy brain, optic nerves, and cochleae. One recent advance is the use of volumetric modulated arc therapy (VMAT). Using this technique, the radiation source rotates around the patient in a continuous arc, with the beam shape varying fluidly. This approach produces a rapid treatment time, while allowing surrounding normal structures to be "carved out" from the high dose region, sparing toxicity. In a comparative study on ten HGG patients, VMAT plans reduced retina and optic nerve doses compared to standard intensity-modulated radiation therapy, with reduced treatment time (Shaffer). Because of these and similar findings, we have adopted VMAT as a standard treatment approach for HGG.

Another promising area is the use of particle beam therapy. This approach generally involves accelerating protons or heavier ions such as carbon to high speeds using a cyclotron or synchrotron. A precisely shaped beam is then directed at the tumor. Whereas X-rays deposit radiation dose all the way through the patient, both protons and carbon ions slow down as they travel through tissue, depositing very little dose past the tumor. Carbon ions also have a potential biological advantage, because they produce a different microscopic structure of DNA damage compared to X-rays and protons which may be more damaging to tumor cells.

Proton Therapy

Since proton therapy is radiobiologically equivalent to photon therapy within a factor of 1.1, its advantages lie in its improved physical dose distribution. The conformality of a radiation treatment is roughly defined as the total volume receiving high radiation dose divided by the volume of the target (usually a tumor). With the recent improvements in precision and dose shaping of X-ray therapy, the conformality of proton and photon plans are generally similar. The main difference is that the integral radiation dose (total amount of energy deposited in the body) is dramatically lower with protons because they stop in the target instead of partially continuing through like photons. In a study on six patients with a variety of brain tumors, proton therapy plans had similar conformality to photon plans, but integral dose was much lower: the volume within the 30% isodose line was around half that of the photon plans (Baumert).

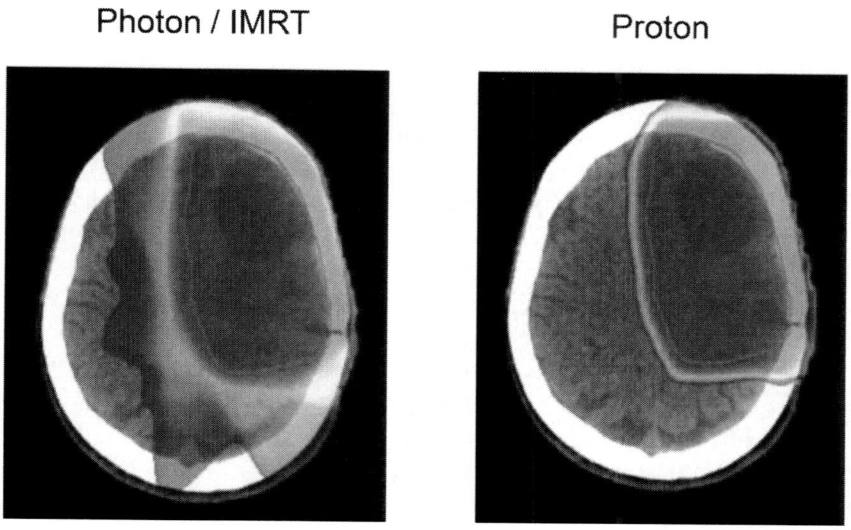

Figure 3. Comparison of photon and proton plans for a patient with a glioma of the left frontal lobe. Target volume outlined in green, radiation dose distribution in colorwash (red=high dose, blue=low dose). While the high dose region is similar, there is more low-dose spillage with the photon plan. Courtesy of Jason Rockhill.

What is the advantage of reducing integral dose to the brain? Holding the prescribed dose constant but reducing the volume of healthy brain exposed to low-to-intermediate doses of radiation could reduce cognitive effects of therapy or reduce the rate of secondary malignancies (Merchant, Chung). These endpoints may be less relevant for the HGG population compared to children with more curable brain tumors. Conversely, it is possible that proton therapy could enable safe dose escalation or concurrent use with targeted agents. Holding the dose to surrounding brain constant, dose to the tumor could be increased. A recent Japanese phase I/II trial explored this concept (Mizumoto). Twenty patients with GBM were treated with a twice-daily regimen consisting of combined photon and proton treatments. Dose was escalated to 96.6 Gy(RBE) (the Gy(RBE) designation means that biologically effective dose was the same as 96.6 Gy of photon irradiation). Toxicity was similar to standard photon treatment, and survival rates were promising with 2-year overall survival of 45.3% and median survival of 21.6 months. While these results appear to be better than those achieved with standard chemoradiation (median survival 14.6 months in the landmark Stupp trial), we would caution that the Japanese study population was small (20 patients) and may have been more favorable: for instance, tumor size was limited to 4 cm. Furthermore, dose escalation to 90 GyE with protons has been previously published by Massachusetts General Hospital and showed high rates of radionecrosis so this strategy was abandoned (Fitzek).

Carbon Ion Therapy

Carbon ion therapy shares advantages in physical dose distribution with proton beam therapy; but because of the dense tracks of DNA damage produced by carbon ions, there may also be a radiobiological advantage in tumor cell kill. *In vitro* experiments showed that GBM cell lines were up to 1.74 times as sensitive to carbon ion irradiation compared to X-rays, especially if p53 was mutated as it is in many GBMs (Iwadate). The first results of carbon ion treatment of HGG were reported in 2007 with a phase I/II Japanese trial (Mizoe). This was a dose escalation trial where the dose of a carbon ion boost was gradually increased in successive cohorts of patients. The final cohort was treated to a total dose of 74.8 Gy(RBE). Dose of the carbon ion boost had a striking impact on overall survival, with median survival time of 7, 19, and 26 months in the low-, middle-, and high-dose groups ($p = 0.0031$). In this trial and in the Japanese proton therapy trial, the outdated chemotherapy drug nimustine was used along with radiation. When radiation is given along with the current standard of care drug, temozolomide, results could change. Therefore, we eagerly await the results of an ongoing phase II trial from Heidelberg University (Combs). Patients are being randomized to carbon ion versus proton boost with concurrent temozolomide. The investigators are targeting an ambitious sample size of 150.

These trials all use standard MRI anatomic imaging for target delineation. Given the promising results of particle beam treatment, a natural question is whether its effectiveness could be increased even further by use of advanced imaging modalities. This topic is only beginning to be explored. In a study from the University of Regensburg in Germany, FET PET studies were obtained in three GBM patients (Rickhey). An optimal radiation dose distribution was calculated based on the expected density of active tumor cells from the FET PET scan. It was found that treatment with protons could better approximate the ideal dose distribution compared to photons, with an added bonus of lower doses to normal structures. Much work needs to be done before this approach is ready for the clinic. As an example of the challenges faced, the authors point out that "no experimental or clinical data were available that mapped the SUV [standardized uptake value] to the presence of tumor cells".

Conclusion

Radiation therapy is an essential part of standard of care treatment for HGG. Despite this, outcomes with standard of care treatment are disappointing, with many recurrences centered inside the high dose radiation region. Advanced highly focused forms of radiation therapy such as carbon ion treatment may enable more effective tumor cell kill with equivalent toxicity rates to standard X-ray therapy. As our ability to precisely distribute radiation dose improves, use of advanced imaging to identify biologically distinct tumor regions will become more useful.

References

Baumert BG, Norton IA, Lomax AJ, Davis JB. Dose conformation of intensity-modulated stereotactic photon beams, proton beams, and intensity-modulated proton beams for intracranial lesions. *Int. J. Radiat. Oncol. Biol. Phys.*, 2004 60(4), 1314-24.

Brandsma D, Stalpers L, Taal W, et al. Clinical features, mechanisms, and management of pseudoprogression in malignant gliomas. *Lancet Oncol.* 2008 9(5), 453-61.

Cao Y, Nagesh V, Hamstra D, et al. The extent and severity of vascular leakage as evidence of tumor aggressiveness in high-grade gliomas. *Cancer Res.*, 2006 66(17), 8912-7.

Chan JL, Lee SW, Fraass BA, et al. Survival and failure patterns of high-grade gliomas after three-dimensional conformal radiotherapy. *J. Clin. Oncol.*, 2002 20(6), 1635-42.

Chaumeil MM, Ozawa T, Park I, et al. Hyperpolarized 13C MR spectroscopic imaging can be used to monitor Everolimus treatment in vivo in an orthotopic rodent model of glioblastoma. *Neuroimage*, 2012 59(1), 193-201.

Chen W, Cloughesy T, Kamdar N et al. Imaging proliferation in brain tumors with 18F-FLT PET: comparison with 18F-FDG. *J. Nucl. Med.*, 2005 46(6), 945-52.

Chung CS, Yock TI, Nelson K, et al. Incidence of second malignancies among patients treated with proton versus photon radiation. *Int. J. Radiat. Oncol. Biol. Phys.*, 2013 87(1), 46-52.

Claes A, Idema AJ, Wesseling P. Diffuse glioma growth: a guerilla war. *Acta Neuropathol.,* 2007 114(5), 443-58.

Combs SE, Kieser M, Rieken S, et al. Randomized phase II study evaluating a carbon ion boost applied after combined radiochemotherapy with temozolomide versus a proton boost after radiochemotherapy with temozolomide in patients with primary glioblastoma: the CLEOPATRA trial. *BMC Cancer*, 2010 10, 478.

Fitzek MM, Thornton AF, Rabinov JD, et al. Accelerated fractionated proton/photon irradiation to 90 cobalt gray equivalent for glioblastoma multiforme: results of a phase II prospective trial. *J. Neurosurg.*, 1999 91(2), 251-60.

Galbán CJ, Chenevert TL, Meyer CR, et al. Prospective analysis of parametric response map-derived MRI biomarkers: identification of early and distinct glioma response patterns not predicted by standard radiographic assessment. *Clin. Cancer Res.*, 2011 17(14), 4751-60.

Kelly PJ, Daumas-Duport C, Kispert DB. Imaging-based stereotaxic serial biopsies in untreated intracranial glial neoplasms. *J. Neurosurg.*, 1987 66(6), 865-74.

Holdsworth CH, Corwin D, Stewart RD et al. Adaptive IMRT using a multiobjective evolutionary algorithm integrated with a diffusion-invasion model of glioblastoma. *Phys. Med. Biol.*, 2012 57(24), 8271-83.

Iwadate Y, Mizoe J, Osaka Y, et al. High linear energy transfer carbon radiation effectively kills cultured glioma cells with either mutant or wild-type p53. *Int. J. Radiat. Oncol. Biol. Phys.*, 2001 50(3), 803-8.

Merchant TE, Kiehna EN, Li C, et al. Modeling radiation dosimetry to predict cognitive outcomes in pediatric patients with CNS embryonal tumors including medulloblastoma. *Int. J. Radiat. Oncol. Biol. Phys.*, 2006 65(1), 210-21.

Mizoe JE, Tsujii H, Hasegawa A, et al. Phase I/II clinical trial of carbon ion radiotherapy for malignant gliomas: combined X-ray radiotherapy, chemotherapy, and carbon ion radiotherapy. *Int. J. Radiat. Oncol. Biol. Phys.*, 2007 69(2), 390-6.

Mizumoto M, Tsuboi K, Igaki H, et al. Phase I/II trial of hyperfractionated concomitant boost proton radiotherapy for supratentorial glioblastoma multiforme. *Int. J. Radiat. Oncol. Biol. Phys.*, 2010 77(1), 98-105.

Pauleit D, Floeth F, Hamacher K et al. O-(2-[18F]fluoroethyl)-L-tyrosine PET combined with MRI improves the diagnostic assessment of cerebral gliomas. *Brain*, 2005 128(Pt 3), 678-87.

Piroth MD, Holy R, Pinkawa M, et al. Prognostic impact of postoperative, pre-irradiation (18)F-fluoroethyl-l-tyrosine uptake in glioblastoma patients treated with radiochemotherapy. *Radiother. Oncol.*, 2011 99(2), 218-24.

Piroth MD, Pinkawa M, Holy R et al. Integrated boost IMRT with FET-PET-adapted local dose escalation in glioblastomas. Results of a prospective phase II study. *Strahlenther. Onkol.*, 2012 188(4), 334-9.

Rickhey M, Morávek Z, Eilles C et al. 18F-FET-PET-based dose painting by numbers with protons. *Strahlenther. Onkol.*, 2010 186(6), 320-6.

Schwarzenberg J, Czernin J, Cloughesy TF et al. 3'-deoxy-3'-18F-fluorothymidine PET and MRI for early survival predictions in patients with recurrent malignant glioma treated with bevacizumab. *J. Nucl. Med.*, 2012 53(1), 29-36.

Shaffer R, Nichol AM, Vollans E, et al. A comparison of volumetric modulated arc therapy and conventional intensity-modulated radiotherapy for frontal and temporal high-grade gliomas. *Int. J. Radiat. Oncol. Biol. Phys.*, 2010 76(4), 1177-84.

Sherriff J, Tamangani J, Senthil L et al. Patterns of relapse in glioblastoma multiforme following concomitant chemoradiotherapy with temozolomide. *Br. J. Radiol.*, 2013 86(1022), 20120414.

Snuderl M, Fazlollahi L, Le LP. Mosaic amplification of multiple receptor tyrosine kinase genes in glioblastoma. *Cancer Cell*, 2011 20(6), 810-7.

Spence AM, Muzi M, Mankoff DA, et al. 18F-FDG PET of gliomas at delayed intervals: improved distinction between tumor and normal gray matter. *J. Nucl. Med.*, 2004 45(10), 1653-9.

Stupp R, Hegi ME, Mason WP et al. Effects of radiotherapy with concomitant and adjuvant temozolomide versus radiotherapy alone on survival in glioblastoma in a randomised phase III study: 5-year analysis of the EORTC-NCIC trial. *Lancet Oncol.*, 2009 10(5), 459-66.

Swanson KR, Bridge C, Murray JD, Alvord EC Jr. Virtual and real brain tumors: using mathematical modeling to quantify glioma growth and invasion. *J. Neurol. Sci.*, 2003 216(1), 1-10.

Swanson KR, Rostomily RC, Alvord EC Jr. A mathematical modelling tool for predicting survival of individual patients following resection of glioblastoma: a proof of principle. *Br. J. Cancer*, 2008 98(1), 113-9.

Walker MD, Green SB, Byar DP et al. Randomized comparisons of radiotherapy and nitrosoureas for the treatment of malignant glioma after surgery. *N. Engl. J. Med.*, 1980 303(23), 1323-9.

Wallner KE, Galicich JH, Krol G et al. Patterns of failure following treatment for glioblastoma multiforme and anaplastic astrocytoma. *Int. J. Radiat. Oncol. Biol. Phys.*, 1989 16(6), 1405-9.

Zeng QS, Li CF, Zhang K, Liu H, et al. Multivoxel 3D proton MR spectroscopy in the distinction of recurrent glioma from radiation injury. *J. Neurooncol.* 2007 84(1), 63-9.

In: Gliomas: Classification, Symptoms, Treatment and Prognosis ISBN: 978-1-63117-868-9
Editor: David Cory Adamson

Chapter 6

PET Tracers in Glioma Imaging

Giorgio Treglia, [1,*] ***, Marco Salsano*** [2]
and Salvatore Annunziata [3]
[1]Department of Nuclear Medicine, Oncology Institute
of Southern Switzerland, Bellinzona, Switzerland
[2]Institute of Radiology, Catholic University of Rome, Italy
[3]Institute of Nuclear Medicine, Catholic University of Rome, Italy

Abstract

Several positron emission tomography (PET) tracers are available for imaging of gliomas, investigating different metabolic pathways including glucose metabolism, amino acid transportation, proliferation rate, membrane protein metabolism, oxygen metabolism and perfusion. In this chapter we briefly discuss the mechanism of uptake of the different PET tracers used in patients with glioma. Furthermore we summarize the literature data about the diagnostic performance of PET using different tracers in the diagnosis of glioma.

Keywords: PET, glioma, tracers, imaging

PET Tracers in Glioma Imaging

Several positron emission tomography (PET) tracers are available for imaging of gliomas, investigating glucose metabolism, amino acid transportation, proliferation rate, membrane proteins, oxygen metabolism, and perfusion [1-7].

Glucose analogue 2-[^{18}F] fluoro-2-deoxy-D-glucose (^{18}F-FDG) is used to evaluate the increased glucose metabolism in patients with glioma. This PET tracer is transported into the cells by glucose transporter proteins.

[*] Corresponding author: Giorgio Treglia, MD. Department of Nuclear Medicine and PET/CT Center, Oncology Institute of Southern Switzerland, Bellinzona, Switzerland. E-mail: giorgiomednuc@libero.it.

Subsequently it is phosphorylated by the enzyme hexokinase to ^{18}F-FDG-6-phosphate, and so it is trapped into brain cells. The rate of anaerobic glycolysis in gliomas increases with the degree of malignancy and tumor grade. However, the main hypothesis is that ^{18}F-FDG uptake is a marker of the density of viable cells, rather than a marker of proliferation [1, 3-6]. The main pitfalls for using ^{18}F-FDG PET are low ^{18}F-FDG uptake in low grade gliomas, false negative results due to physiological uptake of this tracer in the normal brain and false positive results in benign lesions such as inflammatory processes. Tyler et al. [8] evaluated gliomas of different grades by using ^{18}F-FDG-PET and found that ^{18}F-FDG uptake did not correlate with the size and/or the grade of the tumor, showing the greatest variability in high grade gliomas. Broad areas of necrosis are frequent in high grade gliomas and may explain why ^{18}F-FDG uptake may be poor, in spite of the marked proliferative activity of the neoplasm. However, Di Chiro and Brooks [9] observed high ^{18}F-FDG uptake both in treated and untreated high grade gliomas, and explained the low metabolic rates seen by Tyler et al. in untreated high-grade lesions as technical differences (tissue of comparison, scanning technique, and so on). ^{18}F-FDG PET may have a prognostic value in gliomas as for other brain tumors. In a study by Tralins et al. the volume of glioma lesions defined by ^{18}F-FDG PET were predictive of survival and time of tumor progression [10]. ^{18}F-FDG PET is not sensitive in suspected low-grade gliomas, but may be a valuable tool in the prognostic assessment and helpful for therapeutic decisions. The main role of ^{18}F-FDG PET in high-grade lesions, such as glioblastoma, is not in the initial diagnosis, but in evaluating after treatment and in predicting the effectiveness of therapy [3]. In a recent meta-analysis by Nihashi et al. the authors reported a sensitivity and specificity of 77% and 78%, respectively, regarding ^{18}F-FDG PET for recurrent glioma diagnosis [11].

The search for novel PET tracers to image brain tumors has been intensive in the past few decades due to the sub-optimal sensitivity and specificity of ^{18}F-FDG PET in this setting (Table 1). Amino acid transportation and protein synthesis are enhanced in gliomas, allowing the use of radiolabeled amino acids in PET imaging, like ^{11}C-methionine (^{11}C-MET), and aromatic amino acid analogues, like ^{18}F-fluorotyrosine (^{18}F-TYR), ^{18}F-fluoroethyltyrosine (^{18}F-FET), ^{18}F-fluoromethyltyrosine (^{18}F-FMT), and ^{18}F-fluorodopa (^{18}F-DOPA) [4, 5, 7]. Limits of these amino acid PET tracers are: unspecific amino acid uptake due to damage of the blood-brain barrier and inter-individual variability in amino acid uptake. Advantages consist in high-contrast images (due to low uptake in normal brain tissue) and differentiation between low- and high-grade gliomas with dynamic analysis.

The elevation of methionine metabolism in proliferative cells versus normal tissue is, in most cases, markedly higher than the elevation of glucose uptake and metabolism in patients with glioma. Consequently, ^{11}C-MET PET has higher sensitivity and localization precision than ^{18}F-FDG PET [12].

^{18}F-FET is advantageous over ^{18}F-FDG in showing markedly higher uptake in low- and high-grade gliomas and it is more accurate in delineating the outlines of the tumor. Nevertheless ^{18}F-FET has a rather limited specificity in differentiating tumors from other non-neoplastic lesions. Recent comparisons indicate that ^{11}C-MET and ^{18}F-FET appear to be equally useful PET tracers in gliomas with a sensitivity of 91% and a specificity of 100% [13].

^{18}F-DOPA has been tested in brain tumor patients, in particularly in newly diagnosed and recurrent gliomas. This PET tracer displays positive features regarding the delineation of the tumor volume, determination of proliferative activities and tumor grading [12].

Table 1. Sensitivity, specificity, advantages and limitations of the most used PET tracers in glioma imaging

PET tracer	Metabolic function assessed	Sensitivity	Specificity	Main advantages	Main limitations
FDG	glucose metabolism	70-86%	74-97%	prognostic information	physiological uptake in the normal brain and uptake in benign lesions such as inflammatory processes
MET	amino acid transportation and protein synthesis	79-91%	75-100%	low uptake in normal brain and differentiation between low- and high-grade gliomas	unspecific uptake due to damage of the blood-brain barrier
FET		71-93%	88-100%		
DOPA		77-98%	62-89%		
FLT	nucleotide metabolism (proliferation)	79-84%	63-88%	low uptake in normal brain and differentiation between low- and high-grade gliomas	unspecific uptake due to damage of the blood-brain barrier
Choline	membrane protein metabolism	92%	88%	low uptake in normal brain	physiological uptake in choroid plexus, venous sinuses, and pituitary gland

Source: FDG = fluorodeoxyglucose; MET = carbon-methionine; FET = fluoroethyltyrosine; DOPA = fluorodihydroxyphenylalanine; FLT = fluorothymidine.
Table adapted by the paper of Gulyas and Halldin [12].

Recently, a tracer to investigate the proliferation rate of tumor cells has been validated: ^{18}F-fluorothymidine (^{18}F-FLT) [1, 7]. Thymidine is transported into the cells and phosphorylated by thymidine kinase (TK)-1 to thymidine nucleotides, which are taken up during DNA synthesis. Uptake of ^{18}F-FLT correlate with TK-1 activity. ^{18}F-FLT uptake in normal brain is low, due to the low proliferation rate of normal neurons, astrocytes (cell of origin of astrocytomas), and oligodendroglia (cells of origin of oligodendrogliomas). Clinical studies demonstrated that ^{18}F-FLT is an attractive imaging biomarker in brain tumors, especially in high-grade gliomas, for its superiority compared to ^{11}C-MET [14]. Limitations of this tracer are its blood-brain barrier penetration characteristics, and its limited tumor contour delineation ability.

In tumors as gliomas, cell membrane proliferation is increased. Choline is a component of the cell membrane, so radiolabelled choline may be useful for imaging in glioma allowing to distinguish high-grade gliomas, metastases, and benign lesions. ^{11}C-choline uptake is high in some brain structures (such as choroid plexus, venous sinuses, and pituitary gland), reducing the contrast of lesions in these sites [2, 3].

More recently, oxygen metabolism and perfusion have been proposed as pathways to study brain tumors [2, 3].

Tumor hypoxia is caused by tumor growth and insufficient perfusion. Nitroimidazole derivatives such as ^{18}F-fluoromisonidazole (^{18}F-FMISO) and ^{18}F-fluoroazomycinarabinoside (^{18}F-FAZA) are trapped in hypoxic cells. These tracers are reduced, reoxidized, and cleared from tissue in normal cells but not in hypoxic cells. ^{18}F-FMISO uptake was observed in high-grade gliomas. Limits of these tracers are the low contrast and slow uptake in malignant tissue. ^{15}O-labeled H2O is another promising tracer to investigate brain perfusion and lesions with neoangiogenesis such as gliomas, but to date this PET tracer has not been used routinely.

In a recent study, Shi et al. assessed the utility of a perfusion tracer ^{13}N-ammonia in the evaluation of untreated gliomas, comparing the results with that of ^{18}F-FDG PET. The sensitivity and specificity of predicting high-grade gliomas were respectively 83% and 93% for ^{18}F-FDG and 94% and 94% for ^{13}N-ammonia. ^{13}N-Ammonia was superior to ^{18}F-FDG not only in separating low-grade gliomas from high-grade ones but also in the detection of high-grade gliomas for better tumor to normal gray matter contrast [15].

Conclusion

^{18}F-FDG is the most used PET tracer in oncology, nevertheless this radiopharmaceutical has several limitations in evaluating gliomas. Other PET tracers assessing different metabolic pathways could be useful in this setting. In the current era of a growing number of available PET tracers, glioma imaging has moved beyond diagnosis towards functional characterization of tumors.

Therefore, it could be relevant to compare PET tracers with different uptake mechanisms not only to establish a superior diagnostic performance of a specific radiopharmaceutical but also to evaluate matched or mismatched findings, to identify possible advantages of a multi-disciplinary approach or to obtain prognostic information.

Conflict of interest: The authors declare that they have no conflicts of interest.

References

[1] Enslow, M. S., Zollinger, L. V., Morton, K. A., et al. Comparison of 18F-fluorodeoxyglucose and 18F-fluorothymidine PET in differentiating radiation necrosis from recurrent glioma. *Clin. Nucl. Med.* 2012;37:854-61.

[2] Jacobs, A. H., Kracht, L. W., Gossmann, A., et al. Imaging in neurooncology. *NeuroRx.* 2005;2:333-47.

[3] La Fougère, C., Suchorska, B., Bartenstein, P., et al. Molecular imaging of gliomas with PET: opportunities and limitations. *Neuro Oncol*. 2011;13:806-19.

[4] Becherer, A., Karanikas, G., Szabó, M., et al. Brain tumour imaging with PET: a comparison between [18F]fluorodopa and [11C]methionine. *Eur. J. Nucl. Med. Mol. Imaging*. 2003;30:1561-7.

[5] Götz, I., Grosu, A. L. [(18)F]FET-PET Imaging for Treatment and Response Monitoring of Radiation Therapy in Malignant Glioma Patients - A Review. *Front Oncol.* 2013;3:104.

[6] Chen, W., Cloughesy, T., Kamdar, N., et al. Imaging proliferation in brain tumors with 18F-FLT PET: comparison with 18F-FDG. *J. Nucl. Med.* 2005;46:945-52.

[7] Ullrich, R., Backes, H., Li, H., et al. Glioma proliferation as assessed by 3'-fluoro-3'-deoxy-L-thymidine positron emission tomography in patients with newly diagnosed high-grade glioma. *Clin. Cancer Res.* 2008;14:2049-55.

[8] Tyler, J. L., Diksic, M., Villemure, J. G., et al. Metabolic and hemodynamic evaluation of gliomas using positron emission tomography. *J. Nucl. Med.* 1987;28:1123-33.

[9] Di Chiro, G., Brooks, R. A. PET-FDG of untreated and treated gliomas. *J. Nucl. Med.* 1988;29:421-3.

[10] Tralins, K. S., Douglas, J. G., Stelzer, K. J., et al. Volumetric analysis of 18F-FDG PET in gliobalstoma multiforme: prognostic information and possible role in definition of target volumes in radiation dose escalation. *J. Nucl. Med.* 2002;43:1667-73.

[11] Nihashi, T., Dahabreh, I. J., Terasawa, T. Diagnostic accuracy of PET for recurrent glioma diagnosis: a meta-analysis. *AJNR Am. J. Neuroradiol.* 2013;34:944-5.

[12] Gulyás, B., Halldin, C. New PET radiopharmaceuticals beyond FDG for brain tumor imaging. *Q. J. Nucl. Med. Mol. Imaging.* 2012;56:173-90.

[13] Grosu, A. L., Astner, S. T., Riedel, E., et al. An Interindividual Comparison of O-(2-[(18)F] Fluoroethyl)-L-Tyrosine (FET)- and L-[Methyl-(11)C]Methionine (MET)-PET in Patients With Brain Gliomas and Metastases. *Int. J. Radiat. Oncol. Biol. Phys.* 2011; 81:1049-58.

[14] Hatakeyama, T., Kawai, N., Nishiyama, Y., et al. 11C-methionine (MET) and 18F-fluorothymidine (FLT) PET in patients with newly diagnosed glioma. *Eur. J. Nucl. Med. Mol. Imaging.* 2008;35:2009-17.

[15] Shi, X., Liu, Y., Zhang, X., et al. The comparison of 13N-ammonia and 18F-FDG in the evaluation of untreated gliomas. *Clin. Nucl. Med.* 2013;38:522-6.

In: Gliomas: Classification, Symptoms, Treatment and Prognosis ISBN: 978-1-63117-868-9
Editor: David Cory Adamson

Chapter 7

The Role of Genomic Instability and Tumor Suppressors' Alterations in Glioma Pathogenesis

Vedrana Milinkovic and Nikola Tanic*
University of Belgrade, Institute for Biological Research "Sinisa Stankovic",
Department of Neurobiology, Belgrade, Republic of Serbia

Abstract

Glioblastoma multiforme (GBM) is the most common and malignant type of brain tumor in adults and is characterized by diffuse infiltration throughout the brain parenchyma, robust angiogenesis, intense resistance to apoptosis, propensity for necrosis, and genomic instability. Tumor heterogeneity, present in GBM samples, is thought to arise from clonal evolution, in which the expansion and acquisition of mutations during tumor progression promote genetic variability. The majority of GBM (WHO grade IV) develop *de novo* (primary GBM) without clinical or histological evidence of a less malignant precursor lesion, while others, progressing from low-grade diffuse astrocytoma or anaplastic astrocytoma (AA), represent rare secondary GBM. Despite a similar histological appearance, primary and secondary GBM are distinct tumor entities that originate from different precursor cells containing different genetic alterations. Epidermal growth factor receptor (*EGFR*) amplification and *PTEN* mutations are genetic alterations typical of primary GBM, whereas *p53* mutations are early and frequent genetic alterations in the pathway leading to secondary GBM. On the other hand, LOH 10q and alterations of $p16^{INK4a}$/RB1 pathway seem to be important in the development of both primary and secondary GBM. The unique decisive genetic signpost of secondary GBM is *IDH1* mutations, that are absent in primary GBM, and represent earliest detectable genetic alteration in precursor low-grade diffuse astrocytomas and in oligodendrogliomas.

* Corresponding author: Dr Nikola Tanic. Institute for Biological Research "Sinisa Stankovic", Department of Neurobiology, Laboratory for Molecular Neurobiology, Bulevar Despota Stefana 142,11060 Belgrade, Serbia. E-mail: nikolata@ibiss.bg.ac.rs, nikolata@sbb.rs; tel.: +381 11 2078 410; Fax: +381 11 2761 433.

Furthermore, a significant level of genomic instability and heterogeneity detected in glial tumors suggest that they evolve along a multitude of pathways rather than a single defined pathway. An extensive level of genomic instability accompanied with genetic and epigenetic alterations in tumor suppressors and oncogenes involved in major signaling pathways lead to development and progression of both GBM subtypes. Two distinct forms of genomic instability that probably encompass most characterized malignances, including gliomas, have been identified: chromosomal instability (CIN) and micro-satellite instability (MIN). Although, CIN and MIN are thought to be mutually exclusive in cancer, in this chapter we will introduce an intriguing concept that both types of genomic instability play an important role in glioma pathogenesis. Besides impact of genomic instability on patients' outcome, we also focus on alteration of *p53*, *PTEN*, *p16* and *EGFR* and summarize recent studies that correlate these findings with disease outcome. We also present our findings on the most frequent genetic alterations in malignant gliomas with a current literature overview. Specifically, our results showed that *p53* alterations were more frequently present in patients with lower grade tumors and younger age. On the other hand, aberrant *PTEN* and *EGFR* were significantly associated with high grade tumors, and were often present in the group of elderly patients. *p53* mutations, *EGFR* amplification and *PTEN* mutations show inverse association with each other, and were not associated with prognosis of GBM patients.

Moreover, histopathological subtype (lower grade) represents a certain positive predictor in glioma.

Introduction

Gliomas are the most common type of primary brain tumor, accounting for 32% of all CNS tumors and 80% of malignant CNS tumors (Kleihues and Sobin 2000). Gliomas are classified according to their presumed cell of origin and extent of brain infiltration (circumscribed or diffusely infiltrating) and include astrocytomas, oligodendrogliomas, and ependymomas. The most common type of glioma is astrocytoma, which account for about 76 % of gliomas. Glioblastoma multiforme (GBM) is a highly malignant, rapidly progressive astrocytoma, characterized by extensive intra- and inter-tumor heterogeneity, diffuse infiltration throughout the brain parenchyma, robust angiogenesis, intense resistance to apoptosis and propensity for necrosis. GBMs account for 17.1% of brain and other central nervous (CNS) system tumors and constitute 60-70% of all gliomas (CBTRUS 2010). They are more common among men than woman (male:female ratio: 1.58:1) and twice as common in Caucasians versus African-Americans (CBTRUS 2010). Due to its complexity GBM is one of the most difficult malignant tumors to treat. Despite progress in diagnosis, surgery and chemotherapy, the median survival time of patients suffering from GBM is approximately 15 months (Stupp, Mason et al. 2005) and the five year survival rate is less than 5% (CBTRUS, 2010). Although GBM represent a rare tumor type, the number of deaths is comparable to more prevalent tumors, due to its high mortality rates (Wen and Kesari 2008).

Glioblastoma multiforme tumors can be classified according to several criteria:

a) Histopathology (according to World Health Organization, WHO) - conventional GBM (93%), giant cell GBM (5%) and gliosarcoma (2%);
b) Pathogenesis - primary GBM (90%) and secondary GBM (10%);

c) Gene expression - (I) classical, (II) mesenchymal, (III) proneural or (IV) neural type of GBM;
d) Genomic analysis - subgroups harboring specific mutations and/or altered gene dosage/chromosome number.

Different criteria are often overlapped with the aim to identify specific molecular subtypes of GBM that would enable us to predict response to treatment and patient outcome. Histological characterization of glial tumors is widely used in diagnosis and therapy, although this subjective method cannot accurately predict behavior of tumor cells in response to therapy. However, molecular biological studies of gliomas are paving the way for an improved classification system, one in which response to a specific therapy can be predicted for each individual patient. Molecular approaches lead to detection of gene and chromosome copy number alterations and identification of specific point mutations in oncogenes and tumor suppressor genes, important for initiation and progression of different glioma subtypes (Dahlback, Brandal et al. 2009). Development of whole genome sequencing methods and microarrays enabled numerous gene expression studies, leading to integrated molecular classification of glial tumors. Large-scale gene expression profile studies in GBM have demonstrated that transcriptional profiles reflect the underlying tumor biology and can be used to predict tumor classification (eg, being a surrogate for pathological grading), response to treatment and patient outcome (Sulman et al. 2009).

Histopathological Characterization of Gliomas

Histological classification and grading criteria for glial neoplasms are well established. They are based on morphologic evidences of cellular differentiation and on the presence or absence of histopathological features, such as cellularity, nuclear pleomorphism, mitotic activity, endothelial cell proliferation and necrosis (Furnari, Fenton et al. 2007). Malignant gliomas arise from glial cells that support nerve cells of the brain, or their precursors, and diffusely invade surrounding brain, making curative surgical resection almost impossible. Diffuse gliomas are classified on their morphological appearance and similarity to astrocytes (astrocytomas), oligodendrocytes (oligodendrogliomas) or ependymal cells (ependymomas) and graded on a scale of I–IV with increasing malignancy, according to the World Health Organization (WHO) classification (Louis, Ohgaki et al. 2007). Grade I tumors are biologically benign, displaying low proliferative potential and the possibility of cure following surgical resection alone. Grade II (diffuse) tumors are low-grade malignancies that may follow long clinical courses, with 5 to 8 year median survival, and some of these neoplasms may progress to higher grades of malignancy. Grade III (anaplastic) tumors exhibit histological evidence of malignancy, including increased focal or dispersed anaplasia, cell proliferation, nuclear atypia and mitotic activity. The more aggressive nature of grade III tumors results in shorter survival times, often less than 3 years. Grade IV tumors are characterized by advanced cytologically malignant features, such as microvascular proliferation and necrosis, and as they are resistant to radio/chemotherapy, they are generally lethal. Therefore, the type and grade of the tumor, as well as its localization, are currently recognized as the major factors determining patient prognosis. GBMs, classified as grade IV gliomas, are significantly more proliferative, invasive, and angiogenic compared to grade II and grade III astrocytomas (Brat and Van Meir 2004).

The majority of GBM cases (>90%) are primary GBM that develop rapidly *de novo*, without clinical or histological evidence of a less malignant precursor lesion. They affect mainly the elderly population and have a characteristic genetic signature (Ohgaki and Kleihues 2007). The majority of patients with primary GBM (68%) have a clinical history of less than three months, presenting with a very rapid development of clinical symptoms. On the other hand, secondary GBM develop slowly through progression from low-grade diffuse astrocytoma (WHO grade II) or anaplastic astrocytoma (WHO grade III). The diagnosis of secondary GBM requires clinical (neuroimaging) or histological (biopsy) evidence of an evolution from a less malignant astrocytoma. Secondary GBM represent a rare disease (5-10% of all GBM) at a population level. The incidence rate of low-grade and anaplastic astrocytomas is approximately two to three times higher than that of secondary GBM (CBTRUS; *http://www.cbtrus.org*). This may be explained at least in part by the fact that a significant fraction of patients with low-grade or anaplastic astrocytoma succumb to the disease before progression to GBM occurs. Although histologically similar, primary and secondary GBM represent distinct tumor entities in terms of genetic alterations and affected signaling pathways.

The WHO classification has shown considerable utility to date in the clinical arena. For instance, tumors with higher WHO grades tend to follow a more aggressive clinical course, and astrocytomas behave more poorly than grade-matched oligodendrogliomas (Ohgaki, Dessen et al. 2004; Ohgaki and Kleihues 2005). Nevertheless, considerable variability in biological behaviour still exists within individual diagnostic categories, speaking to a greater degree of complexity on the molecular level than can be appreciated by conventional histopathology (Huse, Phillips et al. 2011). Furthermore, malignant gliomas typically contain both neoplastic and stromal tissues, which contribute to their histological heterogeneity.

Molecular Genetics of Malignant Gliomas

The classification of malignant gliomas is moving from a morphology-based guide to a system built on molecular criteria. A limited set of molecular abnormalities have been repeatedly linked to the pathogenesis of the different glioma variants over time, and recent large-scale investigations (Parsons, Jones et al. 2008) including that of The Cancer Genome Atlas (TCGA), have comprehensively catalogued those genomic alterations associated with GBM (Huse and Holland 2010).

Some of these events characterize specific glioma subclasses, while others appear to operate more broadly across the spectrum of diffuse gliomas. The ongoing characterization of the genetic alterations in glioma tumor cells is revealing considerable variability among tumors of the same type and grade. Heterogeneity in glioma tumors is also found within individual tumors, perhaps as a reflection of certain hypoxic conditions or breakdown of the blood-brain barrier (Gladson, Prayson et al. 2010).

Gliomas, like all other tumors, subsequently acquire genetic alterations during the process of malignant transformation. DNA copy number alterations, such as chromosomal and gene deletions, amplifications and gains, LOH and point mutations occur during tumor initiation and progression leading to morphologic changes and alterations in regulation of major signaling pathways (Parsons, Jones et al. 2008).

These molecular alterations are thought to affect gene expression either through overexpression of large amplified regions, or inactivation of genes in deleted regions (Bralten, Kloosterhof et al. 2010). Finally, these genetic alterations seem to modify crucial cellular processes and often result in deregulation of metabolic key pathways affecting growth signaling and cell cycle control (Kanu, Hughes et al. 2009). Genome-scale gene expression profiling using microarray technology has revealed distinct molecular subtypes within GBM. Comprehensive genetic screens have shown that genetic loss is scattered across the entire genome, affecting nearly all chromosomes at frequencies ranging from 2% to 80% (Kanu, Hughes et al. 2009). Particularly, common regions of loss include areas on 1p, 6q, 9p, 10p, 10q, 13q, 14q, 15q, 17p, 18q, 19q, 22q and Y (Kim, Mohapatra et al. 1995; Mohapatra, Bollen et al. 1998; Nishizaki, Ozaki et al. 1998; Collins 2004; Vranova, Necesalova et al. 2007). Loss of heterozygosity (LOH) on chromosome 10 is the most frequent genetic alteration in GBM, occurring in 60% to 80% of cases (Ohgaki and Kleihues 2007). Many GBMs appear to have lost an entire copy of chromosome 10, but several LOH studies have suggested at least three distinct loci to be deleted (e.g., 10p14-p15, 10q23-24, distal to 10q25), supporting the finding of multiple tumor suppressor genes, including *PTEN*, mapped at these loci. Furthermore, DNA profiling identified differences in molecular abnormalities observed between primary and secondary GBM (Figure 1). Most primary GBMs show loss of the entire chromosome 10, whereas partial loss of 10q is observed in secondary GBMs. Besides, epidermal growth factor receptor (*EGFR*) amplification and *PTEN* mutations are genetic alterations typical of primary GBM, whereas *p53* mutations are early and frequent genetic alterations in the pathway leading to secondary GBM (Ohgaki and Kleihues 2007). The most common EGFR mutant type–variant 3 (EGFRvIII) is due to an in-frame deletion of exons 2–7, and it is constitutively active in EGFR-mediated signal-transduction pathways, leading to cell proliferation and survival advantages (Ohgaki and Kleihues 2007) (Van Meir, Hadjipanayis et al. 2010).

The deletion in *PTEN* results in increased protein kinase B/mammalian target of rapamycin (AKT/mTOR) activity, which promotes cell survival, proliferation, and invasion (Louis 2006). Recently, *ERBB2* mutations have also been identified as a recurrent event in primary GBMs. In contrast, secondary GBM are characterized by the occurrence of early detected mutations in the *p53* tumor suppressor gene on chromosome 17p, especially those involving codons 248 and 273 or G:C→A:T mutations at CpG sites (Ohgaki, et al., 2004), abnormalities in the p16 and retinoblastoma (RB) pathways, and loss of heterozygosity of chromosome 10q. Furthermore, Parsons et al. (2008) identified specific recurrent mutations in the active site of isocitrate dehydrogenase 1 (*IDH1*).

Mutations in this gene occurred in a large fraction of young patients and in most patients with secondary GBMs and were associated with an increase in overall survival, and could be used as a reliable marker of secondary GBM. LOH of 10q typically co-presents with any of the other genetic alterations in GBM. In contrast, *TP53* mutations, *EGFR* amplification, and *PTEN* mutations show inverse associations with each other, whereas there is a positive correlation between *p16/INK4a* deletion and *EGFR* amplification (Okamoto, Di Patre et al. 2004).

It has become clear from different genetic profiles recognized within GBM that the underlying molecular characteristics of the tumor are essential to understand its variability and to identify potential therapeutic targets. However, they do not by themselves predict patient outcome or response to treatment.

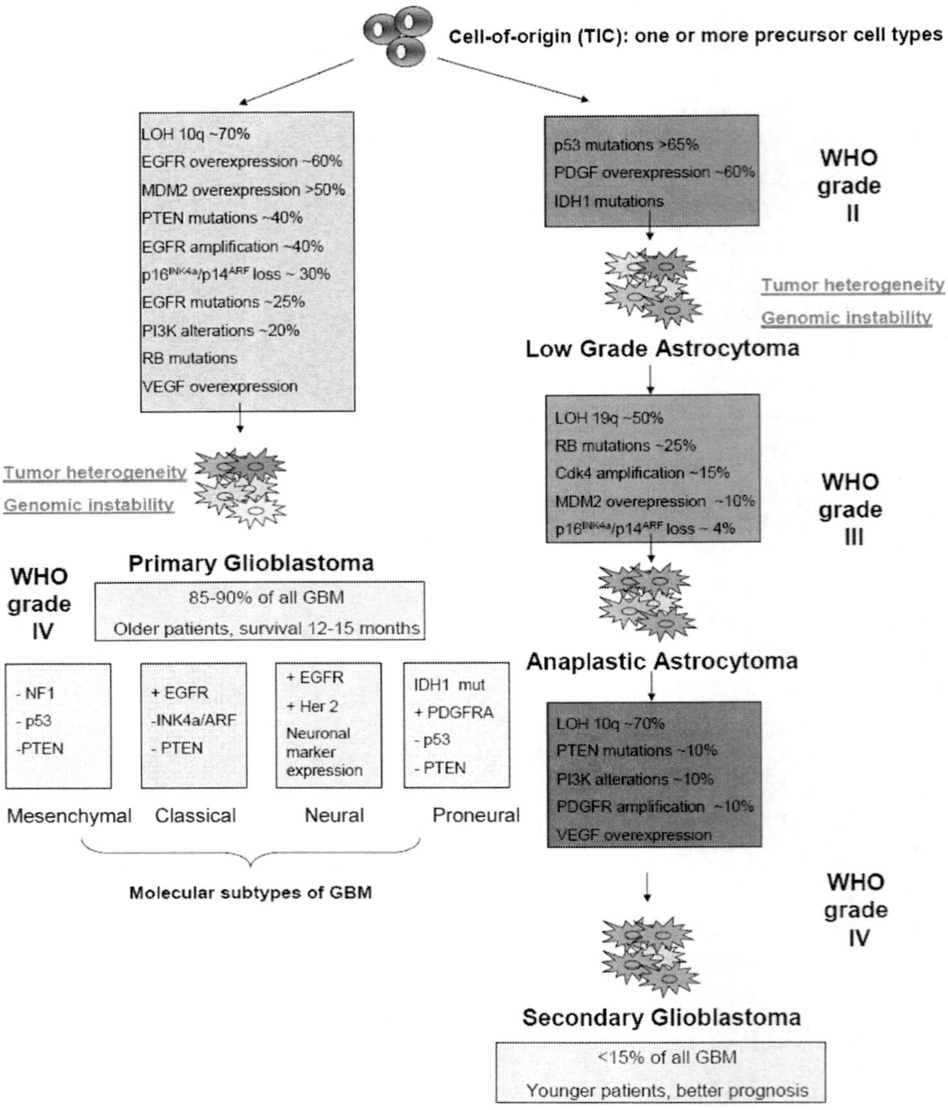

Figure 1. Genetic alterations during the pathogenesis of primary and secondary glioblastomas (GBM). Left - the most frequent molecular alterations in the pathway leading to primary GBM. Primary GBMs develop *de novo*, from tumor initiating cells (TIC) of different origin. LOH 10q is present in approximately 70% of this GBM subtype, followed by EGFR and MDM2 overexpression, PTEN mutations and EGFR amplification. p53 mutations are infrequent in primary GBM. Recent integrated genomic analysis has defined four subtypes of primary GBMs (mesenchymal, classical, neural, and proneural) with specific molecular alterations and transcriptome signatures. Right - basic steps in progression of secondary GBM. Secondary GBM develop through progression from lower-grade astrocytomas, with IDH1 and p53 mutations that appear to be common early events in this pathway. In addition to these alterations, RB mutations, LOH 19q, Cdk4 and PDGFR amplifications, as well as alterations in PI3K signaling are frequently detected in secondary GBMs.

Thus, in the past few years, efforts have been made to further characterize GBM into specific molecular subclasses, defined by combinations of over- or under-expressed genes with a potential impact on survival. Consequently, four GBM subtypes (Classical, Messenchymal, Proneural, and Neural) were identified and characterized by aberrations in gene expression of *EGFR, NF1*, *PDGFRα*, and *ERBB2* genes (Verhaak, Hoadley et al. 2010). Each subtype harbors different mutations, genomic and transcript alterations.

The first subtype has a profile characteristic of highly proliferative cells and is labeled classical. The tumors in this group demonstrate uniform gains on chromosome 7, accompanied by losses on chromosome 10 (93%) and frequent focal losses on chromosome 9p21.3 (95%) (Van Meir, Hadjipanayis et al. 2010).

The classical subtype is also characterized by amplification of (or activating mutations in) *EGFR* and *CDKN2A* (*p16*), and loss of PTEN. Genes involved in pathways highly active in neural stem and progenitor cells (including the Notch and Sonic hedgehog pathway) are highly expressed in the classical subtype (Bar, Chaudry, hedgehog pathway inhibition, 2004). The patients afflicted are typically older, but have best therapeutic response to concurrent radiation/temozolomide treatment compared to other subtypes.

The messenchymal subclass is associated with poor overall survival, and has frequent inactivation of the *NF1* (37%), *p53* (32%), and *PTEN* (32%) genes. These tumors respond to aggressive chemoradiation therapies including Ras, PI3K, and angiogenesis inhibitors. This group is defined by an expression profile associated with mesenchyme and angiogenesis (Van Meir, Hadjipanayis et al. 2010).

The third subtype, termed proneural, has an expression profile reminiscent of gene activation in neuronal development. This includes a high level of expression of oligodendrocytic and proneural development genes. The proneural subtype harbor mutations in genes classically associated with secondary GBMs, including *p53*, *IDH1/2* and *PDGFR*.

Clinically, this subtype typically affects younger patients and is associated with improved overall survival (Phillips, Kharbanda et al. 2006).

The fourth subtype, called neural, is less well defined and has gene expression signatures that are most similar to those found in normal brain tissue. This subtype has elevated levels of neural markers such as *NEFL*, but has no unique alterations that could distinguish it from other classes, although elevated rates of *ERBB2* mutations are observed (Agnihotri, Burrell et al. 2013).

Tumor Heterogeneity and Genomic Instability in GBM

With advances in genomic profiling and sequencing technology, we are beginning to understand the landscape of the genetic events that accumulate during the neoplastic process. GBM are highly cellular and vascularized tumors, very resistant to radio- and chemotherapy, and can diffusely and deeply infiltrate the normal brain parenchyma precluding total surgical resection. The pathology of GBM is that of a highly heterogeneous tumor (as indicated by the old descriptor *multiforme*), which includes a variety of cancer cell types. Some of these cell types have differentiated stellar morphology and expression of markers such as GFAP and S100, whereas others have small and rounded undifferentiated cells mixed with stromal elements such as microvascular cell proliferation, reactive astrocytes, microglia and other immune infiltrates. The heterogeneity of GBM was previously understood as a heterogeneous mix of highly motile tumor cells at different stages in their genetic progression towards malignancy, admixed with stromal elements. Genetic analyses have confirmed that a single astrocytoma could contain different cell populations that are hierarchically organized in the number of genetic alterations they contain, the earliest being remnants of a precursor cell population from which the rest of the tumor is derived (Hadjipanayis and Van Meir 2009). Tumor heterogeneity, present in GBM samples, is thought to arise from clonal evolution, in which the expansion and acquisition of mutations during tumor progression promote genetic variability. The picture emerging suggests that most GBMs evolve along a multitude of pathways rather than a single defined pathway.

Furthermore, this could be one of the main reasons for resistance to therapy and, for short survival of the patients. Although it is widely accepted that gliomas, like other cancers, develop as a consequence of the accumulation of genetic alterations, their exact number and nature remains an issue of debate (Stratton, Campbell et al. 2009). Nevertheless, it is clear that CNS carcinogenesis requires multiple disruptions to the normal cellular circuitry (TCGA 2008). Extensive intra-tumor genetic heterogeneity detected in primary human glial tumors is suggestive of the overall high rate of change in the genomes of these tumors (Misra, Chattopadhyay et al. 2000). Misra et al. (2000) hypothesize that some altered clones, which manifest as zones of heterogeneity in a solid tumor, may accumulate changes at loci known to influence tumor behavior, and thus clinical outcome.

The mutator phenotype, also referred to as genomic instability, refers to the increased mutation rate that occurs in neoplastic cells. The induction of the genomic instability phenotype is emerging to be a crucial early event in carcinogenesis that enables an initiated cell to evolve into a cancer cell by achieving a greater proliferative capacity and genetic plasticity, which can overcome resistance in a localized toxic environment and suboptimal supply of micronutrients (Loeb 1991; Loeb 2001; Loeb, Loeb et al. 2003). Genomic instability is present in all stages of cancer, from precancerous lesions to advanced cancers, and plays a fundamental role in the pathogenesis of a wide variety of solid cancers (Gorgoulis, Vassiliou et al. 2005; Negrini, Gorgoulis et al. 2010). Two distinct forms of genomic instability, chromosomal (CIN) and microsatellite (MIN), may be manifestations of a mutator phenotype (Bielas, Loeb et al. 2006; Klein 2006). Some authors also refer to point mutation instability (PIN, SNI), as a third type of genomic instability present in cancer cells (Klein 2006). Chromosomal instability is characterized by multiple gains and losses at specific chromosome regions, and may be measured as an abnormal number of chromosomes or shifts in the total nuclear DNA content. Loss of tumor suppressor genes and amplification of oncogenes appears to be central to the development of tumors with CIN (Breivik and Gaudernack 1999). In GBM, CIN could be observed as amplification of *EGFR* oncogene, frequently present in this tumor type, as well as loss of tumor suppressor genes, like *PTEN* and *p16*.

Microsatellite instability is recognized as genome-wide alterations in repetitive DNA sequences (Lothe 1997). MIN is caused by defects in the nucleotide mismatch repair (MMR) machinery, which in addition to correcting mismatched nucleotides, also repairs insertions/deletions in repeated DNA sequences. Defects in MMR pathways cause a general increase in the mutational rate. MIN is related to frameshift mutations in cancer genes harboring repetitive nucleotide sequences, such as *PTEN*, *TGFβR-II*, *IGFIIR*, and *BAX* (Ionov, Peinado et al. 1993; Thibodeau, Bren et al. 1993; Kong, Suzuki et al. 1997; Rampino, Yamamoto et al.

1997). In hereditary syndromes, such as the hereditary nonpolyposis colorectal cancer (HNPCC), an extensive level of MSI is attributed to germline mutations in MMR genes, mainly MLH1 and MSH2.

However, in sporadic malignancies, MIN without mutations of those genes could be identified in colorectal, nonsmall cell lung (NSCLC), head and neck, gastric, and prostate cancers (Lothe, Peltomaki et al. 1993; Renault, Calistri et al. 1996; Watanabe, Imai et al. 1996; Markovic, Stojsic et al. 2008). In GBM, MIN has been detected as well, with frequencies ranging from 5–50% (Martinez, Schackert et al. 2005; Milinkovic, Bankovic et al. 2012).

According to Martinez et al. (2005), in these sporadic tumors, MIN is not associated with mutations of the MMR system but to MLH1 promoter hypermethylation-mediated silencing.

Unusually, MIN and CIN both contribute to the total level of genomic instability in gliomas (Milinkovic, Bankovic et al. 2012). Contrary to these findings, many authors propose that MIN and CIN phenotypes are mutually exclusive and that most cancers can be classified in one of these categories (Lengauer, Kinzler et al. 1998; Breivik 2001)). This discrepancy might be the result of different methods used to screen genomes.

DNA fingerprinting methods, such as RAPD (Random Amplified Polymorphic DNA) and AP-PCR (Arbitrarily Primed Polymerase Chain Reaction), could be good methods of choice for detection and quantification of genomic instability. They are rapid and simple procedures that examine the whole genome and detect the propensity of a tumor to undergo genomic rearrangements (Peinado, Malkhosyan et al. 1992; Perucho 1996). AP-PCR DNA fingerprinting is an efficient tool to quickly and easily screen a very large number of loci for possible DNA alterations in cancer cells. It has several advantages. Firstly, minor amounts of template DNA are sufficient for analysis. Secondly, it allows for the screening of anonymous regions of a genome without any prior knowledge of its structure. Thirdly, two types of DNA alterations could be detected in single reactions, i.e., chromosomal rearrangements (manifesta-tions of CIN) and random mutations dispersed over the genome (manifestations of MIN). And fourthly, the possibility of reamplification, cloning and sequencing of variant bands enables the rapid identification of the sequences probably linked to tumor progression (Tanic, Milasin et al. 2009; Bankovic, Stojsic et al. 2010; Milinkovic, Bankovic et al. 2013).

The mutator phenotype hypothesis proposes that genomic instability occurs early during tumor formation, as a result of mutations in genes that maintain genomic stability in normal cells. Instability promotes mutations in other genes, oncogenes and tumor suppressor genes, providing the tumor cell with a selective growth advantage (Vogelstein, Kinzler, 2002). Having in mind that tumor evolution through natural selection depends on two essential elements, the availability of genetic variation and selection pressure, it could be said that genomic instability accelerates the somatic evolutionary process by promoting genetic variations in the organism. Extensive genomic instability is thus expected in early phases of cancer progression. Accordingly, it is expected that the level of genomic instability decreases with the increasing histological grade of tumor (during tumor progression) as shown in NSCLC samples (Markovic, Stojsic et al. 2008). The presence of a significant level of genomic instability in high grade gliomas, with similar values in all histological subtypes, looks contradictory to the expectation. However, primary GBM are not progressive forms of grade III astrocytoma, they develop *de novo*, and therefore, they comprise higher levels of genomic instability than expected (Milinkovic, Bankovic et al. 2012). Thus, a decrease in the level of genomic instability should be expected in secondary GBM samples. Taking this into consideration, inactivation of tumor suppressor genes may represent one of the important steps in the malignant transformation of cells which are driven by an increasing genomic instability through the early inactivation of the DNA MMR genes.

The Role of Tumor Suppressor Gene Alterations in GBM

The typical genetic alterations in glioma target pathways governing cellular proliferation, cell survival (apoptosis and necrosis), invasion and angiogenesis. Molecular progression of gliomas, like many tumors, involves the accumulation of genetic and epigenetic alterations that result in the loss of tumor suppressor gene function (PTEN, p53, INK4a/p16, Rb), or activation of oncogenic pathways (Ras, PI3-kinase, EGFR, CDK4, MDM2) (Furnari, Fenton et al. 2007). Identified genetic alterations are frequently and specifically present in different GBM subtypes. Integrative analyses of common genetic alterations in the GBM genome led to identification of a highly interconnected network of aberrations, including three major pathways: RTK (receptor tyrosine kinases) signaling, and the p53 and RB tumor suppressor pathways (TCGA 2008).

Here, we briefly highlight alterations in these pathways, emphasizing presence of genetic alterations characteristic for GBM subtypes.

P53 Pathway in Gliomas

The TP53 pathway is composed of hundreds of genes and their protein products respond to a wide variety of intrinsic and extrinsic stress signals. These stress signals all impact upon the cellular homeostatic mechanisms that monitor and control the fidelity of DNA replication, chromosome segregation and cell division. (Vogelstein, Lane et al. 2000). Responses to stress include apoptosis, cellular senescence or cell cycle arrest. p53 is often referred to as the "guardian of the genome" (Lane 1992), since it functions as a transcriptional regulator of more than 150 genes, regulating crucial cellular processes (Levine, Hu et al. 2006). Following DNA damage, p53 is activated and induces expression of cell cycle checkpoint proteins, leading to prevention of the propagation of cells with unstable genomes, predominantly by halting the cell cycle in the G1 phase, or by initiating a program of apoptosis or proliferative arrest (Gasco, Shami et al. 2002; Rozan and El-Deiry 2007). Once p53 is activated in response to a stress signal it gains the ability (and increased concentration) to bind to p53-responsive DNA sequence elements in the genome. It has become clear that different types of stress signals as inputs result in different genes being transcribed under p53 control (Zhao, Gish et al. 2000). The best characterized downstream effector of TP53 is the *p21* gene, whose protein product inhibits cyclin-dependent kinases (CDKs) that regulate cell cycle entry and progression. The *p53* gene is transcribed constitutively, and the mRNA is translated to TP53 protein.

However, the TP53 protein is notoriously unstable, which is due to changeable degradation processes that occurs in ubiquitin-dependent and ubiquitin-independent systems of proteasomes (Brooks and Gu 2006). Ubiquitin ligase MDM2, protein product of a p53-

activated gene, is the best studied negative regulator of p53. The increase of TP53 activity leads to upregulation of MDM2, and respectively, to accelerated degradation of TP53 in 26S proteasomes. Therefore, the Mdm2 and p53 proteins form an autoregulatory feedback loop, which controls the activities of p53 (Chumakov 2007). The $p14^{ARF}$ binds to MDM2 and inhibits MDM2-mediated p53 degradation and transactivational silencing (Stott, Bates et al. 1998). $p14^{ARF}$ is also negatively regulated by TP53. MDM4 (also called MDMX) also regulates p53 activity, by inhibiting *p53* transcription and enchasing the ubiquitin ligase activity of MDM2.

p53 and/or other genes from its network are mutated in a wide variety of cancers. Thus, most cancers appear to select for a loss of function of the p53 pathway. Similarly, inactivation of the TP53 network is considered to be an early event in pathogenesis of secondary GBM, resulting from alterations in *p53, MDM2, MDM4* or $p14^{ARF}$, predominantly (Louis 1994).

There is an increased incidence of gliomas in patients with Li-Fraumeni syndrome, a familiar cancer-predisposition syndrome associated with germline *p53* mutations (Malkin, Li et al. 1990). This finding confirms the importance of p53 inactivation in pathogenesis of malignant gliomas.

Inactivation of the TP53 pathway plays a crucial role in the development of secondary GBM. *p53* mutations are the first detectable genetic alteration in two-thirds of precursor low-grade diffuse astrocytomas. This incidence is similar to that in anaplastic astrocytomas and derived secondary GBM. *p53* mutations also occur in primary GBM, but at a lower frequency (less than 30% of cases) (Ohgaki, Dessen et al. 2004; Milinkovic, Bankovic et al. 2012). There is a difference in distribution of *p53* mutations in primary and secondary GBM. More than one half (57%) of all detected mutations in secondary GBM are in hot-spot codons 248 and 273. On the other hand, distribution of mutations is less uniform in primary GBM. Furthermore, G:C → A:T mutations at CpG sites are significantly more frequent in secondary than primary GBM. In GBM, *p53* inactivation may also occur through the loss of chromosome 17p, as well as by amplification or overexpression of *p53*'s negative regulators MDM2 and MDM4, which suppress its transcriptional activity (Zheng, Ying et al. 2008). According to TCGA, TP53 signaling is altered in 87% of analyzed GBM samples. Overall inactivation of the p53 pathway occur in the form of $p14^{ARF}$ deletions (55%), amplifications of *MDM2* (11%) and *MDM4* (4%), in addition to mutations of *p53* itself (TCGA 2008). According to the same source, genetic lesions in *p53* are mutually exclusive of those in *MDM2* or *MDM4*, but not of those in $p14^{ARF}$.

However, methylation of $p14^{ARF}$ causing decreased or no expression, is another mechanism that has been shown to be involved in GBM pathogenesis (Collins 2004).

Although p53 is one of the most important regulators of genome integrity (Morris 2002), mutated *p53* is not associated with higher genomic instability, as would have been expected (Milinkovic, Bankovic et al. 2012). In that study, the correlation of *p53* alterations with the level of genomic instability in anaplastic astrocytoma and primary GBM was analyzed.

According to the frequency of *p53* alterations which is significantly higher in AA compared to primary GBM samples, inactivation of this tumor suppressor could be one of the early events, contributing considerably to genomic instability in early phases of multi-step secondary GBM progression. However, according to available data, the impact of *p53* on development of genomic instability in primary GBM is not of that importance. It is likely that inactivation of other regulators of genomic stability, like PTEN, might be responsible for the high level of genomic instability detected in primary GBM.

PTEN Signaling in Gliomas

The *PTEN* gene, also known as *MMAC1* or *TEP1*, is a tumor suppressor gene located on the long arm of chromosome 10 (10q23). It is involved in the regulation of many important cellular functions, including cell-cycle progression, cell migration and spreading, and cell growth and apoptosis (Di Cristofano and Pandolfi 2000). The *PTEN* promoter carries regulatory elements and binding sites for many transcriptional factors, including TP53, TGFβ (tumor growth factor β), and Egr1 (early growth response 1 transcriptional factor). Because TP53 induces *PTEN* transcription and PTEN protects TP53 from degradation, both proteins cooperate in a positive feedback loop to control the cellular response to stress, DNA damage, and cancer (Mayo, Dixon et al. 2002). Furthermore, the *PTEN* promoter is rich in CpG-dinucleotides, supporting a role of DNA methylation in transcriptional regulation of this gene (Stambolic, MacPherson et al. 2001).

Most of the tumor-suppressive properties of PTEN are dependant on its lipid phosphatase activity, which inhibits the phosphatidylinositol-3'-kinase (PI3K)/Akt signaling pathway through dephosphorylation of phosphatidylinositol-(3,4,5)-tri phosphate (PIP_3). PIP_3 functions as a second messenger molecule that is important for the activation of protein kinase B/Akt, leading to translocation of Akt to the plasma membrane (Vanhaesebroeck and Alessi 2000). In addition, PIP_3 activates PDK, which phosphorylates Akt on threonine 308 position. The phosphorylation of Thr308 activates the protein kinase activity of Akt, especially in tumor samples (Vincent, Elder et al. 2011) Akt is one of the most important serine-threonine kinases which phosphorylates a variety of substrates, and thereby regulates important cellular processes, including cell-cycle progression, cell growth, cell survival, cell motility and adhesion, translation of mRNA into protein, glucose metabolism, and angiogenesis (Knobbe, Merlo et al. 2002). PTEN functions as a key negative regulator of the Akt signaling pathway by dephosphorylating PIP3 and lowering its physiological level, and thus inhibits cell proliferation. The additional function of PTEN as a dual-specificity protein phosphatase may also play a role in tumor pathogenesis, especially in regulation of cellular migration and invasion. PTEN may directly dephosphorylate and thereby inactivate FAK (focal adhesion kinase) by means of its protein phosphatase activity (Tamura, Gu et al. 1998). PTEN also may inhibit the integrin-mediated and growth factor-mediated activation of MAPK (mitogen-activated protein kinase) pathway. This also seems to involve the phosphatase activity of PTEN against protein substrates, such as the adaptor protein Shc (Src homology domain-containing transforming protein) (Gu, Tamura et al. 1999).

The PTEN gene is mutated in 15-40% of primary GBM, but rare in secondary GBM (Ohgaki and Kleihues 2009). The mutations detected in gliomas are distributed along the entire gene. More than a half of detected mutations result in the introduction of premature stop codons and the translation of truncated proteins (Knobbe, Merlo et al. 2002). Missense mutations generally affect conserved residues where substitution leads to structurally altered proteins with impaired functions. In addition to nonsense and missense mutations, several mutations resulting in aberrantly spliced transcripts have been detected.

PTEN aberrations are detectable in a low fraction (<10%) of anaplastic astrocytomas and anaplastic oligodendrogliomas (Sasaki, Zlatescu et al. 2001), but either rare or absent in WHO grade I and II gliomas.

On the other hand, LOH 10q is the most frequent genetic alteration in both primary and secondary GBM with similar frequencies (60 to 80%). Several LOH studies identified at least three commonly deleted loci, i.e., 10p14-p15, 10q23-24 (*PTEN*), and 10q25-pter, suggesting the presence of several tumor suppressor genes that may play significant roles in the pathogenesis of GBM (Ichimura, Schmidt et al. 1998). LOH 10q typically co-presents with any of the other genetic alterations in GBM. In contrast to NSCLC (Andjelkovic, Bankovic et al. 2011), *PTEN* gene alterations in GBM do not correlate with *p53* mutations (Duerr, Rollbrocker et al. 1998). These observations suggest that LOH 10q in combination with one or two other genetic alterations may contribute to the development of both primary and secondary GBM. In the evolution of secondary GBM, *p53* mutation seems to be an early event, while LOH 10q seems to be a late event. Conversely, the sequence of genetic alterations during the development of primary GBM is still unknown.

Besides frequent inactivation of the *PTEN* lipid phosphatase tumor suppressor gene, 86% of the GBM samples harbor at least one genetic event in the core RTK/PI3K pathway (TCGA 2008). About two-thirds (63%) of primary GBM and one-third of secondary GBM show alterations in at least one of *EGFR*, *PTEN* or *PIK3CA* genes (Kita, Yonekawa et al. 2007). Constitutive activation of PI3K and MAPK signaling pathways lead to proliferation of the cancer cells independently of growth factor signals, achieving one of the hallmarks of cancer (Hanahan and Weinberg 2011). Furthermore, amplification and overexpression of the *EGFR* and *PDGFRA* (platelet-derived growth factor receptor –A) genes also contribute to aberrant Akt activity in these tumors. With respect to gliomas, inactivation of PTEN signaling, either by mutation, deletion, or loss of expression, or by aberrations of other genes involved in the PTEN/PI3K/Akt signaling pathway, appears to be important for the malignant progression to GBM.

Retinoblastoma Signaling Pathway and P16 Alterations in Gliomas

RB tumor suppressor pathway is the third major pathway involved in the pathogenesis of gliomas. This pathway consists of several proteins: the cyclin-dependent kinase inhibitors (CDKN), the cyclin D-dependent protein kinases (cdk4, cdk6), the E2F-family of transcripttion factors, and the RB-family (RB, p107, p130) (Knudsen and Wang 2010). RB signaling pathway has an important role in the cell cycle control, regulating G1/S transition. One of the negative regulators of RB signaling pathway is the Ink4-family of proteins, $p16^{INK4a/CDKN2A}$, $p15^{INK4b}$, $p18^{INK4c}$, and $p19^{INK4d}$ which are small heat-stable proteins containing the AKN (ankyrin repeat) domain. Each of the Ink4 proteins can bind to and inhibit the activity of Cdk4 and Cdk6. The Ink4 proteins compete with the D-cyclins for Cdk4/6 to prevent the formation of the active kinase complex that phosphorylates pRB (Knudsen and Wang 2010). Namely, the role of $p16^{INK4a}$ is to check the cell cycle in early G1 phase and inhibit further transition to the cell cycle from G1 to S phase as a component of a multiprotein regulatory complex. During G1 phase, Cdk4 and Cdk6 form complexes with cyclin D1 which in turn phosphorylate the RB protein family resulting in additional phosphorylation by cyclin E/Cdk complexes. These inhibitory phosphorylations of RB cause release of the E2F transcription factor from RB/E2F complexes. Otherwise, RB inhibits this transcriptional factor (Weinberg 1995). E2F is a transcription factor that initiates transcription of genes required for S phase such as DNA polymerase, thymidine kinase, and dihydrofolate reductase (Lukas, Petersen et al. 1996). Action of $p16^{INK4a}$ inhibits binding of Cdk4/6 with cyclin D1 which leaves RB, and RB-related proteins like p107 and p103, un-phosphorylated and E2F bound to RB and therefore inactive (Serrano, Hannon et al. 1993). Thus p16^{INK4a} is an important tumor suppressor gene which regulates gene expression at different levels by modifying functional equilibrium of transcription factors, and consequently of miRNAs, and also by binding to post-transcriptional regulators (hnRNP C1/C2 and hnRNP A2/B1) (Souza-Rodrigues, Estanyol et al. 2007). The role of p16^{Ink4a} in cell growth can also be attributed by irreversible repression of the *hTERT* (human telomerase) gene by increasing the amount of histone H3 bound to the hTERT promoter (Bazarov, Van Sluis et al. 2010). Therefore, p16^{INK4a} induction results in repression of telomerase and, thus, telomere shortening.

p16^{Ink4a} is a potent tumor suppressor, whose loss of function was detected in many malignancies.

Structural and functional alterations of this gene are the second most common genetic alterations in cancer cells, following the *p53* tumor suppressor inactivation (Baylin, Herman et al. 1998). Loss of heterozygosity (LOH) and homozygous deletions of *p16^{INK4a}* gene, as well as hypermethylation of its promoter are important mechanisms which have been shown to result in loss of *p16^{Ink4a}* expression and promote p16-related neoplasms (Agarwal 2012). Mutations in *p16* encoding gene have also been reported in many cancer types including GBM (Agarwal 2012).

The recent report from The Cancer Genome Atlas Research Network (TCGA) showed that RB signaling pathway was altered in 77% of analyzed GBM samples. The most frequently present alteration in this signaling pathway were *p16^{INK4a}* homozygous deletion or mutations (52%), followed by *p15^{INK4b}* homozygous deletion (47%), *p18^{NKk4c}* homozygous deletion, *Cdk4* amplification (18%), *RB* mutation or homozygous deletion (11%), cyclin D2 (*CCND2*) amplification (2%), and *Cdk6* amplification (1%) (TCGA 2008). Additionally, single nucleotide polymorphism in the *p16^{Ink4a}* gene has been identified as risk factors for glioma development (Shete, Hosking et al. 2009). The p16^{Ink4a}/RB pathway seems to be important in evolution of both primary and secondary GBM. As already mentioned, loss of normal RB function may result from altered expression of any of the *RB*, *p16^{INK4a,}* or *CDK4* genes. Homozygous deletions of *p16^{Ink4a}* gene, *Cdk4* amplifications, and loss of RB were largely mutually exclusive (Ohgaki and Kleihues 2009). Homozygous *p16^{INK4a}* deletions were more frequent in primary than in secondary GBM, but there was no significant difference in the overall frequency of *p16^{INK4a}* alterations (homozygous deletion and promoter methylation) (Nakamura, Watanabe et al. 2001). Promoter methylation of the *RB* gene was significantly more frequent in secondary (43%) than in primary GBM (14%) (Nakamura, Yonekawa et al. 2001). Alterations in the *p16^{INK4a}/Cdk4/RB* pathway were rare (4%) in oligodendrogliomas, but frequent (65%) in anaplastic oligodendrogliomas (Watanabe, Yokoo et al. 2001). There was a significant correlation between loss of RB expression and promoter methylation of the *RB* gene in GBM. *RB* promoter methylation was not detected in low-grade and anaplastic astrocytoma, indicating that it is a late event during astrocytoma progression (Ohgaki and Kleihues 2007).

The importance of the inactivation of the RB pathway in glioma progression is evidenced by the near-universal and mutually exclusive alteration of RB pathway effectors and inhibitors in both primary and secondary GBM. However, numerous *in vitro* and *in vivo* assays have demonstrated that the neutralization of this pathway alone is insufficient to abrogate cell cycle control to the extent needed for cellular transformation, suggesting that other important cell cycle regulation pathways complement its activities in preventing gliomagenesis (Furnari, Fenton et al. 2007).

A positive correlation between *p16*^{INK4a} deletion and *EGFR* amplification was demonstrated in gliomas (Ohgaki, Dessen et al. 2004), suggesting complementary action of *EGFR/PTEN/Akt* signaling pathway in the progression of primary GBM. In support of this, Andjelkovic et al. (Andjelkovic, Bankovic et al. 2011) reported the cooperation of aberrant *p16*^{INK4a} and altered PTEN in pathogenesis of non-small cell lung cancer. On the other hand, alterations in p53 signaling together with altered RB pathway may lead to secondary GBM progression.

p16^{INK4a} has an important role in maintaining genomic stability. This tumor suppressor cooperates with p21 in regulation of mitotic spindle and uniform chromosome segregation during mitosis.

Inactivation of this gene causes aneuploidy due to centrosome dysfunction and formation of multipolar mitotic spindles during replication (McDermott, Zhang et al. 2006). However, impact of *p16*^{INK4a} inactivation on the level of genomic instability has not been shown in gliomas so far.

Conclusion

During the past decade, much progress has been made in our understanding of the origin, biology, and genetics of gliomas. Complex genetic and epigenetic events cause inactivation of critical pathways that regulate several key aspects of cellular function. These cellular functions can be categorized as self-sufficiency in growth signaling, evasion of apoptosis, insensitivity to anti-growth signals, tissue invasion, and limitless replicative potential and angiogenesis. The picture emerging from the latest reports suggests that most GBMs evolve along a multitude of pathways in response to differing selective pressures to achieve the various cancer phenotypes. However, complex interactions that occur during gliomagenesis, as well as extensive intra- and inter-tumoral heterogeneity represent barriers for successful prevention, precise diagnose and efficient therapy of this malignant disease. Therapeutic targeting of pathways altered in malignant astrocytomas has had limited success so far, and in most centers, the first line therapy for GBMs is still the cytotoxic agent temozolomide (TMZ) and radiotherapy. Further analyses of genetic alterations present in glioma cancer cells of different grades will lead to identification of additional signaling pathways and novel targets for therapy. Identification of potential biomarkers for early glioma detection and response to therapy could improve patients' outcome.

References

Agarwal, P., F. M. L. Kabir, (2012). "Tumor Suppressor Gene p16/INK4A/CDKN2A and Its Role in Cell Cycle Exit, Differentiation, and Determination of Cell Fate“, *Tumor Suppressor Genes,* Dr. Yue Cheng (Ed.), ISBN: 978-953-307-879-3.

Agnihotri, S., K. E. Burrell, et al. (2013). "Glioblastoma, a brief review of history, molecular genetics, animal models and novel therapeutic strategies." *Arch. Immunol. Ther. Exp.* (Warsz.) 61(1): 25-41.

Andjelkovic, T., J. Bankovic, et al. (2011). "Concurrent alteration of p16 and PTEN tumor suppressor genes could be considered as potential molecular marker for specific subgroups of NSCLC patients." *Cancer Biomark.* 10(6): 277-286.

Andjelkovic, T., J. Bankovic, et al. (2011). "Coalterations of p53 and PTEN tumor suppressor genes in non-small cell lung carcinoma patients." *Transl. Res.* 157(1): 19-28.

Bankovic, J., J. Stojsic, et al. (2010). "Identification of genes associated with non-small-cell lung cancer promotion and progression." *Lung Cancer* 67(2): 151-159.

Baylin, S. B., J. G. Herman, et al. (1998). "Alterations in DNA methylation: a fundamental aspect of neoplasia." *Adv. Cancer Res.* 72: 141-196.

Bazarov, A. V., M. Van Sluis, et al. (2010). "p16(INK4a) -mediated suppression of telomerase in normal and malignant human breast cells." *Aging Cell* 9(5): 736-746.

Bielas, J. H., K. R. Loeb, et al. (2006). "Human cancers express a mutator phenotype." *Proc. Natl. Acad. Sci. US* 103(48): 18238-18242.

Bralten, L. B., N. K. Kloosterhof, et al. (2010). "Integrated genomic profiling identifies candidate genes implicated in glioma-genesis and a novel LEO1-SLC12A1 fusion gene." *Genes Chromosomes Cancer* 49(6): 509-517.

Brat, D. J. and E. G. Van Meir (2004). "Vaso-occlusive and prothrombotic mechanisms associated with tumor hypoxia, necrosis, and accelerated growth in glioblastoma." *Lab. Invest.* 84(4): 397-405.

Breivik, J. (2001). "Don't stop for repairs in a war zone: Darwinian evolution unites genes and environment in cancer development." *Proc. Natl. Acad. Sci. US* 98(10): 5379-5381.

Breivik, J. and G. Gaudernack (1999). "Genomic instability, DNA methylation, and natural selection in colorectal carcinogenesis." *Semin. Cancer Biol.* 9(4): 245-254.

Brooks, C. L. and W. Gu (2006). "p53 ubiquitination: Mdm2 and beyond." *Mol. Cell* 21(3): 307-315.

Chumakov, P. M. (2007). "Versatile functions of p53 protein in multicellular organisms." *Biochemistry (Mosc.)* 72(13): 1399-1421.

Collins, V. P. (2004). "Brain tumours: classification and genes." *J. Neurol. Neurosurg. Psychiatry* 75 Suppl. 2: ii2-11.

Dahlback, H. S., P. Brandal, et al. (2009). "Genomic aberrations in 80 cases of primary glioblastoma multiforme: Pathogenetic heterogeneity and putative cytogenetic pathways." *Genes Chromosomes Cancer* 48(10): 908-924.

Di Cristofano, A. and P. P. Pandolfi (2000). "The multiple roles of PTEN in tumor suppression." *Cell* 100(4): 387-390.

Duerr, E. M., B. Rollbrocker, et al. (1998). "PTEN mutations in gliomas and glioneuronal tumors." *Oncogene* 16(17): 2259-2264.

Furnari, F. B., T. Fenton, et al. (2007). "Malignant astrocytic glioma: genetics, biology, and paths to treatment." *Genes Dev.* 21(21): 2683-2710.

Gasco, M., S. Shami, et al. (2002). "The p53 pathway in breast cancer." *Breast Cancer Res.* 4 (2): 70-76.

Gladson, C. L., R. A. Prayson, et al. (2010). "The pathobiology of glioma tumors." *Annu. Rev. Pathol.* 5: 33-50.

Gorgoulis, V. G., L. V. Vassiliou, et al. (2005). "Activation of the DNA damage checkpoint and genomic instability in human precancerous lesions." *Nature* 434(7035): 907-913.

Gu, J., M. Tamura, et al. (1999). "Shc and FAK differentially regulate cell motility and directionality modulated by PTEN." *J. Cell Biol.* 146(2): 389-403.

Hadjipanayis, C. G. and E. G. Van Meir (2009). "Brain cancer propagating cells: biology, genetics and targeted therapies." *Trends Mol. Med.* 15(11): 519-530.

Hanahan, D. and R. A. Weinberg (2011). "Hallmarks of cancer: the next generation." *Cell* 144(5): 646-674.

Huse, J. T. and E. C. Holland (2010). "Targeting brain cancer: advances in the molecular pathology of malignant glioma and medulloblastoma." *Nat. Rev. Cancer* 10(5): 319-331.

Huse, J. T., H. S. Phillips, et al. (2011). "Molecular subclassification of diffuse gliomas: seeing order in the chaos." *Glia* 59(8): 1190-1199.

Ichimura, K., E. E. Schmidt, et al. (1998). "Distinct patterns of deletion on 10p and 10q suggest involvement of multiple tumor suppressor genes in the development of astrocytic gliomas of different malignancy grades." *Genes Chromosomes Cancer* 22(1): 9-15.

Ionov, Y., M. A. Peinado, et al. (1993). "Ubiquitous somatic mutations in simple repeated sequences reveal a new mechanism for colonic carcinogenesis." *Nature* 363(6429): 558-561.

Kanu, O. O., B. Hughes, et al. (2009). "Glioblastoma Multiforme Oncogenomics and Signaling Pathways." *Clin. Med. Oncol.* 3: 39-52.

Kim, D. H., G. Mohapatra, et al. (1995). "Chromosomal abnormalities in glioblastoma multiforme tumors and glioma cell lines detected by comparative genomic hybridization." *Int. J. Cancer* 60(6): 812-819.

Kita, D., Y. Yonekawa, et al. (2007). "PIK3CA alterations in primary (de novo) and secondary glioblastomas." *Acta Neuropathol.* 113(3): 295-302.

Kleihues, P. and L. H. Sobin (2000). "World Health Organization classification of tumors." *Cancer* 88(12): 2887.

Klein, C. A. (2006). "Random mutations, selected mutations: A PIN opens the door to new genetic landscapes." *Proc. Natl. Acad. Sci. US* 103(48): 18033-18034.

Knobbe, C. B., A. Merlo, et al. (2002). "Pten signaling in gliomas." *Neuro Oncol.* 4(3): 196-211.

Knudsen, E. S. and J. Y. Wang (2010). "Targeting the RB-pathway in cancer therapy." *Clin. Cancer Res.* 16(4): 1094-1099.

Kong, D., A. Suzuki, et al. (1997). "PTEN1 is frequently mutated in primary endometrial carcinomas." *Nat. Genet.* 17(2): 143-144.

Lane, D. P. (1992). "Cancer. p53, guardian of the genome." *Nature* 358(6381): 15-16.

Lengauer, C., K. W. Kinzler, et al. (1998). "Genetic instabilities in human cancers." *Nature* 396(6712): 643-649.

Levine, A. J., W. Hu, et al. (2006). "The P53 pathway: what questions remain to be explored?" *Cell Death Differ.* 13(6): 1027-1036.

Loeb, L. A. (1991). "Mutator phenotype may be required for multistage carcinogenesis." *Cancer Res.* 51(12): 3075-3079.

Loeb, L. A. (2001). "A mutator phenotype in cancer." *Cancer Res.* 61(8): 3230-3239.

Loeb, L. A., K. R. Loeb, et al. (2003). "Multiple mutations and cancer." *Proc. Natl. Acad. Sci. US* 100(3): 776-781.

Lothe, R. A. (1997). "Microsatellite instability in human solid tumors." *Mol. Med. Today* 3 (2): 61-68.

Lothe, R. A., P. Peltomaki, et al. (1993). "Genomic instability in colorectal cancer: relationship to clinicopathological variables and family history." *Cancer Res.* 53(24): 5849-5852.

Louis, D. N. (1994). "The p53 gene and protein in human brain tumors." *J. Neuropathol. Exp. Neurol.* 53(1): 11-21.

Louis, D. N. (2006). "Molecular pathology of malignant gliomas." *Annu. Rev. Pathol.* 1: 97-117.

Louis, D. N., H. Ohgaki, et al. (2007). "The 2007 WHO classification of tumours of the central nervous system." *Acta Neuropathol.* 114(2): 97-109.

Lukas, J., B. O. Petersen, et al. (1996). "Deregulated expression of E2F family members induces S-phase entry and overcomes p16INK4A-mediated growth suppression." *Mol. Cell. Biol.* 16(3): 1047-1057.

Malkin, D., F. P. Li, et al. (1990). "Germ line p53 mutations in a familial syndrome of breast cancer, sarcomas, and other neoplasms." *Science* 250(4985): 1233-1238.

Markovic, J., J. Stojsic, et al. (2008). "Genomic instability in patients with non-small cell lung cancer assessed by the arbitrarily primed polymerase chain reaction." *Cancer Invest.* 26 (3): 262-268.

Martinez, R., H. K. Schackert, et al. (2005). "Low-level microsatellite instability phenotype in sporadic glioblastoma multiforme." *J. Cancer Res. Clin. Oncol.* 131(2): 87-93.

Mayo, L. D., J. E. Dixon, et al. (2002). "PTEN protects p53 from Mdm2 and sensitizes cancer cells to chemotherapy." *J. Biol. Chem.* 277(7): 5484-5489.

McDermott, K. M., J. Zhang, et al. (2006). "p16(INK4a) prevents centrosome dysfunction and genomic instability in primary cells." *PLoS Biol.* 4(3): e51.

Milinkovic, V., J. Bankovic, et al. (2012). "Genomic instability and p53 alterations in patients with malignant glioma." *Exp. Mol. Pathol.* 93(2): 200-206.

Milinkovic, V., J. Bankovic, et al. (2013). "Identification of Novel Genetic Alterations in Samples of Malignant Glioma Patients." *PLoS One.* 8(12): e82108.Misra, A., P. Chattopadhyay, et al. (2000). "Extensive intra-tumor heterogeneity in primary human glial tumors as a result of locus non-specific genomic alterations." *J. Neurooncol.* 48(1): 1-12.

Mohapatra, G., A. W. Bollen, et al. (1998). "Genetic analysis of glioblastoma multiforme provides evidence for subgroups within the grade." *Genes Chromosomes Cancer* 21(3): 195-206.

Morris, S. M. (2002). "A role for p53 in the frequency and mechanism of mutation." *Mutat. Res.* 511(1): 45-62.

Nakamura, M., T. Watanabe, et al. (2001). "p14ARF deletion and methylation in genetic pathways to glioblastomas." *Brain Pathol.* 11(2): 159-168.

Nakamura, M., Y. Yonekawa, et al. (2001). "Promoter hypermethylation of the RB1 gene in glioblastomas." *Lab. Invest.* 81(1): 77-82.

Negrini, S., V. G. Gorgoulis, et al. (2010). "Genomic instability--an evolving hallmark of cancer." *Nat. Rev. Mol. Cell Biol.* 11(3): 220-228.

Nishizaki, T., S. Ozaki, et al. (1998). "Investigation of genetic alterations associated with the grade of astrocytic tumor by comparative genomic hybridization." *Genes Chromosomes Cancer* 21(4): 340-346.

Ohgaki, H., P. Dessen, et al. (2004). "Genetic pathways to glioblastoma: a population-based study." *Cancer Res.* 64(19): 6892-6899.

Ohgaki, H. and P. Kleihues (2005). "Population-based studies on incidence, survival rates, and genetic alterations in astrocytic and oligodendroglial gliomas." *J. Neuropathol. Exp. Neurol.* 64(6): 479-489.

Ohgaki, H. and P. Kleihues (2007). "Genetic pathways to primary and secondary glioblastoma." *Am. J. Pathol.* 170(5): 1445-1453.

Ohgaki, H. and P. Kleihues (2009). "Genetic alterations and signaling pathways in the evolution of gliomas." *Cancer Sci.* 100(12): 2235-2241.

Okamoto, Y., P. L. Di Patre, et al. (2004). "Population-based study on incidence, survival rates, and genetic alterations of low-grade diffuse astrocytomas and oligodendrogliomas." *Acta Neuropathol.* 108(1): 49-56.

Ostrom, Q. T., H. Gittleman, et al. (2013), "CBTRUS Statistical Report: Primary Brain and Central Nervous System Tumors Diagnosed in the United States 2006-2010". *Neuro-Oncol.* 15(sup. 2): ii1 – ii56.

Parsons, D. W., S. Jones, et al. (2008). "An integrated genomic analysis of human glioblastoma multiforme." *Science* 321(5897): 1807-1812.

Peinado, M. A., S. Malkhosyan, et al. (1992). "Isolation and characterization of allelic losses and gains in colorectal tumors by arbitrarily primed polymerase chain reaction." *Proc. Natl. Acad. Sci. US* 89(21): 10065-10069.

Perucho, M. (1996). "Cancer of the microsatellite mutator phenotype." *Biol. Chem.* 377(11): 675-684.

Phillips, H. S., S. Kharbanda, et al. (2006). "Molecular subclasses of high-grade glioma predict prognosis, delineate a pattern of disease progression, and resemble stages in neurogenesis." *Cancer Cell* 9(3): 157-173.

Rampino, N., H. Yamamoto, et al. (1997). "Somatic frameshift mutations in the BAX gene in colon cancers of the microsatellite mutator phenotype." *Science* 275(5302): 967-969.

Renault, B., D. Calistri, et al. (1996). "Microsatellite instability and mutations of p53 and TGF-beta RII genes in gastric cancer." *Hum. Genet.* 98(5): 601-607.

Rozan, L. M. and W. S. El-Deiry (2007). "p53 downstream target genes and tumor suppression: a classical view in evolution." *Cell Death Differ.* 14(1): 3-9.

Sasaki, H., M. C. Zlatescu, et al. (2001). "PTEN is a target of chromosome 10q loss in anaplastic oligodendrogliomas and PTEN alterations are associated with poor prognosis." *Am. J. Pathol.* 159(1): 359-367.

Serrano, M., G. J. Hannon, et al. (1993). "A new regulatory motif in cell-cycle control causing specific inhibition of cyclin D/CDK4." *Nature* 366(6456): 704-707.

Shete, S., F. J. Hosking, et al. (2009). "Genome-wide association study identifies five susceptibility loci for glioma." *Nat. Genet.* 41(8): 899-904.

Souza-Rodrigues, E., J. M. Estanyol, et al. (2007). "Proteomic analysis of p16ink4a-binding proteins." *Proteomics* 7(22): 4102-4111.

Stambolic, V., D. MacPherson, et al. (2001). "Regulation of PTEN transcription by p53." *Mol. Cell* 8(2): 317-325.

Stott, F. J., S. Bates, et al. (1998). "The alternative product from the human CDKN2A locus, p14(ARF), participates in a regulatory feedback loop with p53 and MDM2." *EMBO J.* 17 (17): 5001-5014.

Stratton, M. R., P. J. Campbell, et al. (2009). "The cancer genome." *Nature* 458(7239): 719-724.

Stupp, R., W. P. Mason, et al. (2005). "Radiotherapy plus concomitant and adjuvant temozolomide for glioblastoma." *N. Engl. J. Med.* 352(10): 987-996.

Sulman, E. P., M. Guerrero, et al. (2009) "Transcription profiling of brain tumors: tumor biology and treatment stratification". In: Van Meir, E. G., ed. *CNS Cancer: Models,*

Markers, Prognostic Factors, Targets and Therapeutic Approaches. 1st ed. NewYork: Humana Press (Springer); 529-552.

Tamura, M., J. Gu, et al. (1998). "Inhibition of cell migration, spreading, and focal adhesions by tumor suppressor PTEN." *Science* 280(5369): 1614-1617.

Tanic, N., J. Milasin, et al. (2009). "Genomic instability and tumor-specific DNA alterations in oral leukoplakias." *Eur. J. Oral Sci.* 117(3): 231-237.

TCGA (2008). "Comprehensive genomic characterization defines human glioblastoma genes and core pathways." *Nature* 455(7216): 1061-1068.

Thibodeau, S. N., G. Bren, et al. (1993). "Microsatellite instability in cancer of the proximal colon." *Science* 260(5109): 816-819.

Van Meir, E. G., C. G. Hadjipanayis, et al. (2010). "Exciting new advances in neuro-oncology: the avenue to a cure for malignant glioma." *CA Cancer J. Clin.* 60(3): 166-193.

Vanhaesebroeck, B. and D. R. Alessi (2000). "The PI3K-PDK1 connection: more than just a road to PKB." *Biochem. J.* 346 Pt 3: 561-576.

Verhaak, R. G., K. A. Hoadley, et al. (2010). "Integrated genomic analysis identifies clinically relevant subtypes of glioblastoma characterized by abnormalities in PDGFRA, IDH1, EGFR, and NF1." *Cancer Cell* 17(1): 98-110.

Vincent, E. E., D. J. Elder, et al. (2011). "Akt phosphorylation on Thr308 but not on Ser473 correlates with Akt protein kinase activity in human non-small cell lung cancer." *Br. J. Cancer* 104(11): 1755-1761.

Vogelstein, B., D. Lane, et al. (2000). "Surfing the p53 network." *Nature* 408(6810): 307-310.

Vogelstein, B. and K. W. Kinzler, (2002) *"The genetic basis of human cancer";* McGraw, Hill: New York, 2002.

Vranova, V., E. Necesalova, et al. (2007). "Screening of genomic imbalances in glioblastoma multiforme using high-resolution comparative genomic hybridization." *Oncol. Rep.* 17 (2): 457-464.

Watanabe, M., H. Imai, et al. (1996). "Microsatellite instability in latent prostate cancers." *Int. J. Cancer* 69(5): 394-397.

Watanabe, T., H. Yokoo, et al. (2001). "Concurrent inactivation of RB1 and TP53 pathways in anaplastic oligodendrogliomas." *J. Neuropathol. Exp. Neurol.* 60(12): 1181-1189.

Weinberg, R. A. (1995). "The retinoblastoma protein and cell cycle control." *Cell* 81(3): 323-330.

Wen, P. Y. and S. Kesari (2008). "Malignant gliomas in adults." *N. Engl. J. Med.* 359(5): 492-507.

Zhao, R., K. Gish, et al. (2000). "The transcriptional program following p53 activation." *Cold Spring Harb. Symp. Quant. Biol.* 65: 475-482.

Zheng, H., H. Ying, et al. (2008). "p53 and Pten control neural and glioma stem/progenitor cell renewal and differentiation." *Nature* 455(7216): 1129-1133.

In: Gliomas: Classification, Symptoms, Treatment and Prognosis ISBN: 978-1-63117-868-9
Editor: David Cory Adamson

Chapter 8

Signaling Pathways and Therapeutic Targets in GBM

Cristina Trejo-Solís*[*]*, Isabel Anaya-Rubio and Julio Sotelo
Departamento de Neuroinmunología, Instituto Nacional de Neurología y Neurocirugía
"Manuel Velasco Suárez", D.F, México

Abstract

Glioblastoma (GBM) is the most common and aggressive primary malignant cancer of the central nervous system. Despite technological advances in surgical management and combined regimens of radiotherapy with new generation chemotherapy agents, the median survival rate of GBM patients is 14 months. The lethality of GBM is due to a highly mutated genome with opportunistic deletions of tumor suppressor genes and the amplification and/ or mutational hyper-activation of tyrosine kinase receptors. These genetic changes affect signaling pathways controlling cell cycle progression, cellular proliferation, survival, migration, invasion, apoptosis and angiogenesis. It is critical to explore novel diagnostic and therapeutic strategies that target these pathways to improve malignant glioma treatments in the future. This chapter reviews the most common and important signaling pathways that are highly mutated or deregulated in GBM, focusing specifically on growth factors and their receptors [e.g., epidermal growth factor receptor (EGFR), platelet-derived growth factor receptor (PDGFR) and vascular endothelial growth factor receptor (VEGFR)] and the intracellular effector molecules downstream of these growth factors [e.g., RAS/RAF/MAPK, PI3K/PTEN/AKT/mTOR and PKC]. In addition, some of the most promising therapeutic approaches targeting these pathways in GBM are discussed, including multi-targeted kinase inhibitors, monoclonal antibodies, vaccines and microRNAs.

[*] Correspondence should be addressed to Cristina Trejo Solis; trejosolis@yahoo.com.mx.

Abbreviations

EGF	Epidermal Growth Factor
PDGF	Platelet-Derived Growth Factor
VEGF	Vascular Endothelial Growth Factor
EGFR	Epidermal Growth Factor Receptor
PDGFR	Platelet-Derived Growth Factor Receptor
VEGFR	Vascular Endothelial Growth Factor Receptor
MAPK	Mitogen Activated Protein Kinase
RTK	Protein tyrosine kinase
PI3K	Phosphoinositol 3 Kinase
PIP2	Phosphatidyl-Inositol-4, 5-Bisphosphate
PIP3	Phosphatidyl-Inositol 3,4,5-Triphosphate
PDK 1	Phosphoinositide-Dependent Protein Kinase 1
PTEN	Phosphatase and Tensin Homolog
mTOR	Mammalian Target of Rapamycin
PLC	Phospholipase C
PKC	Protein Kinase C
DSBs	DNA double-strand breaks
DNA-PKcs	DNA-dependent protein kinase catalytic subunit
SHP-2	Protein Tyrosine Phosphatase
ECM	Extra-Cellular Matrix
HIF-1	Hypoxia-Inducible Factor-1
DAG	Diacylglycerol
STAT	Signal Transducer and Activator of Transcription
FOXO	Forkhead

Introduction

Gliomas are the most frequent cancer of the central nervous system, accounting for approximately 80% of all malignant primary brain tumors. Gliomas are derived from glial cells and include tumors of astrocytic, oligodendroglial, ependymal or mixed origin. The World Health Organization (WHO) classifies gliomas into prognostic grades ranging from I to IV [1]. The most malignant and aggressive astrocytic glioma, glioblastoma multiforme (GBM; WHO grade IV), constitutes more than 50% of all gliomas, with a global incidence rate of 2-5 per 100,000 people per year in Western Europe and North America [2]. GBM significantly impacts the life of the affected patients due to its poor prognosis with a median survival time of less than two years after diagnosis [3]. GBM lethality is due to characteristics such as a high growth rate, extreme invasiveness and intrinsic resistance to current therapies. Even novel treatments have not substantially improved the survival rate of GBM patients to date. Therefore, the use of personalized medicine using knowledge of the essential molecular mechanisms involved in tumor survival provides new hope.

Primary or "de novo" GBM represents the majority of cases; this tumor type arises without any prior evidence of a lower-grade precursor lesion and more commonly affects elderly patients (mean age, 62 years). Secondary GBMs progress from lower-grade gliomas and are the tumor type typically found in younger patients (median age, 45 years).

Phenotypically, primary and secondary GBM are indistinguishable. However, both GBM subtypes display distinct genetic abnormalities suggesting that their malignant transformation occurs through different genetic pathways. Primary GBM is associated with epidermal growth factor receptor (EGFR) overexpression and mutation, loss of heterozygosity at 10q, mutation of the phosphatase and tensin homology (PTEN) gene, deletion of the $p16^{INK4a}$ gene, amplification of MDM2 or MDM4 and over-expression or mutation in the p53 gene [4]. Secondary GBM is related to mutations in the p53 gene (65%), loss of heterozygosity at 10q and 17p, over-expression of the platelet-derived growth factor receptor (PDGFR) and abnormalities of the $p16^{INK4a}$ and Rb pathways [5]. Although distinct genetic alterations may be used to distinguish primary and secondary GBM, these changes are not mutually exclusive, and similar molecular pathways may be affected, resulting in progressively uncontrolled proliferation, loss of normal cell cycle control mechanisms, diminished ability to undergo apoptosis in response to genotoxic agents, failure of DNA repair mechanisms, increased genetic instability and regulation of growth factor signaling pathways [4,5].

This chapter explains the most common and important signaling pathways that are highly mutated or deregulated in GBM, focusing specifically on growth factors and their receptors [EGFR, PDGFR, VEGFR] and intracellular effector molecules that are downstream of these growth factors [RAS/RAF/mitogen-activated protein kinase (MAPK), PI3K/PTEN/AKT/mTOR and PKC]. Some of the most promising therapeutic approaches attempting to target these pathways in GBM are discussed, including multi-targeted kinase inhibitors, monoclonal antibodies, vaccines and microRNAs.

Tyrosine Kinases in GBM

Receptor protein tyrosine kinases (RTKs) mediate the effect of growth factors and sustain the communication between signals outside the cell surface and inside cell compartments [6]. They are divided into receptor and non-receptor tyrosine kinases, which initiate signaling processes through the phosphorylation/dephosphorylation (activation/deactivation) of a variety of downstream proteins including members of the RAS/RAF/MAPK pathway, the phosphoinositol 3 kinase (PI3K)/PTEN/AKT pathway and PKC [7]. The most prevalent mutations in GBM include those found in RTKs such as EGFR, PDGFR and VEGFR. Gene overexpression or deletion results in aberrations in signal transduction leading to the development of the tumor phenotype characterized by altered differentiation, increased proliferation and survival, resistance to apoptosis, sustained angiogenesis, tissue invasion and metastases (Figure 1) [6,7].

The Epidermal Growth Factor and its Receptor

The EGFR is a tyrosine kinase cell surface receptor that induces cellular proliferation, survival, migration and invasion and inhibits apoptosis in gliomas [8]. The EGFR is abnormally activated in 70% of solid cancers and is amplified or over-expressed in up to 60% of primary GBMs [9]. EGFR amplification is the most common genetic abnormality in high-grade gliomas [10]. EGFR is a membrane-bound glycoprotein with a molecular weight of

160-180 kD and is a member of the ERBB family, which also comprises the ERBB-2, -3 and -4 receptors. EGFR is composed of an extracellular ligand-binding domain, a hydrophobic transmembrane region and a cytoplasmic domain with intrinsic tyrosine kinase activity, tyrosine residues and regulatory motifs [11]. EGFR activation is elicited through the binding of its ligands, including epidermal growth factor (EGF), transforming growth factor-α (TNFα), amphiregulin and others, to its extracellular domain. Ligand binding triggers EGFR dimerization, activation and autophosphorylation of several tyrosine residues in the carboxy-terminal region of the intracellular domain [12]. These phosphorylated residues serve as docking sites for a number of proteins, resulting in the activation of intracellular signaling pathways. The main pathways activated in response to EGFR and ERBB2 phosphorylation include MAPK, PI3K/AKT, signal transducer and activator of transcription (STAT) and SRC tyrosine kinase, which are associated with cell proliferation and survival (Figure 1) [13].

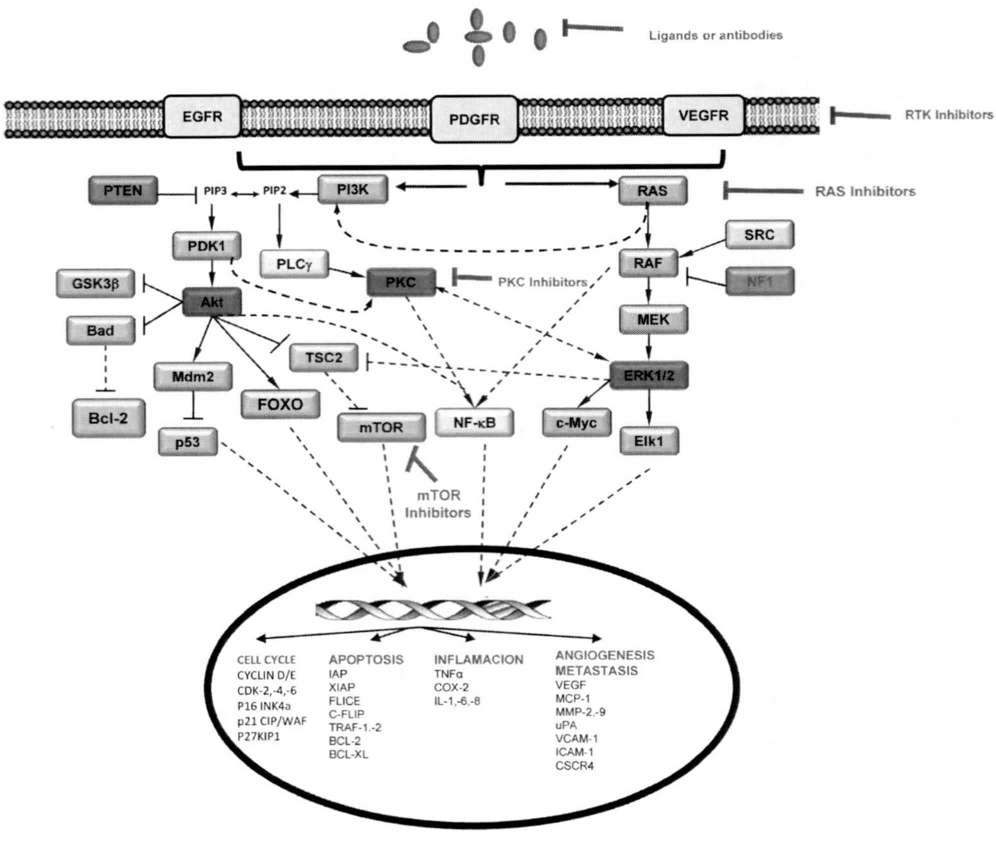

Figure 1. Relevant glioma signaling pathways and potential targets for molecular therapeutic agents. EGFR, PDGFR and VEGFR are receptor tyrosine kinase (RTKs). In glioblastoma, 40-60 % of cases exhibit EGFR amplification and high EGFR protein expression levels. PDGFR and VEGFR also are overexpressed at transcriptional levels in GBM. These TKIs-mediated signal transduction pathways such as RAS/RAF/MAPKs, PI3K/AKT/mTOR and PKC, which activate transcription factors (NF-κB, c-myc, FOXO, ELK-1, p53) that regulate the expression of genes that control cellular processes such as proliferation, cell cycle, apoptosis, metabolism, inflammation, angiogenesis, invasion and metastasis.

The EGF/EGFR Pathway in GBM

EGFR is rarely detectable in normal glial cells but is highly expressed in human gliomas due to amplification of the ERB-1 gene, the first major molecular genetic alteration identified in human gliomas. Approximately 40% of all GBM cases present with EGFR amplification, and 30% of GBMs show the presence of a constitutively activated EGFR mutant known as EGFRvIII (EGFR type III, de2-7, ΔEGFR) [14,15], generated by the genomic deletion of exons 2 to 7 of the EGFR gene, which is part of the extracellular domain of the receptor. This mutant is an EGFR variant unable to bind its ligand and signals constitutively [16]. There are additional missense mutations in the EGFR extracellular domain in GBM that are oncogenic and mutually exclusive to EGFRvIII [17]. EGFR amplification and EGFRvIII are associated with high-grade malignancy and may provide prognostic information; they have been suggested as indicators of poor survival in GBM [18]. In addition, EGFRvIII has been reported to be an indicator of poor response to radiation therapy and chemotherapy [19].

Previous studies have suggested that EGFRvIII is more tumorigenic than wild-type EGFR due to the altered signaling kinetics because the cytoplasmic (signaling) domain is the same for both receptors [20]. Ligand binding to the wild-type EGFR results in rapid internalization of the receptor followed by its dephosphorylation and degradation or recycling [21]. Because EGFRvIII does not bind EGF, its internalization is slow, promoting a state of low–level continuous signaling from activated receptors at the membrane [20]. Increased membrane persistence of activated receptor is known to favor mitogenic signaling [22]. The altered kinetics of EGFRvIII activation may result in a distinct set of downstream signals compared with the wild-type EGFR. Several lines of evidence indicate that ligand-activated EGFR and EGFRvIII stimulate both the RAS/RAF/MAPK and the PI3K/AKT pathways [23]. However, EGFRvIII may preferentially activate the PI3K/AKT pathway [24], and the activation of this pathway may be more robust that wild-type EGRF, leading to the activation of mammalian target of rapamycin (mTOR), the forkhead (FOX) transcription factor family and S6 [25]. Another consequence of EGFRvIII activation of PI3K/AKT is increased proliferation and cell cycle progression mediated by a decrease in the levels of $p27^{KIP1}$, a cyclin-dependent kinase (CDK) inhibitor that binds and inactivates CDK2/cyclin E complexes and thereby inhibits the transition of cells from the G_1 phase to the S phase [26]. Recently, EGFRvIII has been shown to activate mTORC2 via the PI3K/AKT pathway, which in turn leads to the stimulation of the NF-κB pathway and chemotherapy resistance [27]. It has been reported that EGFRvIII contributes to the radioresistance of glioma-relevant cells and tumors by promoting the repair of DNA double-strand breaks (DSBs) through hyperactivation of the DNA-dependent protein kinase catalytic subunit (DNA-PKcs) via the PI3K/AKT pathway, while EGFR may respond to radiation-induced DNA damage in a direct manner [28]. Radiation induces EGFR translocation to the nucleus (in addition to its activation by phosphorylation), where it stimulates DNA-PKcs kinase activity [29]. It has been reported that EGFRvIII signaling via PI3K/AKT may be facilitated by association with deletion or mutations of the PTEN gene, which occur in approximately 40% of GBM samples that express EGFRvIII [30].

Several studies have shown that EGFR and EGFRvIII work cooperatively with kinases to enhance GBM tumorigenicity. EGFR and EGFRvIII expression induces the activation of SRC and FYN kinases through physical association and through phosphorylating them at their active site, promoting GBM tumor growth and motility [31]. It has been reported that patients with amplified or mutated EGFR show high SRC and FYN levels and that the inhibition of both kinases may increase the efficacy of anti-EGFR targeting therapies [31]. In addition, it has been shown that EGFRvIII induces the phosphorylation of dedicator of cytokinesis1 (DOCK180) at tyrosine residues Y722 by the SRC kinases family and that p-DOCK180Y722 is co-expressed with EGFRvIII and p-SRCY418 in clinical GBM specimens. Such co-expression correlates with an extremely poor prognosis [31]. DOCK1 is a guanine nucleotide exchange factor (GEF) that activates Rac1 and controls several cellular functions including cell motility, survival and proliferation [33]. Targeting the SFK-p-DOCK180Y722-Rac1 signaling pathway also offers a novel target as a therapeutic strategy in GBM with EGFRvIII overexpression [33]. Other studies have shown an important role for JNK activation in EGFRvIII signaling [34] and that myristoylated alanine-rich protein kinase C substrate contributes to EGFRvIII-mediated invasiveness [35].

The enhanced tumorigenicity of GBM cells expressing EGFR and EGFRvIII is also associated with enhanced angiogenesis via VEGF upregulation [36]. It has been reported that EGFRvIII promotes angiogenesis because it increases the expression of angiogenic factors such as IL-8 and VEGF. This overexpression appears mediated at the transcriptional level by NF-κB, as blocking the NF-κB pathway abrogates tumor angiogenesis with a concomitant reduction in tumor formation [36].

Platelet-Derived Growth Factor and its Receptor

The overexpression of PDGF and its receptor PDGFR plays an important role in cancer development through the autocrine stimulation of cancer cells and angiogenesis. PDGF is a potent mitogen for glial cells, vascular smooth muscle cells, and fibroblasts. It exists as a disulphide-linked dimer of four homologous polypeptide chains: PDGF-A; PDGF-B; PDGF-C and PDGF-D. PDGF binds to two receptor tyrosine kinases (PDGFRα and PDGFRβ), which are transmembrane glycoproteins with five immunoglobulin-like repeats in the extracellular domain [37]. PDGF-A, PDGF-B and PDGF-C bind to PDGFRα, while PDGF-B and PDGF-D bind to PDGFRβ. Ligand binding (PDGF-AA, -BB, -CC,-DD and the heterodimer PDGF-AB) leads to receptor homo- or heterodimerization and autophosphorylation and propagation of intracellular signals including MAP kinase, PI3K/AKT and JAK/STAT resulting in changes in cellular behavior, such as proliferation, survival, angiogenesis, migration and invasion [38, 39].

The PDGF/PDGFR Pathway in Gliomas

One of the most common cellular defects found in brain tumors is the presence of a PDGF/PDGFR autocrine loop. The importance of PDGF signaling in malignant gliomas has been demonstrated in several models. PDGFR autocrine stimulation in the brain of neonatal mice results in astrocytoma formation [40] and PDGF overexpression in either neural progenitor or differentiated astrocytes leads to the formation of gliomas with oligodendroglial and oligoastrocytic features [41], suggesting a role for PDGF and PDGFR in the early stages and progression of glioma tumors. It has been reported that PDGFRα overexpression and gene amplification occurs mostly in lower-grade gliomas as well as secondary GBMs [42,

43]. The coordinated genomic analysis of a large cohort of clinical GBM specimens showed that the gene encoding PDGFRα was amplified in approximately 13% of the total analyzed GBMs, placing itself as third of the top 11 amplified genes in GBM [44].

Overexpression of PDGFRα and its ligand, PDGF-A, in clinical gliomas is associated with a poor prognosis and a shorter patient survival time [45], whereas PDGF-B and PDGFRβ have been found in hyperplastic tumor endothelial cells in GBM [46], suggesting a PDGF role in glioma angiogenesis [47]. In addition, it has been reported that PDGFRβ induces GBM stem cell renewal, survival, tumor growth and invasion [48]. In addition to PDGFR-A and –B, Lokker et al. identified the ligands –C and –D. They also found that PDGF-C is ubiquitously expressed in GBM cells and tissue, but its expression is low or absent in normal adult and fetal brains. PDGF-D was expressed in 10 of 11 GBM cell lines and in 3 of 5 primary brain tumor samples [38].

Although activation of the PDGF/PDGFR-specific pathway involves tumor progression of malignant GBM, the molecular mechanisms by which PDGFRs promote GBM growth and invasion remain largely unknown. However, it has been reported that inhibition of PDGFR kinase activity correlates with a decrease in p-ERK and p-AKT levels, likely as a result of decreased signaling through MAPK and P13K pathways, respectively [38]. In particular, PI3K has been identified as the major effector of PDGFα signaling *in vitro* and *in vivo* [49]. Liu et al. demonstrated that the specific activation of PDGFRα signaling by PDGF-A in cooperation with the loss of tumor suppressor $p16^{INK4a}$ is required for gliomagenesis [50]. Furthermore, it has been shown that CDK4/6/pRB signaling is required for PDGFRα-induced tumorigenesis, and the non-receptor protein tyrosine phosphatase SHP-2 is a critical linker between the PI3K/AKT/mTOR pathway and PDGFRα in the formation of glioma *in vitro*, in mice and in clinical GBM specimens [51]. Recently, it has been reported that dynamin 2 (Dyn2), a large GTPase, mediates PDGFRα-SHP-2-promoted GBM growth and invasion, suggesting that PDGF-A activation of PDGFRα induces Dyn2 association with PI3K and SHP-2 and activates SHP-2 and SRC, leading to SRC-dependent tyrosine phosphorylation of Dyn2. Dyn2 activation stimulates its downstream effectors AKT, ERK 1/2, Rac and Cdc42, resulting in increased glioma growth and invasion [44]. Furthermore, it has been reported that PDGF-A stimulation of PDGFRα induces Src-dependent p-Y at DOCK 180Y181, leading to the formation of the DOCK180/CrkII/p130 complex and activation of the GTPase Rac1 signaling, thereby promoting glioma cell growth, survival and invasion [52]. It has been reported that genetic and pharmacological targeting of PDGFRβ attenuates GBM stem cell self-renewal, survival, tumor growth and invasion [52]. Ding et al. found that PDGFRβ stimulation promotes the specific recruitment of integrin $\alpha_v\beta_3$-containing focal adhesions in vitronectin–adherent cells and induces migration through a LYN kinase-mediated pathway [53] and also found that the engagement of different integrins alters the identity of the Src members activated upon stimulation with PDGF [53]. In addition, Guo et al. showed that PDGF-B stimulates human U87MG tumor angiogenesis through a paracrine pathway. PDGF-B enhances glioma angiogenesis and growth by stimulating VEGF expression in the tumor endothelium, which increases endothelial cell (EC) mitogenesis by promoting pericyte recruitment into growing vessels, thus facilitating vessel assembly. The authors hypothesize that in low-grade gliomas, overexpression of PDGF-B in tumor cells and PDGFRβ in ECs [54] might be part of an angiogenic switch that upregulates VEGF and enhances vessel growth, thus promoting glioma progression. During the later stages of glioma development, hypoxia and increased expression of other growth factors or genes in tumors enhance VEGF expression, which in turn results in vigorous blood vessel growth [55]. Other reports support that PDGFR-B may also act through a paracrine mechanism in promoting tumor growth and angiogenesis. *In vitro,* PDGF-B stimulates cell proliferation and cord/tube formation of vascular ECs that express PDGFR but has no effect on PDGFRβ-negative ECs [56]. Stimulation of fibroblasts and ECs by PDGF-B increases VEGF expression through the AKT signaling pathway in these cells [57]. In addition, PDGF-C has been reported to induce angiogenic activity indirectly, via VEGF upregulation, and directly, via PDGFRα activation [58]. These observations, along with the fact that PDGFRα and PDGFRβ are expressed in astrocytomas and glioma ECs [59], point to PDGF-C as a potentially important mediator of brain tumor progression. Di Tomaso et al. reported that overexpression of PDGF-C changes the morphology and function of brain vessels, rendering them more stable and less sensitive to anti-VEGFR2 inhibition [60].

Vascular Endothelial Growth Factor and Its Receptor

Angiogenesis is a normal feature in growth, development and wound repair and involves endothelial cell proliferation, extra-cellular matrix (ECM) degradation, sprout and tubule formation and pericyte recruitment. This process is, in part, driven by the expression of the regulatory protein VEGF, which functions as a survival factor for endothelial cells and stimulates the endothelial production of urokinase–type plasminogen activator (uPA), which induces the conversion of plasminogen to plasmin, causing the breakdown of ECM components and leading to ECM remodeling [61,62]. In addition, VEGF increases microvascular permeability through fenestrae induction in endothelial cells and transendothelial cell transport involving vesiculovacuolar organelles, which eventually form the transendothelial cell pore [61, 62]. The result of VEGF signaling in tumors is the production of immature, highly permeable blood vessels with the subsequent poor maintenance of blood-brain barrier (BBB) and parenchymal edema [61, 63]. VEGF comprises a family of six secreted dimeric glycoproteins of approximately 40 kDa (VEGF-A, -B, -C, -D, -E and placental-derived growth factor) that exhibits its cellular response by binding to the transmembrane tyrosine receptors VEGFR1 (flt-1) and VEGFR2 (Flk-1/KDR). VEGFR contains seven IgG-like repeats in the ligand-binding domain, a single transmembrane domain and a tyrosine kinase domain [61, 62]. VEGFR2 appears to mediate almost all of the known cellular responses to VEGF. The function of VEGFR1 is to modulate VEGFR2 signaling; in addition, VEGFR1 may act as a decoy receptor, sequestering VEGF from VEGFR2 binding [61, 62]. Through receptor dimerization, VEGF leads to a cascade of different signaling pathways with various cell-regulating effects, such as DNA synthesis and cell growth via MAPK pathway activation. On the other hand, PI3K/AKT pathway activation leads to increased endothelial cell survival, whereas SRC activation can lead to actin cytoskeleton changes and endothelial cell migration [61, 62].

Many types of human tumor cells express VEGF, often at elevated levels. This is mostly due to various environmental stimuli (e.g., hypoxia, cytokines, sex hormones, growth factors, chemokines) and genetic or epigenetic changes in tumor cells (e.g., mutant p53, VHL, PTEN-suppressor genes) or activated oncogenes (e.g., RAS, SRC, EGFR and PDGFR) [61-64].

Hypoxia is an important VEGFR inducer because it stabilizes hypoxia-inducible factor (HIF)-1α and HIF-2α, which promote metabolic changes to sustain continued tumor growth.

Specifically, HIF-1α and HIF-2α have the following effects: (1) block VEGF proteolysis by ubiquitin, allowing its accumulation [65], (2) upregulate GLUT-1 receptors to increase glucose uptake from blood [66], (3) up-regulate carbonic anhydrase IX (CAIX) to stabilize pH in hypoxic conditions, making the environmental tolerable for continued proliferation [67] and (4) sensitize endothelial cells to angiogenic signals [68]. The above events result in the growth of additional vessels to supply nutrients needed to support continued tumor growth. These adaptive responses make tumor cells particularly resistant to various treatment modalities.

The VEGF/VEGFR Pathway in GBM

The vascularization level, measured as plasma vascular space, was found to be 11 ml/100g in GBM, whereas in normal brain, it is only 2 ml/100g [69]. These data support the knowledge that malignant gliomas are highly angiogenic and are the most vascularized tumors in humans. VEGFR2 mRNA expression is confined to vascular cells only in high-grade gliomas, whereas VEGFR1 mRNA expression was also found in the vascular cells of both low- and high-grade gliomas. Little or no expression of both receptors was observed in the normal brain [61]. A comparison of ligand and receptor expression in gliomas showed a clear correlation between VEGF and VEGFR1 and VEGFR2 levels [62]. These findings suggest that the progression of low- to high-grade gliomas is mediated by the coordinated induction of VEGF and VEGF receptors. It has been reported that higher VEGF expression levels in gliomas correlate with the number of lesions and a higher histological grade, although plasma VEGF levels do not correlate with patient survival [63]. In GBM, VEGF mRNA is up to 50-fold overexpressed compared with normal brain tissue [64]. VEGF mRNA expression is remarkably spatially restricted, namely, to perinecrotic (palisading) cells [70].

VEGF protein is detected in VEGF mRNA producing tumor cells, but the largest amount is found in the vasculature [71]. This observation supports the hypothesis of a paracrine mechanism of tumor angiogenesis: VEGF is secreted by tumor cells and bound to endothelial cells, which express VEGF receptors. VEGF expression levels are regulated by the following mechanisms: (1) low oxygen concentrations in growing gliomas induce hypoxia-inducible factor (HIF) up-regulation, which increases VEGF mRNA levels [72], (2) HuR protein upregulation suppresses the posttranscriptional degradation of VEGF-A mRNA under hypoxia, which leads to a further increase in VEGF levels [73], (3) brain-derived neurotrophin factor enhances VEGF expression, increasing HIF-1α expression levels [74], (4) integrin-linked kinase 1 is an important regulator of tumor angiogenesis because it increases VEGF expression by stimulating HIF-1α via AKT phosphorylation on Ser^{473} [75], (5) EGFR signaling stimulates VEGFR gene expression via an HIF-independent mechanism [76] and (6) FoxM1B transcription factor is up-regulated in GBM and stimulates VEGF expression independent of HIF [77].

VEGF induces the activation of different signaling pathways including RAS/RAF/MAPK/, PI3K/AKT and PLC/PKC in GBM through VEGFR2, which regulates cell cycle progression, proliferation, survival, angiogenesis, metastasis and radio-resistance. Kil et al. reported that radiation-induced VEGF in cultured medium collected from irradiated glioma cells enhances tumor motility through VEGF-stimulated SRC and FAK phosphorylation [78]. VEGF also enhances vascular permeability through the MAPK signaling cascade by rearranging cadherin/catenin complexes and perturbing junctions between endothelial cells [79]. Although high VEGF levels facilitate angiogenesis and thereby enable tumor cells to expand, low VEGF levels lead to a reduction in tumor vessel growth and protection of the remaining vessels and concomitantly promote signals for GBM cells to migrate away from these undesirable conditions. Lu et al. demonstrated that VEGF directly and negatively regulates tumor cell migration through enhanced recruitment of protein tyrosine phosphatase 1B (PTP1B) to a MET/VEGFR2 hetero-complex, thereby suppressing HGF-dependent MET phosphorylation and tumor migration [80]. These findings support the hypothesis that combined treatment strategies targeting both VEGF and MET may be used in GBM patients to overcome pro-invasive resistance and prolong survival [80]. Therefore, further research regarding the mechanisms underlying angiogenesis and invasion in GBM is essential for the development of improved therapies.

Signal Transduction Pathways

There are a number of different signal transduction pathways associated with the various receptors mentioned above. In the following paragraphs, two pathways will be discussed in detail: the RAS/RAF/MAPK, PI3K/AKT/mTOR and PKC pathways (Figure 1). These cellular signaling pathways are required for normal cell physiology [5-7]. However, in gliomas, these pathways are overactive due to RTK overexpression and constitutive activation [4-7]. The RAS/MAPK and PI3K/AKT/mTOR pathways, in particular, are involved in tumor resistance to radiotherapy and chemotherapy.

The RAS/RAF/MAPK Pathway

The constitutive activation of the RAS/RAF/MAPK pathway has been detected in GBMs [81, 82]. RAS (Ras, H-, K-, N- isotypes) encodes a protein family of small GTPases that cycle between inactive GDP-bound and active GTP-bound conformations by coupling cell membrane growth factor receptors such as EGFR, EGFRvIII, PDGFR and VEGFR [81,82]. Typically, ligand binding to receptor tyrosine kinases induces receptor dimerization and autophosphorylation of specific tyrosine residues in the C-terminal region. This event generates binding sites for adaptor proteins, e.g., growth factor receptor-bound protein 2 (GRB2), that recruit the GEF Sos at the plasma membrane and in turn activates the membrane-bound RAS by catalyzing GDP to GTP. In its GTP-bound conformation, RAS combines with RAF and mobilizes the inactive protein from the cytoplasm recruiting the Raf kinases (A-RAF, B-RAF and C-RAF) to the plasma membrane [82]. Once the RAS-RAF complex translocates to the cell membrane, RAS activates the serine/threonine kinase function of the RAF isoforms. Upon RAS activation, RAF acts as a MAP kinase kinase kinase (MAPKKK) to activate MEK1 and MEK2, which, in turn, catalyze the activation of the effector ERK 1/2 kinases and their translocation into the nucleus. ERK-2 activates nuclear targets such as topoisomerase II, a cell cycle progression mediator, and transcription factors including cyclic AMP response element binding protein (CREB), estrogen receptor-α (ER-α), IκB/NF-κB, and c-FOS. Activation of these transcription factors results in the expression of oncogenes involved in cell cycle progression, cell growth, angiogenesis and anti-apoptosis (Figure 1) [83]. Although RAF can also be activated by RAS-independent activators, experimental evidence indicates that the RAF-MEK-ERK cascade is a major mediator of RAS-induced oncogenesis. In addition, signal transduction via other pathways such as PI3K and the Ral guanine nucleotide exchange factors (Ral-GEFs) cascades may be important for RAS-induced transformation [84].

The RAS/MAPK Pathway in GBM

Aberrant RAS/RAF signaling has been reported to be important for many tumor types including gliomas. Increased RAS expression and high RAS-GTP levels have been demonstrated in GBM cell lines and tumor specimens [85]. RAS/RAF pathway activation can result from oncogenic mutations of RAS/RAF itself; however, such mutations have only occasionally been reported in gliomas. The Cancer Genome Atlas (TCGA) network reported a 2% mutation rate in RAS genes in 206 GBM samples [86]. Sharman et al. identified one of 21 pilocytic astrocytomas to carry the K-RAS (G13R) mutations but did not detect H-RAS or N-RAS mutations in the tumor cohort [87]. In addition, a lower frequency of BRAF mutations in glioma cell lines and primary specimens has been reported. Davies et al. reported that 4/38 (11%) of glioma cell lines carried the BRAF (V600E) mutation, whereas 0/15 of primary gliomas contained BRAF mutations [88]. A study led by Knobbe et al. examined 94 GBM and found only three tumors (3.2%) with the oncogenic BRAF (V600E) gene [89]. In addition, Bastro et al. reported the presence of the BRAF hot-spot mutation (V600E) in 6% of 34 GBM and 0.1% of 13 anaplastic astrocytoma [90]. These studies indicate that RAS and RAF activation mutations are infrequent events in gliomas; however, extra copies of the RAS/RAF genes have been reported in gliomas. Jeuken et al. reported that 44% of gliomas contained a gain of RAS/BRAF genes, that the gain of BRAF gene is the most frequent (38% of gliomas), and that this gain is more predominant in high-grade glioma [91]. They also reported a copy number gain of the growth factors EGF, PDGF, IGF, FGF, TGF and their receptors in 43 tumors (53%). Furthermore, they found a significant correlation between activated MAPK and copy number gain of these genes, suggesting that RAS/RAF pathway activation in gliomas is achieved by copy number gain rather than through activating RAS/RAF mutations [91].

For a better understanding of the effects of deregulated RAS/RAF signaling on gliomagenesis, a number of studies have utilized oncogenic RAS genes to create cells with increased RAS activity. The results from a transgenic mouse model suggest that activated RAS alone is sufficient to transform normal astrocytes and neuronal precursor cells into malignant gliomas. Ding et al. using a GFAP-driven H-Ras (G12V) transgenic mouse model, showed that high levels of H-RAS (G12V) alone in astrocytes yielded multifocal malignant astrocytomas, and the tumor-bearing mice died within two weeks. Mice with moderate H-RAS (G12V) levels underwent germ-line transmission in which 95% of these mice died from solitary or multifocal low- and high-grade gliomas within 2–6 months. Furthermore, they demonstrated that transgenic astrocytomas are pathologically similar to human astrocytomas with a high mitotic index, nuclear pleomorphism, infiltration, necrosis and increased vascularity [92]. Abel et al. reported that targeting oncogenic K-RAS (G12D) to neural stem cells (NSC) is sufficient to produce marked hyperplasia of the subventricular zone (SVZ). In addition, the targeted mice develop multifocal, infiltrating, intermediate-grade gliomas that often arise near the expanded SVZ. Furthermore, the tumor cells express markers associated with neural progenitor cells including Olig2, Bim-1 and PDGFRα [93].

Others have reported that RAS activation alone may not be sufficient for gliomagenesis, and additional activation of oncogenes or loss of tumor suppressor genes is required for glioma oncogenesis. Holland et al. engineered tissue-specific viral expression vectors to specifically express K-RAS (G12D) and AKT in astrocytes (*via* the promoter for the gene encoding glial fibrillary acidic protein, GFAP) and neural progenitors (*via* the nestin promoter) in mice. Although neither K-RAS (G12D) nor AKT alone was sufficient to induce GBM formation, their combination induced the formation of high-grade gliomas with the histological features of human GBM [94]. It has also been demonstrated that K-RAS (G12D) expression cooperates with the loss of the *INK4a-Arf* locus to induce malignant transformation of astrocytes and neural progenitors into GBM in mice [94]. Furthermore, Lyustikman et al. found that constitutive RAF-1 activation cooperates with *INK4a-Arf* loss or AKT activation to induce gliomagenesis in mice and that RAF-1 tumors are very similar to those induced by K-RAS in incidence and histologic features. Finally, the authors suggest that RAS contributes to human GBM formation in part through RAF signaling [95].

In addition, RAS signaling is required for the maintenance of the GBM malignant phenotype. Blum et al. reported that the RAS inhibition by farnesylthiosalicylic acid (FTS), which directly affects the membrane-bound RAS protein, leads to HIF-1α destabilization in U87 cells. Concomitant with HIF-1α loss, the expression of key enzymes of the glycolysis pathway and other HIF-1α-regulated genes (including VEGF and glucose transporter GLUT1) are transcriptionally downregulated by the FTS treatment. This event leads to glycolysis shutdown, resulting in a dramatic ATP reduction and a severe energy crisis. As a consequence, U87 cell growth was arrested and the cells died [96]. Importantly, the inhibition of active RAS by FTS in these U87 GBM cells also promotes proteasomal degradation of cyclin D1 with a concomitant decrease in phosphorylated Rb protein accompanied by E2F1 downregulation and decreased expression of key E21-regulated genes critical for cell-cycle progression [96]. In addition, RAS inhibition by FTS releases the surviving "brake" in apoptosis and activates the mitochondrial apoptotic pathway: Bad dephosphorylation; Bax activation; cytochrome c release and caspase activation [97]. Blum et al.suggested that down-regulation of E2F1 and HIF-1α represents two distinct arms of the antioncogenic effect of RAS inhibitors in GBM [98].

The PI3K/AKT/mTOR Pathway

In gliomas, abnormal RTK pathway activity is triggered by several mechanisms, such as amplifications, receptor mutations and growth factor over-expression. Three growth factors, EGF, PDGF and VEGF, play important roles in both gliomagenesis and normal central nervous system development. Growth factor binding to their specific RTKs induces RTK dimerization. The dimeric receptor subsequently phosphorylates the intracellular domains of the other, which in turn activates downstream effectors such as RAS and PI3K. RTK pathway activation recruits PI3K to the cell membrane, which then phosphorylates phosphatidyl-inositol-4, 5-bisphosphate (PIP2) to phosphatidyl-inositol 3,4,5-triphosphate (PIP3) to further recruit AKT to the membrane, where AKT can be phosphorylated at Thr308 by phosphoinositide-dependent protein kinase 1 (PDK1) and at Ser473 by the mTOR-rictor complex (mTORC2) for full AKT activation [99]. AKT is a serine-threonine kinase that suppresses apoptosis, drives proliferation and promotes cell growth via the mammalian target of rapamycin (mTOR), which is generally deregulated in a variety of cancers including GBM [100-102]. mTOR is a serine-threonine kinase that exists in two multiprotein complexes, mTORC1 (mTOR with PRAS40, raptor and mLST8/GbL) and mTORC2 (mTOR with rictor, mSINI, protor and mLST8) [103]. mTORC1 plays an important role in regulating protein translation through the phosphorylation of S6 kinases (S6K1 and S6K2), proteins involved in ribosome biogenesis and 4E-binding proteins (4E-BP1), which are a family of proteins involved in repressing the cap-dependent mRNA translation of cyclins, c-myc, Bcl-xl, S6, PDCD4 and others [104,105]. In addition, mTORC1 integrates various inputs, including growth factors, energy status, oxygen and amino acid levels, to regulate cell growth by promoting the biosynthesis of proteins, lipids and organelles as well as limiting catabolic autophagic activity [106]. mTORC2 activation results in phosphorylation of AKT, serum glucorticoid-induced protein kinase (SGK1), and PKCα involved in cell survival, metabolism, proliferation and cytoskeletal organization.

PTEN is a lipid and protein phosphatase and the lipid phosphatase activity is essential for its function as a tumor suppressor [107]. PTEN antagonizes PI3K function by dephosphorylating PIP3 at the D3 position [108]. PI(3,4,5)P3 facilitates AKT translocation to the plasma membrane and induces PDK1 activity, which then phosphorylates and activates AKT [109-111]. Thus, PTEN acts as a major inhibitor of the PI3K/AKT/mTOR pathway, which, when mutated or lost, cannot be compensated for by any other enzyme. PTEN mutations result in constitutive activation of this pathway, which activate multiple targets including GSK3β, $p21^{WAF/CIP}$, $p27^{KIP1}$ and NF-κB [112]. AKT also activates mTOR, which is negatively regulated by suppressor protein tuberous sclerosis complex (TSC1/2) comprising hamartin (TSC1) and tuberin (TSC2). Tuberin is directly phosphorylated by AKT, which disrupts the TSC1/2 complex and stimulates mTOR activity [113].

The PI3K/AKT/mTOR Pathway in GBM

Increased AKT phosphorylation is observed in 85% of GBMs despite the lack of detected PTEN mutations [114]. Loss of heterozygosity or PTEN mutations are found in up to 65% of high-grade gliomas, 25% of primary GBMs and 5% of secondary GBMs [115]. In GBM, reduced PTEN levels and increased AKT activity have been correlated with more aggressive tumor behavior and reduced patient survival time [116]. PTEN loss up-regulates genes involved in the cell cycle (cyclins) and DNA replication (Ki-67, DNA primases) as well as genes involved in stemness, cell differentiation and metabolism of neural stem cells [117]. In PTEN-null GBM cell lines, re-expression of PTEN suppresses proliferation due to G_1 cellular arrest dependent on $p27^{kip1}$expression as opposed to apoptosis induction [118]. Furokawa et al. introduced the wild-type PTEN gene into malignant glioma cell lines, which inactivated Rac and cdc42 (two Rho-family GTP–binding proteins), inhibited MMP-2 and MMP-9 enzyme activity and decreased MMP-2 mRNA expression. This also resulted in a significant reduction of migration and invasion activities of the transfected cells [119]. In addition, it has been reported that PTEN upregulation in gliomas cells and in nude mice tumors down-regulates AKT and PI3K signaling pathways and the expression of several genes, including

AKT, PI3K, JUN, MAPK14, PDK2, PTK2, RAS and RAF. This resulted in the inhibition of migration as well as the wound healing property of the glioma cells; *in vivo,* PTEN upregulation decreases AKT and XAIP levels [120]. It has been proposed that XIAP acts as an E3 ubiquitin ligase for PTEN and promotes AKT activity by regulating PTEN content and compartmentalization [121]. Similarly, reduced *in vivo* tumor growth was also observed upon PTEN reconstitution in GBM due to reduced AKT-dependent angiogenesis [122]. The involvement of AKT in diverse tumorigenic activities suggests that AKT activation alone may be sufficient to induce cancer [123]. AKT activation may contribute by stimulating the secretion of matrix metalloproteinases [124]. Newhart et al. demonstrated, using *in vivo* orthotopic GBM models, a strong correlation between AKT activation and GBM growth rate and invasiveness [125]. In addition to its oncogenic effect, AKT activation in glial tumors also leads to astrocytic differentiation [126].

Several studies have suggested a linear oncogenic pathway of PTEN/AKT/mTOR. PTEN-null tumors have higher AKT and mTOR activity [127] and the mTOR inhibitor rapamycin reduces tumor cell proliferation and growth but has no effect on PTEN-positive tumors, suggesting that mTOR is responsible for the oncogenic effect of PTEN loss [128]. In addition, mTOR is required for cell transformation by PI3K and AKT [129]. Moreover, in human GBMs, mTOR activity correlates with AKT activity raising the possibility that the oncogenic effect of AKT might be achieved through mTOR [130]. Hu et al. reported that mTOR promotes survival and astrocytic characteristics induced by PTEN/AKT signaling in GBM [131]. Moreover, it has been reported that PKCα is a key intermediate linking EGFR signaling to mTOR in a pathway independent of AKT signaling [132]. mTORC1 promotes cell growth and proliferation, activates HIF-1-dependent glycolysis [133], and stimulates angiogenesis in many cancer types [134]. Therefore, mTORC1 is well established as a cancer drug target. It has also been shown that mTORC2 activity is elevated in gliomas and promotes growth and cell motility via rictor overexpression [135]. The combined RNAi-mediated suppression of rictor and EGFR results in complete tumor regression in an orthopedic GBM tumor model [136]

PKC Signaling

Protein kinase C (PKC) is a family of serine/threonine kinases comprising 12 members in mammalian cells [137]. PKCs are divided into three subgroups: first, the *classical or conventional* PKCs (α, βI, βII and γ), which are Ca^{2+} dependent and activated by diacylglycerol (DAG) and phosphatidylserine (PS); second, *novel* PKCs (δ, ε, η, μ and θ), which are Ca^{2+} independent and regulated by DAG and PS; and finally, *atypical* PKCs (ζ and λ /ι), which are Ca^{2+} independent and do not require DAG for activation, although PS can regulated their activity [132-139]. All PKC isoforms are composed of an NH_2-terminal regulatory domain and a COOH-terminal catalytic domain with serine-threonine kinase activity [140]. Both domains contain conserved regions of extended sequence homology and variable regions [141,142]. In the classical PKC isoforms, the regulatory domain contains a Ca^{2+}-binding domain, and in both the classical and novel PKC isoforms, it contains a pseudosubstrate region and a pair of highly conserved zinc fingers (C1 domains) that bind phorbol esters [143].

PKC is activated downstream of transmembrane receptors, including RTKs and phospholipase C (PLC) [143]. PLC is one of the main enzymes involved in PKC activation. PLC cleaves PIP_2 into DAG and IP_3. PKC may participate in mitogenic signaling by activating the RAF/MEK/MAPK pathway. It has been reported that PKC can directly phosphorylate and activate RAF-A [144], although RAS appears to be required to recruit RAF to the membrane [145]. The PKC signaling pathway is involved in diverse cellular function such as proliferation, cell cycle, apoptosis, invasion and angiogenesis [146,147].

PKC Signaling in Glioma

There is substantial evidence to indicate PKC is not mutated nor amplified, the PKC pathway is hyperactivated in gliomas due to the constitutive activation of several growth factor receptors, and the inactivation of negative regulators such as PTEN [148-150], which could lead to activation of PLC and PDK1, two enzymes that play critical roles in PKC activation [150]. The catalytic region of PKC requires phosphorylation events to be catalytically active. The phosphorylation of the activation loop of PKC by PDK1, followed by autophosphorylation on two additional sites, is necessary for the release of newly synthesized PKC into the cytosol and to obtain a catalytically active conformation. PDK1 can phosphorylate all PKC isoforms at the activation loop of the kinase domain; this step is required for PKC to be catalytically active [150-151].

It has been reported that PKC activity is markedly increased in astrocytoma cell lines compared with non-transformed astrocytes, and PKC activity directly correlates with the growth rate [148]. PKC activity is also elevated in astrocytoma specimens [149]. PKC stimulation using phorbol esters resulted in dramatically increased proliferation and S-phase progression, measured by ^{3}H-thymidine incorporation [152]. Tamoxifen, at PKC inhibitory concentrations, has a dramatic effect on glioma cell proliferation and prevents PDGF or serum-induced DNA synthesis [153]. Similarly, the mitogenic effect of serum addition or stimulation with EGF, PDGF or FGF on established glioma cell lines or low passage glioma cells was completely abrogated by PKC inhibition with various inhibitors [149-153]. These results suggest that mitogenic signaling from RTCs in astrocytoma cells is mediated through a PKC-dependent pathway.

Several studies have focused on characterizing the functions of specific PKC isoforms in glioma cell proliferation. PKCα has been implicated in promitogenic and prosurvival signals in glioma cells [154]. Furthermore, Hu et al. reported that PKCα phosphorylation is a pre-requisite for C6 cell migration [154]. In addition, it has been reported that PKCα induces a proliferative response in GBM cells through the phosphorylation and nuclear translocation of the NF-κB p65 subunit [155]. Furthermore, it has been reported that PKCα is the main regulator of ERK 1/2, which is required for FGF expression, a potent mitogen for glioma cell proliferation [156,157]. Lin et al. demonstrated that 12-O- tetradecanoylphosphol-13 acetate (TPA) induces glioma cell migration/invasion through activating PKCα/ERK/NF-κB-dependent MMP-9 expression, suggesting that PKCα protein translocation is an early event that transmits a signal to activate downstream targets, such as ERK and JNK, followed by the activation of NF-κB-dependent MMP-9 activation and migration/invasion in TPA-treated GBM840 cells [158]. Surprisingly, an AKT-independent, PKCα-dependent mechanism that links PI3K with mTORC1 in GBM has been described [132]. Taken together, these results show that PKCα is involved in glioma cell survival, proliferation and migration, whereas PKCγ and PKCδ increase glioma cell anchorage-independent growth [159]. Furthermore, it has been reported that PKC-ζ participates in MMP-9 expression induction by interleukin-1 (IL-1) and tumor necrosis factor-α (TNF-α) via NF-κB in rat C6 cells [160]. In a recent report, PKCη was shown to play a role in the PMA-induced proliferation of glioma cells through an ERK/ELK-1 pathway [161], and PKCε is essential for the survival of glioma cells via AKT [162]. Furthermore, it has been shown that PKCε positively regulates the integrin-dependent adhesion, spreading and motility of human glioma cells through the scaffolding protein receptor for activated C kinase 1 (RACK1) [163]. It has also been reported that PKCι promotes GBM motility by coordinating the formation of a single leading edge lamellipodia and has a role in remodeling the cytoskeleton at the lamellipodia leading edge, promoting Lgl dissociation from non-muscle myosin II. In addition, PKCι is required for the transition of glioma cells through mitosis [164]. Desai et al. reported that PKCι promotes glioma cell survival by phosphorylating and inhibiting the pro-apoptotic BAD protein through the PI3K pathway [165] as well as cell cycle progression and proliferation through PI3K/PKCι/Cdk7/cdk2 signaling [165]. These results suggesting that dysregulation of various PKC isoforms may be involved in gliomagenesis.

Current Treatment Options for Glioblastoma

Standard of Care

Standard therapy for newly diagnosed GBM consists of surgery followed by radiotherapy with concomitant and adjuvant chemotherapy. Complete surgical tumor resection is not possible due to its highly infiltrative growth; however, maximal surgical debulking (optimally > 95%) is performed to maximally reduce tumor size. Subsequent post-operative radiotherapy typically involves the administration of 50 to 60 Gy of irradiation to the whole brain [166]. The main chemotherapeutic agent used for treatment of GBM is temozolomide (TMZ; Temodar®, Temodal®, Shering Plough), an oral alkylating agent with a reasonable penetration of the normal BBB [167]. In circulation, it undergoes rapid conversion to its active derivative 3-methyl-(triazen-1-yl) imidazole-4-carboxamide (MTIC), which exhibits anti-neoplastic activity by adding alkyl groups to DNA, thereby interfering with DNA replication. Furthermore, TMZ causes DNA methylation at the O^6 position of guanine and crosslinks between DNA strands, resulting in cell death [167]. A large randomised clinical trial showed that the median survival in newly diagnosed GBM patients treated with radiation plus TMZ was 14.6 months as opposed to 12.1 months for the radiation-only group [168]. In addition to TMZ, the topoisomerase I inhibitor irinotecan is frequently used to treat GBM patients. Irinotecan has demonstrated efficacy in patients with recurrent GBM, mainly when used in combination with other chemotherapeutic compounds such as TMZ [169].

Despite these optimizations to the adjuvant therapy regimens, the overall survival rate for GBM patients has remained relatively unchanged from ten years ago. Tumors inevitably recur; once they do, life expectancy drastically diminishes, and only limited therapeutic options are available. Major advances in molecular and cell biology have afforded the development of novel second and third line therapies for GBM patients in the realm of target therapy. To date, targeted therapy has been used effectively against breast tumors driven by growth factor receptor dysregulation, and, in the case of GBM, therapies directed against a number of growth factors and receptors (i.e., EGFR, PDGFR, and VEGFR) are in various stages of clinical development. Table 1 lists the current EGFR, PDGFR and VEGFR pathway-targeted agents for the treatment of GBM, which include monoclonal antibodies, tumor –antigen specific vaccines, small molecules inhibitors and microRNAs.

Table 1. Main molecular targeted agents used in the treatment of glioblastoma

Agent class	Agent name
Agent-EGFR antibodies	Cetuximab, ^{125}I-MAb 425, mAb806
Agent-PDGFR antibodies	IB3, IMC-2C5
Agent- VEGFR antibodies	Bevacizumab, aflibercept/VEGF-Trap
EGF vaccines	CDX-110, EGFR-lytic-type peptide
PDGF vaccines	PDGFβ
VEGF vaccines	FLK-1-based DNA, FLK-*salmonella typhimurium*
EGF-TKIs	Erlotinib, gefitinib, lapatanib, PKI166, canertinib, pelitinib
PDGF-TKIs	Imatinib
VEGF-TKIs	Sunitinib, vandetanib, sorafenid, cediranib, vatalanib
EGF- miRNAs	miR-7
PDGF- miRNAs	miR-34a
VEGF- miRNAs	miRNA-205
RAS/RAF/MAPKs TK inhibitors	Tipifarnib, ionofarnib
PI3K/Akt/mTOR TK inhibitors	Rapamycin, temsirolimus, sirolimus, everolimus, AP23573
PKC TK inhibitors	Tamoxifen, enzastaurin

EGF, epidermal growth factor; PDGF, platelet-derived growth factor, VEGF, vascular endothelial growth factor, and their respective receptors EGFR, VEGFR and PDGR; TK, tyrosine kinase.

Targeting Growth Factors in GBM

Monoclonal antibodies. Cancer immunotherapy seeks to manipulate a person's own immune system to recognize and specifically destroy tumor cells, using target-specific antigenic proteins and peptides [170]. Although tumor immunotherapy has shown some success in the treatment of several cancers such as renal cell carcinoma, melanoma, and hematologic cancers, the application of this approach to GBM presents more of a challenge [171]. Limitations include possible hindrance in the drug's ability to cross the BBB and induction of potential autoimmunity, which could lead to severe and undesired effects such as central nervous system toxicity [171]. In the early 1900s, Paul Erhlich was the first to propose the process of using monoclonal antibodies to target tumors, and later, advances in antibody technology afforded the production of human monoclonal antibodies [172]. One method of inhibiting grown factor–mediated signaling is to disrupt receptor-activating ligand binding [171]. Blocking ligand binding to its cognate receptor could normalize the growth rate, induce apoptosis and increase tumor susceptibility to chemotherapeutic agents.

EGF. Monoclonal antibodies, unconjugated and conjugated, directed against wtEGFR and EGFRvIII have been developed for therapeutic use in GBM. The most advanced unconjugated antibody is cetuximab (Erbitux®; Merck), which is a human/murine chimeric monoclonal antibody that binds to the extracellular domain III of EGFR. This interaction partially blocks the ligand-binding domain and sterically hinders the correct extended conformation of the dimerization arm on domain II. Thus, cetuximab prevents EGFR-mediated signal transduction by interfering with ligand binding and EGFR extracellular dimerization with other HER family members [171]. It has been reported that cetuximab induces cell cycle arrest in the G_1 phase of the cell cycle by increasing $p27^{KIP1}$ expression in cancer cell lines and human tumor xenografts. This increased expression leads to the formation of $p27^{KIP1}$-Cdk2 complexes and the prevention of cells from exiting the G_1 phase of the cell cycle [171,173]. Furthermore, cetuximab induces a decrease in the expression of pro-angiogenic factors and inhibition in the invasion and metastatic spread of tumor cells [174,175]. In addition, cetuximab treatment induces the up-regulation of various pro-apoptotic factors such as Bax and the down-regulation of Bcl-2, leading to caspase activation and tumor cell death [176,177]. It has also been suggested that cetuximab binds to and internalizes EGFRvIII. This internalization induces an 80% reduction in the active form of EGFRvIII [178]. Preclinical data suggest that the combination of radiotherapy, TMZ and cetuximab can lead to additive cytotoxic effects in glioma cell lines [178,179]. This combination is currently being explored in an on-going phase I/II trial [180].

With respect to conjugated antibodies, ^{125}I-MAb425 is one of the most advanced radioisotope-conjugated monoclonal anti-EGFR antibodies. Various phase II clinical trials have reported that ^{125}I-MAb 425, either administered alone or combined with radiotherapy or TMZ, significantly improves the median survival in GBM patients [181,182]. Some monoclonal antibodies have been engineered to specifically target EGFRvIII. One such antibody is mAb806, which attenuates receptor autophosphorylation by binding to the short cysteine loop of the extracellular domain that is always exposed in EGFRvIII, and it may also weakly target amplified wtEGFR, which transiently exposes this epitope during the switch from the inactive to the ligand-activated conformation [183]. Pre-clinical data show that systemic administration of mAb806 inhibits the growth of intracranial glioma xenografts and, more weakly, of tumors that express wtEGFR [184]. Mechanistically, *in vivo* mAb806 treatment results in reduced phosphorylation of the constitutively active EGFR and causes down-regulated expression of the apoptotic protector, Bcl-XL [184]. In the clinic, it is well tolerated and displays excellent biodistribution and specificity for its target in GBM patients [185]. These promising results have prompted a phase I clinical trial with a humanized version of mAb806.

PDGF. PDGF and its receptor play important roles in tumorigenesis through stimulating tumor growth and promoting angiogenesis via enhancing pericyte recruitment and vessel maturation. Several antagonistic antibodies to PDGFRs have been developed as potential antitumor agents and have demonstrated promising antitumor activity in both preclinical and clinical settings. Shen et al. have reported the development of antibodies directed against mouse (IB3) and human (IMC-2C5) PDGFRβ that blocks the binding of PDGFR-BB to its receptor. The antibodies also block ligand-stimulated PDGFRβ activation and down-stream signaling molecules including AKT and MAPK p42/44 [186,187]. In animal studies, both antibodies significantly delay growth in various tumor xenograft models [186,187]. The authors have suggested that the efficacy of IB3 and IMC-2C5 is due to its effects on the tumor stroma rather than on the tumor cells directly. Furthermore, they have shown that each antibody enhances the anti-tumor and anti-angiogenic activities of DC101, an antibody directed against VEGFR2 [186,187]. These finding lend great support to the use of PDGFRβ antagonists in combination with other anti-tumor and/to anti-angiogenic agents in the treatment of a broad range of human cancers such as GBM.

VEGF. The use of monoclonal antibodies against the VEGF pathway has played a large role in cancer therapy. Bevacizumab (Avastin, Genentech) is a humanized monoclonal antibody that targets VEGF-A, thereby preventing activation of the VEGFR and the subsequent signaling cascade involved in tumor angiogenesis. In preclinical studies, bevacizumab inhibits angiogenesis and human GBM growth in flank and intracranial xenograft models [188,189]. In tumor xenograft models, bevacizumab administration in combination with RT inhibits tumor growth with an additive effect compared with treatment with bevacizumab or radiation alone [190,191]. The main mechanism by which bevacizumab may enhance the radiation response is by increasing tumor oxygenation through vascular normalization and by improving intratumoral perfusion, as shown in GBM cell lines and in orthotopic U87 GBM xenografts [192,193]. In addition, it has been reported that the combination of bevacizumab with TMZ increases the antitumor efficacy of TMZ in a human GBM orthotopic xenograft model [192]. Bevacizumab received accelerated approval as a monotherapy for the treatment of recurrent GBM in 2009 by the US Food and Drug Administration (FDA) based on radiographic response rates of 26-61% and 6-month progression-free survival rates (PFS6) of 20-50% in two phase II trials. In both studies, bevacizumab administration reduced the peritumoral edema and the need for corticosteroids in the majority of patients. Based on these results, bevacizumab is now widely used in the US for the treatment of recurrent GBM. In general, bevacizumab is well tolerated, with low incidences of intratumoral hemorrhage (2–3%) and only a modest increase in the incidence of venous thromboembolism and bowel perforation [194,195]. Multiple phase II/III clinical trials of bevacizumab in combination with chemotherapy with or without radiation are ongoing in GBM. Despite an initial responsiveness, the beneficial effects of bevacizumab are transient, and GBM inevitably progress during anti-VEGF treatment by adapting and utilizing alternative pathways to sustain tumor growth, all while VEGF signaling remains inhibited [196]. It has been reported that inhibition of VEGF signaling by bevacizumab leads to the activation of MET and a pro-invasive phenotype in mouse models of GBM. Lu et al. demonstrated that VEGF directly and negatively regulates tumor cell invasion through the enhanced PTP1B recruitment to a MET/VEGFR2 hetero-complex, thereby suppressing HGF-dependent MET phosphorylation as well as tumor migration in a hypoxia-independent manner [196]. In addition, Lucio-Eterovic et al. have shown that anti-VEGF therapy (bevacizumab) promotes the expression of multiple pro-angiogenic (fibroblast growth factor (FGFs), interleukins and angiogenin), pro-invasive (metalloproteinase (MMP)-2, MMP-9, MMP-12), and tissue inhibitor of metalloproteinase 1 (TIMP-1) factors, which are important for the degradation of tumor stroma, for the release of VEGF and other pro-angiogenic factors bound to the ECM and for facilitating tumor invasion in an orthotopic glioma model [197]. These findings suggest that the combination of angiogenesis inhibitors with therapies targeting the invasive components of the tumor may produce a more efficacious therapeutic effect in GBM. In addition to bevacizumab, another anti-VEGF agent, Aflibercept /VEGF-Trap, has been developed by incorporating the domains of VEGFR-1 and VEGFR-2 fused to the Fc fragment of IgG1, which acts as a soluble decoy receptor for VEGF. VEGF-Trap has a high affinity for VEGF-A, VEGF-B and placental growth factor (PlGF), which are implicated in pathological angiogenesis [198]. In preclinical studies, VEGF-Trap improved survival in an orthotopic GBM model [199] and enhanced the activity of radiation therapy [200]. A phase I study evaluating VEGF-Trap with radiation therapy and TMZ for patients with newly diagnosed malignant glioma is ongoing. In addition to anti-angiogenesis therapy, IMC-1121B (ramucirumab) is another fully human monoclonal antibody directed against the extracellular domain of VEGFR2, which blocks the interaction of VEGF2 with VEGF and prevents pro-angiogenic signaling [201]. In preclinical studies, IMC-1121B blocked the proliferation and migration of human ECs *in vitro* and has shown efficacy in mouse leukemia models. In phase I dose-escalation studies in patients with solid tumors, the single agent IMC-1121B was tolerated and preliminary evidence of antitumor activity was observed [202]. A phase II trial of ramucirumab is underway for recurrent GBM.

Vaccines. Cancer vaccines represent promising GBM therapies. Vaccination with cytokine-transfected tumor cells, adoptive transfer of tumor-activated T cells, and administration of antigen-pulsed dendritic cell (DC) vaccines have all been associated with enhanced immunity and/or favorable clinical outcomes [203].

The EGFRvIII-specific vaccine (PEP-3-KLH; CDX-110) is a 14-mer peptide (H-Leu-Glu-Glu-Lys-Lys-Gln-Asn-Tyr-Val-Val-Thr-Asp-His-Cys-OH) coupled to keyhole limpet haemocyanin (KLH) directed against a novel glycine epitope at the fusion junction that arises as a consequence of the in-frame deletion of exons 2–7 from the extracellular domain of wtEGFR [203]. The proposed mechanism of action for tumor regression is believed to initiate with peptide capture by the antigen-presenting complex (APC). The peptide is then relocated into the most proximal lymph nodes, where the antigenic peptide is presented to circulating cytotoxic T-lymphocytes (CTLs), which are then activated upon recognition and finally infiltrate the tumor to eliminate the respective cancer cells [204,205]. Rodents with EGFRvIII-positive tumors subcutaneously or intracerebrally showed significant tumor reduction and increased survival rates after administration of dendritic cells (DCs) with the EGFRvIII synthetic peptide conjugated to KLH [206]. A dendritic cell (DC)–based vaccine targeting the EGFRvIII antigen was evaluated in adults with GBM. EGFRvIII-specific immune responses were evident in most patients, with an increase in overall median survival time (22.8 vs. 15.2 months) without severe adverse events [207]. Furthermore, the evaluation of PEP-3-KLH in combination with TMZ showed a significant improvement of PFS (14.2 vs. 7.3 months) and median survival (26 vs. 15.2 months) [203]. From these results, it has been proposed that vaccination with PEP-3-KLH is safe and capable of inducing EGFRvIII-specific immune responses in patients with a newly diagnosed primary GBM.

A vaccine recognizing wtEGFR has also been designed, in which an EGFR-binding peptide is conjugated with a lytic-type peptide containing cationic-rich amino acids that kills the cancer cell through disintegration of the cell membrane [208]. It has been proposed that the EGFR binding moiety of the hybrid peptide binds to EGFR on the cell surface, and then, the lytic moiety of this peptide penetrates to form a pore and disrupt the cell membrane. *In vitro* studies have shown that the EGFR-lytic peptide induces apoptosis in cancer cells and exerts strong cytotoxicity against tyrosine kinase inhibitors-resistant cancer cells. Furthermore, it is effective in suppressing the growth of both breast and pancreatic xenografts [208]. It has been demonstrated that a single replacement of histidine to arginine in the lytic peptide sequence enhances its anticancer activity [209]. These results suggest a potential value for this therapy against GBMs.

The tumor stroma contains several potential therapeutic targets including reactive fibroblasts and pericytes, which over-express PDGFβ in several neoplasms. Kaplan et al. described for the first time a novel strategy for achieving protection against tumor growth and metastasis with an orally delivered murine PDGFRβ (mPDGFRβ)-based DNA vaccine in colon, breast and lung carcinoma. This vaccine suppresses angiogenesis *in vivo* and reduces the intratumoral expression of PDGFβ and NG2 [210]. The authors suggest that this vaccine can be used in tumors that over-express PDGFβ such as gliomas.

Zhou et al. reported an alternative strategy with an oral DNA vaccine that encodes the VEGFR2 (FLK-1) gene, which prevents effective angiogenesis and inhibits tumor growth significantly through $CD8^+$ T cell-mediated immune responses. $CD8^+$ CTLs have the ability to specifically detect and kill antigen-bearing cells. They recognize antigens in the form of 8 to 10 amino acid-long peptides that are presented to T-cell receptors (TCRs) on the cell surface as complexes with major histocompatibility complex (MHC) class I molecules. These peptides, usually referred to as CTL epitopes, are generated in the cell cytosol after proteolytic processing of the antigen by the proteasome [211]. One of the primary aims of tumor vaccines is to induce $CD8^+$ CTL responses against such epitopes to eradicate tumors and prevent relapse. The induction of a more effective antigen-specific immune response by DNA vaccines requires vaccine design optimization including novel approaches for vaccine delivery and effective antigen processing. Such strategies include the use of an oral carrier system with a double-attenuated strain of *Salmonella typhimurium* (*dam; AroA*⁻), which delivers the DNA to secondary lymphoid organs for subsequent transcription, translation and antigen processing [212]. Feng et al. demonstrated that an attenuated *salmonella typhimurium* vaccine strain expressing the FLK gene inhibits GBM growth, reduces vessel density and improves the survival rate in mice. The study also demonstrated that the vaccine could break peripheral immune tolerance in glioma against this self-antigen, kill endothelial cells by the orally administered vaccine and can be used for both prophylactic and therapeutic purposes [213]. In addition, Feng et al. reported that the anti-angiogenic effect and the anti-tumor effect were better with the combination of an orally administered FLK-1-based DNA vaccine and an immunomodulatory interleukin gene (IL-12) than either alone on gliomas, suggesting that the vaccine reduces the tumor environment to a necrotic or apoptotic state. This action may not only serve to reduce the number of viable tumor cells but may also enhance the availability of tumor-associated antigens for the presentation by scavenging APCs. The inclusion of IL-2 activates immune effector cells including dendritic, NK and T cells and also initiates an IFN-γ-induced cytokine cascade, resulting in antiangiogenic and pro-T cell chemotactic generation, which may enhance specific CTLs against the FLK-1-based DNA vaccine. Furthermore, the authors suggest that further studies will be conducted to validate the extendibility of the treatment in other tumor models [214].

Small Molecule Inhibitors

Small molecule tyrosine kinase inhibitors (TKIs) are the most clinically advanced of the EGFR-targeted therapies, and both reversible and irreversible inhibitors are in clinical trials. Some of the reversible inhibitors include erlotinib (Tarceva®/OSI774; Genentech), gefitinib (Iressa®/ZD1839; AstraZeneca), lapatanib (Tykerb®; GlaxoSmithKline) and PKI166 (Novartis); the irreversible inhibitors include canertinib (CI1033; Pfizer/Warner-Lambert) and pelitinib (EKB-569; Wyest-Ayerst) [215]. They act by binding to the catalytic site in the TK domain, competing with ATP. This event inhibits the activating autophosphorylation of the receptor itself and in turn prevents the recruitment of downstream signaling proteins [216]. Of these inhibitors, gefinitib and erlotinib represent the best-explored TKI in the clinic for the treatment of GBM.

In pre-clinical *in vitro* studies, erlotinib inhibits EGF-dependent proliferation of cells at submicromolar concentrations and blocks cell-cycle progression in the G_1 phase [217], inhibits anchorage-independent growth and decreases the expression of EGFR mRNA[218]. In addition, long-term exposure to erlotinib down-regulates the expression of EGFRvIII and the molecular effectors of tumor invasion in glioma cells [219]. Furthermore, erlotinib enhances radiation-induced apoptosis in human solid tumor cell lines and in human tumor xenografts [220]. In a recent randomised phase I/II trial of erlotinib vs. TMZ or carmustine among recurrent GBM patients, the PFS-6 was 11.4% in the erlotinib group compared with 24% in the TMZ and carmustine groups [221], whereas in another phase II trial, the combination of erlotinib with TMZ before and after RT showed an increased median survival (19.1 months) relative to historical controls (14.1 months). Mellinghoff et al. reported that the responsiveness to erlitinib in patients with GBM appears to be dependent on the co-expression of EGFRvIII and the tumor suppressor gene PTEN [222].

Gefitinib as well as erlotinib inhibits the *in vitro* growth of a variety of human cancer cell lines through similar mechanisms [223]. Carrasco-Garcia et al. reported that gefitinib induces G_1 arrest in association with a reduction in the steady-state levels of proteins involved in the G_1 checkpoint (cyclin D1, cyclin D3, cdk6, cdk4 and cdk2) and an increase in cdk inhibitor protein levels ($p27^{KIP1}$ and $p21^{CIP/WAF}$) [224]. This group also reported that gefitinib interrupts EGFR signaling by interacting with ERBB-3, inhibiting the ERK1/2 and AKT activity in glioma cell lines [224]. In addition, it has been reported that stem-like glioma-spheres were sensitive to gefitinib effects, which enhanced radiosensitivity and increased cytotoxicity through the inhibition of EGFR-AKT activation and DNA-PKcs expression, accompanied by enhanced irradiation-induced DNA DSBs/ inhibition of DNA DSB repair [225]. Initial clinical studies have reported that gefitinib is well tolerated at effective doses [226]; however, it induces an acne form of skin rash and diarrhea. In phase I/II studies, 12.7% of GBM patients treated with gefitinib showed a partial tumor regression, although the median times to progression were no better than historic controls [227]. In another study for recurrent GBM, the median progression-free survival was 2 months, the PFS at 6 months was 13%, and the median overall survival (OS) was 10 months, with no observed radiographic response [226]. Another phase II study by the North Central Cancer Treatment Group noted some radiographic responses but no superior survival benefits [227].

The PDGFR inhibitor (Imatinib mesylate (STI571, Gleevec®, Novartis Pharmaceuticals) is a kinase inhibitor of PDGFRα, PDGFRβ, the stem cell factor c-Kit, the non-receptor protein tyrosine kinase C-abl and breast cancer resistance protein (BCRP) [228,229]. Preclinical studies have demonstrated that imatinib inhibits the growth of human GBM cell lines and prolongs the survival of nude mice with intracranial GBM cell implants [229]. Imatinib inhibits growth by cell cycle arrest through disrupting the PDGF receptor autocine loop [230]. Furthermore, it has been reported that imatinib sensitizes human GBM cells to ionizing radiation [231]. It has also been reported that the combination of imatinib and docetaxel has a synergistic antitumor effect on glioma cells by inhibiting proliferation and invasion [232]. Preclinical evidence suggests that imatinib may enhance chemosensitivity by several possible mechanisms, including decreasing interstitial fluid pressure and angiogenesis, affecting DNA repair mechanisms and stromal chemokines [233]. Clinical studies evaluating imatinib as a monotherapy in relapsed GBM showed a minimal clinical benefit with a radiographic response rate of <6% and a PFS-6 of <16% [233]. The low response to treatment could be due to the limited permeability of imitinib into the brain. In mice, only 20% of imitinib crosses the BBB; the other 80% is effluxed by BCRP and P-glycoprotein (PGP) [234]. However, it has been reported that the combination of imatinib mesylate and hydroxyurea shows promising results [234]. These initial results were supported in a phase II trial in patients with recurrent GBM, which reported a PFS-6 of 27% and a median PFS of 14 weeks; 42% of patients had stable radiologic disease at a median follow-up of 58 weeks [235]. The mechanism of action of this combination is still unknown, but it has been shown that imatinib decreases the interstitial tumor pressure and may increase delivery of hydroxyurea into the tumor microenvironment and enhance its antitumor activity, which provides a possible explanation for the initial success associated with this combination [236]. Unfortunately, a phase III trial did not provide further evidence of efficacy [236].

A number of VEGFR inhibitors have been examined: sunitinib (SU11248, Sutent®, Pfizer), which is directed against VEGFR, PDGFR, RET, c-kit and Flt-3; vandetanib (ZD6474, Zactima™, AstraZeneca), directed against VEGFR2, EGFR and RET; sorafenid (Nexavar®, Bayer), directed against VEGFR, PDGF and Raf; cediranib (AZD2171, Zactima™, AstraZeneca), directed against VEGFR, PDGFR and c-Kit and vatalanib (PTK787/ZK 222584, Novartis and Schering), directed against VEGFR1 (Flt-1), VEGFR2 (KDR) and VEGFR3 (Flt-4) and can also inhibit PDGFRβ.

Preclinical studies suggest that sunitinib in an organotypic malignant glioma brain slice model enhances apoptosis and decreases tumor cell proliferation, angiogenesis and invasion through the partial phosphorylation of SRC and FAK, while sunitinib treatment in U87MG intracranial xenografts resulted in growth delay and diminished microvessel density [237]. Chahal et al. demonstrated that sunitinib decreases proliferation and survival of O^6-methylguanine methyltransferase (MGMT)-transfected U87MG cells treated with radiotherapy alone, TMZ alone or the combination, but does not affect U87MG MGMT-negative cells [238]. It has also been shown that sunitinib augments chemotherapy cytotoxicity in a flank xenograft GBM model [239]. Furthermore, it can enhance the intratumoral delivery of TMZ in intracranial malignant glioma models, consistent with vascular normalization. The combined treatment may aggravate pericyte-mediated vascular resistance mechanisms by altering Ang-1-Tie-2 and Dll4/Notch pathways [240]. However, a clinical study of sunitinib in recurrent malignant glioma patients did not observe any objective radiographic responses, which were associated with a median PFS of only 1.6 months [241]. It has also has been reported that the combination of sunitinib and irinotecan in recurrent malignant glioma patients is associated with moderate toxicity and limited anti-tumor activity [242].

It has been reported that vandetanib shows a better inhibition of cell growth and survival in cells that express EGFRvIII through attenuated phosphorylation of STAT 3, AKT, and Bcl-X_L expression. These data showed that vandetanib significantly inhibits growth and angiogenesis of glioma cells that express EGFRvIII by blocking EGFRvIII-activated signaling mediators [243]. Albeit to a lesser extent, vandetanib also suppresses cells that overexpress wtEGFR [243]. The synergistic effect of vandetanib has also been studied. Jane et al. reported that vandetanib synergistically potentiates histone deacetylase inhibitor-induced apoptosis in human glioma cells [244]. Furthermore, Jo et al. reported that the combination of TMZ and vandetanib effectively reduces GBM tumor volume through antiangiogenic and antiproliferative mechanisms [245]. Phase I studies have demonstrated that vandetanib can be safely combined with RT and TMZ in GBM patients [243]. Patients with recurrent GBM and anaplastic gliomas were treated with vandetanib in a phase II trial; PFS-6 was 6.5% in the GBM group and 7.0% in the astrocytic glioma group. The median overall survival was 6.3 months in the GBM group and 7.6 months in the astrocytic glioma group [246].

Sorafenib significantly induces apoptosis through the down-regulation of anti-apoptotic proteins (Bcl-2 and Mcl-1) in human GBM cell lines [247]. It has also been demonstrated that sorafenid reduces proliferation of GBM cultures, and this effect depends, at least in part, on the inhibition of PI3K/AKT and MAPK signaling, both of which are involved in gliomagenesis [247]. In addition Carra et al. demonstrated that sorafenib has a selective action on GBM stem cells, causing enrichment of cultures in differentiated cells, down-regulation of the expression of stemness markers required to maintain malignancy (nestin, Olig2 and Sox2) and reducing cell clonogenic ability *in vitro* and tumorigenic potential *in vivo* [247]. It has also been reported that mice treated with sorafenid showed significant inhibition of glioma cell proliferation, increased apoptosis and autophagy and suppression of angiogenesis *in vivo* [248]. Furthermore, sorafenib inhibits proliferation synergistically in combination with bortezomib, a proteasome inhibitor, and rottlerin, an experimental inhibitor of PKC [249]. A phase II trial found that first-line TMZ and radiotherapy followed by TMZ plus sorafenib is tolerated by patients with GBM, although the preliminary efficacy data for this regimen (median PFS duration, 6 months; 12-month PFS rate, 16%) are similar to the data for standard therapy [250].

Batchelor et al. demonstrated that cediranib achieved a radiographic response rate of 50% and a median PFS of 16 weeks among recurrent GBM patients [251]. Furthermore, using a constellation of sophisticated imaging modalities, the authors demonstrated that patients treated with cediranib exhibited radiographic findings consistent with the hypothesis that antiangiogenic agents can transiently normalize tumor vasculature [252]. However, in both studies, the benefits of cediranib for gliomas are typically transient and followed by an apparent increase in tumor burden [251,252]. In addition, imaging studies suggest that GBM progression may not be visible on contrast enhanced MRI [253]. Moreover, preclinical studies suggest a "wave" or tumor re-vascularization after discontinuation of anti-VEGF therapy, which might accelerate tumor relapse [254-257]. Di Tomaso et al. compared molecular, cellular and vascular parameters in autopsy tissues from recurrent GBM patients treated with cediranib vs. control patients. After cediranib treatment, endothelial proliferation and glomeruloid vessels were decreased and vessel diameters and perimeters were reduced to levels comparable to the unaffected contralateral brain hemisphere. In addition, tumor endothelial cells expressed molecular markers specific to the BBB, indicative of a lack of revascularization despite the therapy discontinuation. Surprisingly, in cediranib-treated GBM, the cellular density in the central area of the tumor was lower than in control cases and gradually decreased toward the infiltrating edge, indicative of a change in growth pattern of recurrent GBMs after cediranib treatment. Finally, cediranib-treated GBM showed high levels of PDGF-C and MET expression and infiltration by myeloid cells, which may potentially contribute to resistance to anti-VEGF therapy. In summary, the authors show that recurrent GBMs switch their growth pattern after anti-VEGF therapy, as characterized by lower tumor cellularity in the central area, decreased pseudopalisading necrosis, and blood vessels with normal molecular expression and morphology, without a second wave of angiogenesis [258].

In preclinical models, vatalanib significantly decreased VEGF-mediated glioma growth by inhibiting neovascularization and proliferation [259]. Furthermore, it has been shown that vatalanib, with other chemotherapeutics, improves the survival time, inhibits the tumor volume, decreases the number of PCNA-positive proliferating cells, increases the number of apoptotic cells and inhibits tumor angiogenesis [260]. In a study of 47 patients with recurrent GBM treated as vatalanib, a partial response of 4% and stability of disease in 56% were obtained [261]. Although the combination of vatalanib with either TMZ or lomustine was well tolerated in phase I/II trials, the anti-tumor efficacy was modest. Among the 51 evaluable patients, 8% had a partial response, and 53% were stable; the median time to progression was 16 weeks for patients in the TMZ group and 10 weeks for patients in the lomustine group [262].

Micro RNAs- miRNAs are highly conserved noncoding RNAs that control gene expression post-transcriptionally through the degradation of target mRNAs or the inhibition of protein translation. miRNAs are now emerging as master regulators that act as either an oncogene or a tumor suppressor or even affect both phases of tumorigenesis. Each miRNA is thought to control the expression of multiple mRNA targets, and they have been shown to be involved in the initiation and progression of human cancer. As they control important processes such as differentiation, cell growth and cell death, miRNAs hold great promise for targeted cancer therapy.

EGF- Low expression levels of miR-7 have been found in GBM compared with the normal brain [263]. Yang et al. reported that miR-7 significantly inhibits glioma cell line proliferation, partially silences EGFR post-transcriptional translation and reduces EGFR activity and function [264]. Furthermore, Kefas et al. reported that GBM cells transfected with miR-7 undergo apoptosis (cleaved poly(ADP-ribose) polymerase) and show reduced invasion through decreased levels of EGFR and upstream regulators of the AKT pathway, insulin receptor substrate 1 (IRS1) and 2 (IRS2). The authors suggest that miR-7 regulates the EGFR and AKT pathways [263]. It has also been suggested that miR-7 may be a useful therapeutic target for overcoming the radio-resistance of human cancers with activated EGFR-PI3K-AKT signaling and that miR-7 could regulate the EGFR and AKT pathways [265]. In addition, miR-7 over-expression inhibits invasion and migration, and miR-7 modulates FAK expression directly by binding the 3'UTR of FAK mRNA. Furthermore, miR-7 represses p-ERK1/2 and p-AKT levels and MMP-2 and MMP-9 expression levels [266]. Animal experiments have shown that neither liposome- or adenovirus-transfected miR-7 can effectively inhibit human malignant glioma growth *in vivo* [267]. These data suggest that miR-7-based gene treatment may be a novel anti-invasion therapeutic strategy for malignant glioma.

PDGF- miR-34a was originally identified as a likely tumor suppressor miRNA and a downstream transcriptional target of p53 [268,269]. Several reports have shown that miR-34a is downregulated in GBM compared with normal brain, and it inhibits cell proliferation, survival, and invasion in adherent glioma cell lines by targeting MET, NOTCH1, NOTCH2 and CDK6 [270-272]. In addition, miR-34a appears to promote differentiation in glioma cells grown in stem-like conditions [273]. Silber et al. demonstrated that the induction of miR-34a inhibits the growth of proneural glioma cells *in vitro* and *in vivo* and that the PDGF-driven miR-34a repression is unlikely to operate solely through a p53-dependent mechanism [274]. However, Li et al. reported that miR-34a expression is higher in wild-type p53 GBM tissues than in mutant p53 GBM tissues [275]. In addition, transient transfection of miR-34a into glioma and medulloblastoma cell lines strongly inhibits cell proliferation, cell cycle progression, survival and invasion by targeting multiple oncogenes [275]. Transient expression of miR-34a in GBM cells strongly inhibited *in vivo* glioma xenograft growth [275].

VEGF- miRNA-205 is significantly down-regulated in glioma cell lines and tissue specimens. Hou et al. showed that the ectopic expression of miRNA-205 induces apoptosis, cell cycle arrest, impairs cell viability, clonability and invasive properties of glioma cells. The authors further demonstrate that miRNA-205 can specifically suppress VEGF expression by directly interacting with the putative miRNA-205 binding site at the 3'-UTR [276]. Therefore, identification of VEGF as a direct target for miRNA-205 may indicate that miRNA-205 is a novel target for glioma therapy

Targeting Downstream Intracellular Effector Molecules

The RAS/RAF/MAPK Pathway

To transmit signals, RAS must attach to the plasma membrane, and this event is dependent upon the post-translational addition of a farnesyl group to the C-terminal amino acid group known as farnesylation/palmitoylation (CKCVLS) of H-RAS signaling (CAAX) box by the enzyme farnesyl-transferase [277,278]. Farnesyl transferase inhibitors (FTIs) block RAS-mediated signaling; they may also inhibit signaling through other pathways requiring farnesylation including Rho B and the PI3K/AKT pathway [279]. Farnesyltransferase inhibitors (FTIs) such tipifarnib (R115777, Zarnestra™; Ortho Biotech Products) and lonafarnib (SCH66336, Sarasar™; Schering-Plough) are the inhibitors more frequently studied in RAS signaling in the clinic for the treatment of GBM.

Tipifarnib- It has been reported that tipifarnib is a radiosensitive that induces postmitotic necrotic cell death of radioresistant glioma cells [280]. However, Delmas et al. reported that tipifarnib reduces HIF1α intracellular levels and MMP-2 activity, leading to intrinsic radioresistance, hypoxia and angiogenesis in glioma cells and glioma xenografts [281]. In a recent phase II trial, tipifarnib showed only modest activity, with a PFS6 of 12% in recurrent GBM and 9% in patients with anaplastic glioma [282], and another study was stopped early due to disease progression in 48% of patients, where tipifarnib administration prior to irradiation in patients with newly diagnosed GBM and residual enhancing disease did not result in survival improvements [283].

Ionofarnib- Glass et al. demonstrated that ionofarnib inhibits viability and anchorage-independent growth in a time- and dose-dependent manner in GBM cell lines through of the down-regulation of phospho-MAPK, whereas EGFR overexpression appears to alter cellular sensitivity to farnesyltransferase inhibitors [284]. In addition, ionofarnib inhibits the growth of human GBM explant xenografts in NOD-SCID mice [284]. Ionofarnib improves the activity of temozolomide and radiation for orthotopic malignant gliomas [285]. A phase I study of ionofarniband TMZ in patients with recurrent GBM reported that 27% of patients who were previously resistant to temozolomide showed a partial response to both treatments with a PFS-6 rate of 38%, a median PFS of 3.9 months, and a median disease-specific survival of 13.7 months [286]. These studies demonstrate that TMZ can be safely combined with a farnesyltransferase inhibitor and that this regimen is active, although the current study cannot determine the relative contributions of the two agents or the contribution of the novel administration schedule [286].

Targeting the PI3K/Akt/mTOR Pathway

LY294002, a PI3K inhibitor, sensitizes glioma cell lines to radiation [287]. Direct AKT inhibitors have been difficult to develop and have not been tested in glioma clinical trials. As an alternative, agents directed at the mTOR pathway have been developed [288]. The classic mTOR inhibitor is rapamycin, initially developed as an immunosuppressant for patients undergoing transplantation. This agent works by forming a complex that binds to mTOR and inhibits its kinase activity, resulting in G_1 cell-cycle arrest [289]. Preclinical studies have shown that rapamycin is cytostatic against xenografts of glioblastoma and medulloblastoma [290]. Compared with PTEN-positive tumors, PTEN-negative tumors appear to be more sensitive to inhibition by rapamycin [289].

mTOR inhibitors- Several inhibitors of the mTOR are being investigated in clinical trials [291,292]. These agents include temsirolimus (CCI-779; Torisel®; Wyeth), sirolimus (Rapamune®; Wyeth), everolimus (RAD001, Certican®; Novartis) and AP23573 (ARIAD).

Temsirolimus is a lipid soluble analogue of rapamycin that inhibits mTOR by binding to immunophilin FK-506 binding protein 12 (FKBP-12), inducing cell cycle arrest and decreasing the growth of several human cancer cell lines [293]. Temsirolimus in a mouse model of PDGF-B-driven, low-grade gliomas demonstrated an antiproliferative effect [294]. Furthermore, Hu et al. demonstrated that mTOR blockage with temsirolimus resulted in regional apoptosis and conversion in the character of the surviving tumor cells from astrocytoma to oligodendroglioma in a mouse model of Akt+KRas-induced GBM. There are other reports that have shown the pro-apoptotic effects of rapamycin [295]; however, there are also data indicating that it promotes cell survival [293]. In a phase II study, temsirolimus administration to patients with progressive GBM was well tolerated, with some objective responses [291]. High levels of phosphorylated ribosomal S6 kinase at baseline appeared to correlate with treatment response. Radiographic improvement was evident in some patients, although the PFS6 was only 7.8% and 2.5% in two studies [291,292]. These studies suggest that temsirolimus has limited activity in glioblastomas as a monotherapy; no obvious subpopulation of patients who could benefit from treatment has been reliably identified.

More recently, based on evidence of the synergism between mTOR inhibitors and EGFR TKIs [296], on-going trials have been exploring such a combination [296,297]. In a phase I study, the combination of gefitinib and sirolimus in malignant gliomas found no significant pharmacokinetic interaction between the two drugs, with a partial radiological response and stable disease noted in 2 and 13 of 34 patients, respectively [296]. Similarly, a study combining gefitinib and everolimus failed to find a survival benefit of this combination compared with historical controls, although a radiological response occurred in a 33% of patients [297].

Targeting the PKC Pathway

There are two PKC inhibitors: tamoxifen (Nolvadex, AstraZeneca) and enzastaurin (LY317615, Eli Lilly).

Tamoxifen- It has been reported that tamoxifen inhibits PKC and has antioestrogenic effects [298]. High tamoxifen doses have demonstrated anti-tumor activity in glioma xenografts [298] but have failed to show benefit in clinical trials [299]. In an attempt to increase clinical efficacy, tamoxifen has been combined with many other standard chemotherapeutic regimens such as low-dose TMZ without clear additional benefit to date [300].

Enzastaurin- Enzastaurin is a PKCβ inhibitor that prevents substrate phosphorylation by competing with the enzyme ATP binding site. This agent has demonstrated antiangiogenic activity as well as anti-tumor activity in U87 glioma xenografts and a variety of other solid tumors [301-303]. In addition, this compound inhibits signaling through the PI3K/AKT signaling pathway, suppresses glycogen synthase kinase 3β phosphorylation, induces apoptosis and inhibits proliferation in several cell lines from a variety of human cancers including gliomas, and has antiangiogenic activity [302]. Furthermore, it has been shown that enzastaurin enhances the efficacy of RT by inhibiting unwanted proinvasive and angiogenic effects and enhances TMZ-induced cell death in GBM cell lines [303]. Enzastaurin was well tolerated as a single agent [304], and preliminary results in adult patients with recurrence reported that 22% of patients achieved objective radiographic responses and 5% achieved stable disease. However, intratumoral hemorrhages were noted in several patients [304]. Based on these encouraging results, a phase III study was initiated in adult patients treated with lomustine and enzastaurin in recurrent GBM; however, it was terminated prematurely due to lack of survival benefit of enzastaurin over the control [305]. In a recent phase II study, it was shown that the combination of enzastaurin with TMZ plus radiation therapy in GBM patients was well tolerated with a historic 15-month survival, making enzastaurin a potentially attractive agent to evaluate in combination with other antiangiogenic and cytotoxic agents in patients with malignant glioma [306].

Conclusion

Gliomas are among the most difficult tumors to treat. Their highly invasive nature leads to recurrence even after aggressive therapy of surgery, radiotherapy and chemotherapy. A promising target for new therapies are tyrosine kinases because they regulate a large range of proteins involved in growth, metabolism and differentiation. The TKRs, EGFR, PDGFR and VEGF are often amplified, overexpressed, and/or mutated in gliomas and play an important role in glioma development. A number of agents including multi-targeted kinase inhibitors, monoclonal antibodies, vaccines and microRNAs have been developed and tested in clinical trials with mixed results.

Despite an initial responsiveness, the benefits are typically only transient, and most tumors eventually progress. In a subset of patients, these tumors recur not as enhancing masses, but with a more infiltrative phenotype resembling gliomatosis.

The negative results reported in the majority of published clinical studies may be explained, at least in part, by this single-target approach. Single-target therapies may provide limited effects, as the restricted passage through the BBB. Furthermore, GBM cells may exhibit significant genetic instability, possibly leading to resistance of single-targeted agents by switching to alternative molecular pathways. To improve on the advances made with these agents, it will be critical to identify the mechanisms that determine intrinsic resistance of subsets of GBMs to these agents as well as the mechanisms that develop during therapy that allows the tumor to eventually progress after an initial response. These mechanisms of ‘‘evasive resistance’’ are thought to include the upregulation of alternative pro-angiogenic signals, such as FGF, ephrins and angiopoietins, leading to revascularization, recruitment of vascular progenitor cells and pro-angiogenic inflammatory cells, such as CD11b monocytes, or by the protection of the tumor vasculature by increasing protective pericyte coverage as well as the co-option of normal vasculature and invasion into surrounding tissue.

Tumor cell resistance to these agents strongly indicates that a multiple target approach that can simultaneously inhibit a variety of molecular pathways, including growth factor receptor signaling pathways, DNA damage repair processes, angiogenesis and invasion, will provide a more favorable future for targeted therapies in GBM.

References

[1] Louis DN, Ohgaki H, Wiestler OD, et al. (2007). The 2007 WHO classification of tumours of the central nervous system. *Acta Neuropathol*, 114, 97–109.

[2] CBTRUS. (2012). *CBTRUS Statistical Report: Primary Brain and Central Nervous System Tumors Diagnosed in the United States in 2004-2008.*

[3] Stupp R, Mason WP, Van den Bent MJ, et al. (2005). Radiotherapy plus concomitant and adjuvant temozolomide for glioblastoma. *N Engl J Med*, 352,987-996

[4] Furnari FB, Fenton T, Bachoo RM, et al. (2007). Malignant astrocytic glioma: genetics, biology, and paths to treatment. *Genes Dev*, 21, 2683–710.

[5] Ohgaki H and Kleihues P. (2007). Genetic pathways to primary and secondary glioblastoma. *Am J Pathol*, 170, 1445–1453.

[6] Haas-kogan DA, Prados MD, Tihan T, et al. (2005). Epidermal Growth Factor Receptor, Protein Kinase B/Akt, and Glioma Response to Erlotinib. *J Natl Cancer Inst*, 97, 880–887.

[7] Schlessinger J. (2000). Cell Signaling by Receptor Tyrosine Kinases. *Cell*, 103, 211-225.

[8] Hynes NE and Lane HA. (2005). ERBB receptors and cancer: the complexity of targeted inhibitors. *Nat Rev Cancer*, 5, 341-354.

[9] Omuro AMP, Faivre S, and Raymond E. (2007). Lessons learned in the development of targeted therapy for malignant gliomas. *Mol Cancer Ther*, 6, 1909–1919.

[10] Ziegler DS, Wright RD, Kesari S, et al. (2008). Resistance of human glioblastoma multiforme cells to growth factor inhibitors is overcome by blockade of inhibitor of apoptosis proteins. *J Cli Invest*, 118, 3109-3122.

[11] Schlessinger J. (2002). Ligand-induced, receptor-mediated dimerization and activation of EGF receptor. *Cell*, 110, 669–672.

[12] Bunn PA Jr, Franklin W. (2002). Epidermal growth factor receptor expression, signal pathway, and inhibitors in non–small cell lung cancer. *Semin Oncol*, 29, 38–44.
[13] Salomon DS, Brandt R, Ciardiello F, et al. (1995). Epidermal growth factor-related peptides and their receptors in human malignancies. *Crit Rev Oncol Hematol*, 19, 183–232.
[14] Aldape KD, Ballman K, Furth A, et al. (2004). Immunohistochemical detection of EGFRvIII in high malignancy grade astrocytomas and evaluation of prognostic significance. *J Neuropathol Exp Neurol,* 63, 700–707.
[15] Sugawa N, Ekstrand AJ, Jamest CD, et al. (1990). Identical splicing of aberrant epidermal growth factor receptor transcripts from amplified rearranged genes in human glioblastomas. *Proc Natl Acad Sci USA,* 87, 8602–8606.
[16] Voldborg BR, Damstrup L, Spang-Thomsen M, et al. (1997). Epidermal growth factor receptor (EGFR) and EGFR mutations, function and possible role in clinical trials. *Ann Oncol,* 8, 1197–1206.
[17] Lee JC, Vivanco I, Beroukhim R, et al. (2006). Epidermal growth factor receptor activation in glioblastoma through novel missense mutations in the extracellular domain. *PLoS Med,* 3, e485.
[18] Vaidyanathan G, Affleck DJ, Bigner DD, et al. (2002). Improved xenograft targeting of tumor-specific anti-epidermal growth factor receptor variant III antibody labeled using N-succinimidyl 4-guanidinomethyl-3-iodobenzoate. *Nucl Med Biol,* 29, 1–11.
[19] Weppler SA, Li Y, Dubois L, et al. (2007). Expression of EGFR variant vIII promotes both radiation resistance and hypoxia tolerance. *Radiother Oncol,* 83, 333–339.
[20] Huang HS, Nagane M, Klingbeil CK, et al. (1997). The Enhanced Tumorigenic Activity of a Mutant Epidermal Growth Factor Receptor Common in Human Cancers Is Mediated by Threshold Levels of Constitutive Tyrosine Phosphorylation and Unattenuated Signaling. *J Biol Chem,* 272, 2927–2935.
[21] Wiley, H. Steven. (2003). Trafficking of the ErbB receptors and its influence on signaling. *Experimental Cell Research,* 284, 78–88.
[22] Di Fiore PP and Gill GN. (1999). Endocytosis and mitogenic signaling. *Curr Opin Cell Biol,* 11, 483–488.
[23] Choe G, Horvath S, Cloughesy TF, et al. (2003). Analysis of the Phosphatidylinositol 3′ -Kinase Signaling Pathway in Glioblastoma Patients in Vivo. *Cancer Res*, 63, 2742–2746.
[24] Moscatello DK, Holgado-Madruga M, Emlet DR, et al. (1998). Constitutive Activation of Phosphatidylinositol 3-Kinase by a Naturally Occurring Mutant Epidermal Growth Factor Receptor. *J Biol Chem,* 273, 200–206.
[25] Narita Y, Nagane M, Mishima K, et al. (2002). Mutant Epidermal Growth Factor Receptor Signaling Down-Regulates p27 through Activation of the Phosphatidylinositol 3-Kinase / Akt Pathway in Glioblastomas. *Cancer Res*, 62, 6764–6769.
[26] Tanaka K, Babic I, Nathanson D, et al. (2011). Oncogenic EGFR signaling activates an mTORC2-NF-κB pathway that promotes chemotherapy resistance. *Cancer Discov,* 1, 524–538.
[27] Mukherjee B, McEllin B, Camacho CV, et al. (2009). EGFRvIII and DNA double-strand break repair: a molecular mechanism for radioresistance in glioblastoma. *Cancer Res,* 69, 4252–4259.

[28] Burma S and Chen DJ. (2004). Role of DNA–PK in the cellular response to DNA double-strand breaks. *DNA Repair,* 3, 909–918.

[29] Smith JS, Tachibana I, Passe SM, et al. (2001). PTEN mutation, EGFR amplification, and outcome in patients with anaplastic astrocytoma and glioblastoma multiforme. *J Nat Cancer Inst,* 93, 1246–1256.

[30] Lu KV, Zhu S, Cvrljevic A, et al. (2009). Fyn and SRC are effectors of oncogenic epidermal growth factor receptor signaling in glioblastoma patients. *Cancer Res,* 69, 6889–6898.

[31] Mizoguchi M, Betensky RA, Batchelor TT, et al. (2006). Activation of STAT3, MAPK, and AKT in malignant astrocytic gliomas: correlation with EGFR status, tumor grade, and survival. *J Neuropathol Exp Neurol,* 65, 1181–1188.

[32] Feng H, Hu B, Jarzynka MJ, et al. (2012). Phosphorylation of dedicator of cytokinesis 1 (Dock180) at tyrosine residue Y722 by Src family kinases mediates EGFRvIII-driven glioblastoma tumorigenesis. *Proc Nat Acad Sci USA,* 109, 3018–3023.

[33] Antonyak, MA, Kenyon LC, Godwin AK, et al. (2002). Elevated JNK activation contributes to the pathogenesis of human brain tumors. *Oncogene,* 21, 5038–5046.

[34] Micallef J, Taccone M, Mukherjee J, et al. (2009). Epidermal growth factor receptor variant III-induced glioma invasion is mediated through myristoylated alanine-rich protein kinase C substrate overexpression. *Cancer research,* 69, 7548–7556.

[35] Wu JL, Abe T, Inoue R, et al. (2004). IkappaBalpha suppresses angiogenesis and tumorigenesis promoted by a constitutively active mutant EGFR in human glioma cells. *Neurol Res,* 26, 785–791.

[36] Bonavia R, Inda MM, Vandenberg S, et al. (2012). EGFRvIII promotes glioma angiogenesis and growth through the NF-κB, interleukin-8 pathway. *Oncogene,* 31, 4054–4066.

[37] Kanakaraj P, Raj S, Khan S, et al. (1991). Ligand-induced interaction between alpha- and beta-type platelet-derived growth factor (PDGF) receptors: role of receptor heterodimers in kinase activation. *Biochemistry*, 30, 1761–1767.

[38] Lokker N A, Sullivan C M, Hollenbach S J, et al. (2002). Platelet-derived Growth Factor (PDGF) Autocrine Signaling Regulates Survival and Mitogenic Pathways in Glioblastoma Cells : Evidence That the Novel PDGF-C and PDGF-D Ligands May Play a Role in the Development of Brain Tumors. *Cancer Res*, 62, 3729–35.

[39] Franke TF, Yang S, Chan TO, et al. (1995). The Protein Kinase Encoded by the Akt Proto-Oncogene Is a Target of the PDGF-activated phosphatidylinositol 3-kinase. *Cell,* 81, 727–736.

[40] Katz AM, Amankulor NM, Pitter K, et al. (2012). Astrocyte-specific expression patterns associated with the PDGF-induced glioma microenvironment. *PloS One*, 7, e32453.

[41] Ishii Y, Matsumoto Y, Watanabe R, et al. (2008). Characterization of neuroprogenitor cells expressing the PDGF beta-receptor within the subventricular zone of postnatal mice. *Mol Cell Neurosci*, 37, 507–518.

[42] Shih AH, Dai C, Rosenblum MK, et al. (2004). Dose-Dependent Effects of Platelet-Derived Growth Factor-B on Glial Tumorigenesis. *Cancer Res*, 64, 4783–4789.

[43] Furnari FB, Fenton T, Bachoo RM, et al. (2007). Malignant astrocytic glioma: genetics, biology, and paths to treatment. *Genes dev*, 21, 2683–26710.

[44] Feng H, Liu KW, Guo P, et al. (2012). Dynamin 2 Mediates PDGFRα-SHP-2-Promoted Glioblastoma Growth and Invasion. *Oncogene*, 31, 2691–2702.
[45] Varela M, Ranuncolo S, Morand A, et al. (2004). EGF-R and PDGF-R, but not bcl-2, overexpression predict overall survival in patients with low-grade astrocytomas. *J Surg Oncol*, 86, 34–40.
[46] Nistér M, Heldin C, Wasteson A, et al. (1982). A platelet-derived growth factor analog produced by a human clonal glioma cell line. *Ann N Y Acad Sci*, 397: 25–33.
[47] Thorarinsdottir H K, Santi M, Mccarter R, et al. (2008). Protein Expression of Platelet-Derived Growth Factor Receptor Correlates with Malignant Histology and PTEN with Survival in Childhood Gliomas. *Clin Cancer Res*, 14, 3386–3394.
[48] Mazzoleni S, Politi LS, Pala M, et al. (2010). Epidermal growth factor receptor expression identifies functionally and molecularly distinct tumor-initiating cells in human glioblastoma multiforme and is required for gliomagenesis. *Cancer research*, 70, 7500–7513.
[49] Cai WW, Chen R, Gibbs RA, et al. (2001). A clone-array pooled shotgun strategy for sequencing large genomes. *Genome research*, 11, 1619–1623.
[50] Liu K, Feng H, Bachoo R, et al. (2011). SHP-2 / PTPN11 mediates gliomagenesis driven by PDGFRA and INK4A / ARF aberrations in mice and humans. *J Cli Invest*, 121, 905–917.
[51] Wu C, O´Rourke DM, Feng G, et al. (2001). The tyrosine phosphatase SHP-2 is required for mediating phosphatidylinositol 3-kinase / Akt activation by growth factors. *Oncogene*, 20, 6018–6025.
[52] Feng H, Hu B, Liu K, et al. (2011). Activation of Rac1 by Src-dependent phosphorylation of Dock180 Y1811 mediates PDGFRα-stimulated glioma tumorigenesis in mice and humans. *J Cli Inv*, 121, 4670–4684.
[53] Ding Q, Stewart J, Olman MA, et al. (2003). The Pattern of Enhancement of Src Kinase Activity on Platelet-derived Growth Factor Stimulation of Glioblastoma Cells Is Affected by the Integrin Engaged. *J Biol Chem*, 278, 39882–39891.
[54] Guo P, Hu B, Gu W, et al. (2003). Platelet-Derived Growth Factor-B Enhances Glioma Angiogenesis by Stimulating Vascular Endothelial Growth Factor Expression in Tumor Endothelia and by Promoting Pericyte Recruitment. *Am J Pathol*, 162, 1083–1093.
[55] Shen J, Vil M, Zhang H, et al. (2007). An antibody directed against PDGF receptor β enhances the antitumor and the anti-angiogenic activities of an anti-VEGF receptor 2 antibody. *Biochem Biophys ResCommun*, 357, 1142–1147.
[56] Li X, and Eriksson U. (2003). Novel PDGF family members: PDGF-C and PDGF-D. *Cytokine Growth Factor Rev*, 14, 91–8.
[57] Cao R, Brakenhielm E, Li X, et al. (2002). Angiogenesis stimulated by PDGF-CC, a novel member in the PDGF family, involves activation of PDGFR- alphaalpha and -alphabeta receptors. *FASEB J*, 16, 1575–1583.
[58] Kilic T, Alberta JA, Zdunek PR, et al. (2000). Intracranial Inhibition of Platelet-derived Growth Factor-mediated Glioblastoma Cell Growth by an Orally Active Kinase Inhibitor of the 2-Phenylaminopyrimidine Class. *Cancer Res*, 60, 5143–5150.
[59] Hermansson M, Nisttrt M, Betsholtzt C, et al. (1988). Endothelial cell hyperplasia in human glioblastoma: Coexpression of mRNA for platelet-derived growth factor (PDGF) B chain and PDGF receptor suggests autocrine growth stimulation. *Proc Natl Acad Sci USA*, 85, 7748–7752.

[60] Di Tomaso E, London N, Fuja D, et al. (2009). PDGF-C induces maturation of blood vessels in a model of glioblastoma and attenuates the response to anti-VEGF treatment. *PloS One*, 4, e5123.

[61] Brem S, Cotran R, and Folkman J. (1972). Tumor angiogenesis: a quantitative method for histologic grading. *J Natl Cancer Inst*, 48, 347–56.

[62] Machein, M, and Plate, K. (2000). VEGF in brain tumors. *J Neurooncol*, 50, 109–20.

[63] Plate KH, Breier G, Millauer B, et al. (1993). Up-Regulation of Vascular Endothelial Growth Factor and Its Cognate Receptors in a Rat Glioma Model of Tumor Angiogenesis *Cancer Res*, 53, 5822–5827.

[64] Forsythe JOA, Jiang B, Iyer NV, et al. (1996). Activation of Vascular Endothelial Growth Factor Gene Transcription by Hypoxia-Inducible Factor 1. *Mol Cell Biol*, 16, 4604–4613.

[65] Keunen O, Johansson M, Oudin A, et al. (2011). Anti-VEGF treatment reduces blood supply and increases tumor cell invasion in glioblastoma. *Proc Natl Acad Sci U S A*, 108, 3749-54

[66] Shibuya M. (2008). Vascular endothelial growth *BMB Rep*, 41, 278-286.

[67] Korkolopoulou P, Perdiki M, Thymara I, Boviatsis E, et al. (2007). Expression of hypoxia *Hum Pathol*, 38, 629-638

[68] Giatromanolaki A, Koukourakis MI, Sivridis E, et al. (2110). Expression of hypoxia *Cancer Res*, 6, 7992-7998.

[69] Papadopoulos MC, Saadoun S, Davies DC, et al. (2001). Emerging molecular mechanisms of brain *Br J Neurosurg*, 15, 101-108.

[70] Plate K, Breier G, Weich H, et al. (1992). Vascular endothelial growth factor is a potential tumour angiogenesis factor in human gliomas in vivo. *Nature*, 359, 845–458.

[71] Meister B, Grünebach F, Bautz F, et al. (1999). Expression of vascular endothelial growth factor (VEGF) and its receptors in human neuroblastoma. *Eur J Cancer*, 35, 445–449.

[72] Levy AP, Levy NS, Goldberg MA. (1996). Hypoxia-inducible Protein Binding to Vascular Endothelial Growth Factor mRNA and Its Modulation by the von Hippel-Lindau Protein. *J Biol Chem*, 271, 25492–25497.

[73] Goldberg-Cohen I, Furneauxb H, and Levy AP. (2002). A 40-bp RNA element that mediates stabilization of vascular endothelial growth factor mRNA by HuR. *J Biol chem*, 277, 13635–13640.

[74] Nakamura K, Martin KC, Jackson JK, et al. (2006). Brain-derived neurotrophic factor activation of TrkB induces vascular endothelial growth factor expression via hypoxia-inducible factor-1alpha in neuroblastoma cells. *Cancer Res*, 66, 4249–4255.

[75] Tan C, Cruet-hennequart S, Troussard A, et al. (2004). Regulation of tumor angiogenesis by integrin-linked kinase (ILK). *Cell*, 5, 79–90.

[76] Khong TL, Thairu N, Larsen H, et al. (2013). Identification of the angiogenic gene signature induced by EGF and hypoxia in colorectal cancer. *BMC Cancer*, 13, 518-525.

[77] Zhang Y, Zhang N, Dai B, et al. (2008). FoxM1B transcriptionally regulates vascular endothelial growth factor expression and promotes the angiogenesis and growth of glioma cells. *Cancer Res*, 68, 8733–8742.

[78] Kil WJ, Tofilon PJ, and Camphausen K. (2012). Post-radiation increase in VEGF enhances glioma cell motility in vitro. *Radiat oncol, 7,25-30.*

[79] Seebach J, Mädler H, Wojciak-Stothard B, et al. (2005). Tyrosine phosphorylation and the small GTPase rac cross-talk in regulation of endothelial barrier function. *Thromb Haemost*, 94, 620–629.

[80] Lu KV, Chang JP, Parachoniak CA, et al.(2012). VEGF inhibits tumor cell invasion and mesenchymal transition through a MET/VEGFR2 complex. *Cancer cell*, 22, 21–35.

[81] Lo HW. (2010). EGFR-targeted therapy in malignant glioma: novel aspects and mechanisms of drug resistance. *Curr Mol Pharmacol*, 3, 37–52.

[82] Castellano E, and Downward J. (2011). RAS Interaction with PI3K: More Than Just Another Effector Pathway. *Genes Cancer*, 2, 261–74.

[83] Boettner B, and Van Aelst L. (2002). The role of Rho GTPases in disease development. *Gene*, 286, 155–174.

[84] Malumbres M, and Barbacid M. (2003). RAS oncogenes: the first 30 years. *Nat Rev Cancer*, 3, 459–465.

[85] Guha A, Feldkamp MM, Lau N, et al. (1997). Proliferation of human malignant astrocytomas is dependent on Ras activation. *Oncogene*, 15, 2755–2765.

[86] Cancer Genome Atlas Research Network. (2008). Comprehensive genomic characterization defines human glioblastoma genes and core pathways. *Nature*, 455, 1061–1068.

[87] Sharma M, Zehnbauer B, Watson M, et al. (2005). RAS pathway activation and an oncogenic RAS mutation in sporadic pilocytic astrocytoma. *Neurology*, 65, 1335–1336.

[88] Davies H, Bignell GR, Cox C, et al. (2002). Mutations of the BRAF gene in human cancer. *Nature*, 417, 949–954.

[89] Knobbe CB, Reifenberger J, and Reifenberger G. (2004). Mutation analysis of the Ras pathway genes NRAS, HRAS, KRAS and BRAF in glioblastomas. *Acta neuropathol*, 108, 467–470.

[90] Basto D, Trovisco V, Lopes JM, et al. (2005). Mutation analysis of B-RAF gene in human gliomas. *Acta neuropathol*, 109, 207–210.

[91] Jeuken J, Van den Broecke C, Gijsen S, et al. (2007). RAS/RAF pathway activation in gliomas: the result of copy number gains rather than activating mutations. *Acta neuropathol*, 114, 121–133.

[92] Ding H, Roncari L, Shannon P, et al. (2001). Astrocyte-specific Expression of Activated p21-ras Results in Malignant Astrocytoma Formation in a Transgenic Mouse Model of Human Gliomas. *Cancer Res*, 61, 3826-3836.

[93] Abel TW, Clark C, Bierie B, et al. (2009). GFAP-Cre-Mediated Activation of Oncogenic K-ras Results in Expansion of the Subventricular Zone and Infiltrating Glioma. *Mol Cancer Res*, 7, 645–653

[94] Holland EC, Celestino J, Dai C, et al. (2000). Combined activation of Ras and Akt in neural progenitors induces glioblastoma formation in mice. *Nature Genetics*, 25, 55–57.

[95] Lyustikman Y, Momota H, Pao W, et al. (2008). Constitutive Activation of Raf-1 Induces Glioma Formation in Mice. *Neoplasia* 10, 501-510.

[96] Blum R, Jacob-Hirsch J, Amariglio N, et al. (2005). Ras Inhibition in Glioblastoma Down-regulates Hypoxia-Inducible Factor-1 α, Causing Glycolysis Shutdown and Cell Death. *Cancer Res*, 65, 999–1006.

[97] Blum R, Jacob-Hirsch J, Rechavi G, et al. (2006). Suppression of survivin expression in glioblastoma cells by the Ras inhibitor farnesylthiosalicylic acid promotes caspase-dependent apoptosis. *Mol Cancer Ther*, 5, 2337–2347.

[98] Blum R, and Kloog Y. (2005). Tailoring Ras-pathway—Inhibitor combinations for cancer therapy. *Drug Resist Updat*, 8, 369–380.

[99] Alessi DR, Andjelkovic M, Caudwell B, et al. (1996). Mechanism of activation of protein kinase B by insulin and IGF-1. *EMBO J*, 15, 6541–6551.

[100] Jacinto E, and Hall MN. (2003). Tor signalling in bugs, brain and brawn. *Nat Rev Mol Cell Biol*, 4, 117–126.

[101] Sabatini DM. (2006). mTOR and cancer: insights into a complex relationship. *Nate Rev Cancer*, 6, 729–734.

[102] Dowling RJO, Topisirovic I, Fonseca BD, et al. (2010). Dissecting the role of mTOR: lessons from mTOR inhibitors. *Biochim Biophys Acta*, 1804, 433–439.

[103] Sonenberg N, and Gingras, AC. (1998). The mRNA 5′ cap-binding protein eIF4E and control of cell growth. *Curr Opin Cell Biol*, 10, 268–275.

[104] De Benedetti A, and Graff JR. (2004). eIF-4E expression and its role in malignancies and metastases. *Oncogene*, 23, 3189–3199.

[105] Laplante M, and Sabatini DM. (2009). mTOR signaling at a glance. *J cell sci*, 122, 3589–3594.

[106] Myers MP, Pass I, Batty IH, et al. (1998). The lipid phosphatase activity of PTEN is critical for its tumor supressor function. *Proc Natl Acad Sci USA.*, 95, 13513–13518.

[107] Stambolic V, Suzuki A, De Pompa L, et al. (1998). Negative Regulation of PKB / Akt-Dependent Cell Survival by the Tumor Suppressor PTEN. *Cell*, 95, 29–39.

[108] Stokoe D, Stephens L, Copeland T, et al. (1997). Dual role of phosphatidylinositol-3,4,5-trisphosphate in the activation of protein kinase B. *Science*, 277, 567–570.

[109] Stephens L, Anderson K, Stokoe D, et al. (1998). Protein kinase B kinases that mediate phosphatidylinositol 3,4,5-trisphosphate-dependent activation of protein kinase B. *Science*, 279, 710–714.

[110] Vanhaesebroeck B, and Alessi DR. (2000). The PI3K – PDK1 connection/: more than just a road to PKB. *Biochem J*, 346, 561–576.

[111] Vivanco I, and Sawyers CL. (2002). The phosphatidylinositol 3-Kinase AKT pathway in human cancer. *Nat Rev Cancer*, 2, 489–501

[112] Manning BD, Tee AR, Logsdon MN, et al. (2002). Identification of the Tuberous Sclerosis Complex-2 Tumor Suppressor Gene Product Tuberin as a Target of the Phosphoinositide 3-Kinase/Akt Pathway. *Mol Cell*, 10, 151–162.

[113] Tohma Y, Gratas C, Biernat W, et al. (1998). PTEN (MMAC1) mutations are frequent in primary glioblastomas (de novo) but not in secondary glioblastomas. *J Neuropathol Exp Neurol*, 57, 684–689.

[114] Chakravarti A, Delaney MA, Noll E, et al. (2001). Prognostic and Pathologic Significance of Quantitative Protein Expression Profiling in Human Gliomas. *Clin Cancer Res.*, 7, 2387–2395.

[115] Groszer M, Erickson R, Scripture-Adams D, et al. (2001). Negative regulation of neural stem/progenitor cell proliferation by the Pten tumor suppressor gene in vivo. *Science*, 294, 2186–2189.

[116] Furnari FB, Huang HS, and Cavenee WK. (1998). The Phosphoinositol Phosphatase Activity of PTEN Mediates a Serum-sensitive G 1 Growth Arrest in Glioma Cells *Cancer Res*, 58, 5002–5008.

[117] Gottschalk AR, Basila D, Wong M, et al. (2001). p27 Kip1 Is Required for PTEN-induced G 1 Growth Arrest *Cancer Res*, 61, 2105–2111.

[118] Dasari VR, Kaur K, Velpula KK, et al. (2010). Upregulation of PTEN in glioma cells by cord blood mesenchymal stem cells inhibits migration via downregulation of the PI3K/Akt pathway. *PloS One*, 5, e10350.

[119] Furukawa K, Kumon Y, Harada H, et al. (2006). PTEN gene transfer suppresses the invasive potential of human malignant gliomas by regulating cell invasion-related molecules. *Int J Oncol*, 29, 73-81.

[120] Van Themsche C, Leblanc V, Parent S, et al. (2009). X-linked inhibitor of apoptosis protein (XIAP) regulates PTEN ubiquitination, content, and compartmentalization. *J Biol Chem*, 284, 20462–20466.

[121] Wen S, Stolarov J, Myers MP, et al. (2001). PTEN controls tumor-induced angiogenesis. *Proc Natl Acad Sci U S A*, 98, 4622–4627.

[122] Testa JR, and Bellacosa A. (2001). AKT plays a central role in tumorigenesis. *Proc Natl Acad Sci U S A*, 98, 10983–10985.

[123] Thant A, Nawa A, Kikkawa F, et al. (2000). Fibronectin activates matrix metalloproteinase-9 secretion via the MEK1-MAPK and the PI3K-Akt pathways in ovarian cancer cells. *Clin Exp Metastasis*, 18, 423–428.

[124] Uhrbom L, Dai C, Celestino JC, et al. (2002). Ink4a-Arf Loss Cooperates with KRas Activation in Astrocytes and Neural Progenitors to Generate Glioblastomas of Various Morphologies Depending on Activated Akt. *Cancer Res.*, 62, 5551–5558.

[125] Neshat MS, Mellinghoff IK, Tran C, et al. (2001). Enhanced sensitivity of PTEN-deficient tumors to inhibition of FRAP¯mTOR. *Proc Natl Acad Sci U S A*, 98, 10314–10319.

[126] Podsypanina K, Lee RT, Politis C, et al. (2001). An inhibitor of mTOR reduces neoplasia and normalizes p70¯S6 kinase activity in Pten+/- mice. *Proc Natl Acad Sci U S A*, 98, 10320–10325.

[127] Aoki M, Blazek E, and Vogt PK. (2001). A role of the kinase mTOR in cellular transformation induced by the oncoproteins P3k and Akt. *Proc Natl Acad Sci U S A*, 98, 136–141.

[128] Choe G, Horvath S, Cloughesy TF, et al. (2003). Analysis of the Phosphatidylinositol 3 ′ -Kinase Signaling Pathway in Glioblastoma Patients in Vivo. *Cancer Res*, 63, 2742–2746.

[129] Schmelzle T, and Hall MN. (2000). TOR, a Central Controller of Cell Growth. *Cell*, 103, 253–262.

[130] Castedo M, Ferri KF, and Kroemer G. (2002). Mammalian Target of Rapamycin (mTOR): Pro- and Anti-Apoptotic. *Cell Death Differ*, 9, 99–100.

[131] Hu X, Pandolfi PP, Li Y, et al. (2005). mTOR Promotes Survival and Astrocytic Characteristics Induced by Pten/Akt Signaling in Glioblastoma. *Neoplasia*, 7, 356–368.

[132] Fan Q, Cheng C, Knight ZA, et al. (2009). EGFR signals to mTOR through PKC and independently of Akt in glioma. *Sci Signal.*, 2, ra4.

[133] Majumder P, Febbo P, Bikoff R, et al. (2004). mTOR inhibition reverses Akt-dependent prostate intraepithelial neoplasia through regulation of apoptotic and HIF-1-dependent pathways. *Nat Med*, 10, 594–601.

[134] Inoki K, Corradetti MN, and Guan KL. (2005). Dysregulation of the TSC-mTOR pathway in human disease. *Nat Genet*, 37, 19–24.

[135] Masri J, Bernath A, Martin J, et al. (2007). mTORC2 activity is elevated in gliomas and promotes growth and cell motility via overexpression of rictor. *Cancer research*, 67, 11712–11720.

[136] Verreault M, Weppler SA, Stegeman A, et al. (2013). Combined RNAi-mediated suppression of Rictor and EGFR resulted in complete tumor regression in an orthotopic glioblastoma tumor model. *PloS One*, 8, e59597.

[137] Stabel S, and Parker PJ. (1991). Protein kinase C. *Pharmacol Ther*, 51, 71–95.

[138] Johannes F, Prestle J, Eis S, et al. (1994). PKCu Is a Novel, Atypical Member of the Protein Kinase C Family ". *J Biol Chem*, 269, 6140–6148.

[139] Newton AC. (1995). Protein kinase C. Seeing two domains. *Curr Biol*, 5, 973–976.

[140] Burns DJ, and Belly RM. (1991). Protein Kinase C Contains Two Phorbol Ester Binding Domains. *J Bol Chem.*, 266, 18330–18338.

[141] Newton AC. (1995). Protein Kinase C/: Structure, Function, and Regulation. *J Biol Chem*, 270, 28495–284998.

[142] Hurley JH, Newton AC, Parker PJ, et al. (1997). Taxonomy and function of C1 protein kinase C homology domains. *Protein Sci*, 6, 477–480.

[143] Kolch W, Heidecker G, Kochs G, et al. (1993). Protein kinase Cα activates RAF-1 by direct phosphorylation. *Nature*, 364, 249–252.

[144] Marais R, Light Y, Mason C, et al. (1998). Requirement of Ras-GTP-Raf complexes for activation of Raf-1 by protein kinase C. *Science*, 280, 109–112.

[145] Nishizuka Y. (1984). The role of protein kinase C in cell surface signal transduction and tumour promotion. *Nature*, 308, 693–698.

[146] Nishizuka Y. (1988). The molecular heterogeneity of protein kinase C and its implications for cellular regulation. *Nature*, 334, 661–665.

[147] Couldwell W, Uhm J, Antel J, et al. (1991). Enhanced protein kinase C activity correlates with the growth rate of malignant gliomas in vitro. *Neurosurgery*, 29, 880–886.

[148] Couldwell W, Antel J, and Yong V. (1992). Protein kinase C activity correlates with the growth rate of malignant gliomas: Part II. Effects of glioma mitogens and modulators of protein kinase C. *Neurosurgery*, 31, 717–724.

[149] Le Good J, Ziegler W, Parekh D, et al. (1998). Protein kinase C isotypes controlled by phosphoinositide 3-kinase through the protein kinase PDK1. *Science*, 281, 2042–2045.

[150] Dutil EM, Toker A, and Newton AC. (1998). Regulation of conventional protein kinase C isozymes by phosphoinositide-dependent kinase 1 (PDK-1). *Curr Biol,* 8,1366–1375.

[151] Baltuch G, and Yong V. (1996). Signal transduction for proliferation of glioma cells in vitro occurs predominantly through a protein kinase C-mediated pathway. *Brain Res*, 710, 143–149.

[152] Pollack IF, Randall MS, Kristofik MP, et al. (1990). Effect of Tamoxifen on DNA Synthesis and Proliferation of Human Malignant Glioma Lines in Vitro. *Cancer Res*, 50, 7134–7138.

[153] Bredel M and Pollack I. (1997). The role of protein kinase C (PKC) in the evolution and proliferation of malignant gliomas, and the application of PKC inhibition as a novel approach to anti-glioma therapy. *Acta Neurochir (Wien)*, 139, 1000–1013.

[154] Hu J, Wang X, Zhou J, et al. (2010). Activation of PKCα is required for migration of C6 glioma cells. *Acta Neurobiol Exp (Wars)*, 70, 239–245.

[155] Mut M, Amos S, and Hussaini IM. (2010). PKC alpha phosphorylates cytosolic NF-kappaB/p65 and PKC delta delays nuclear translocation of NF-kappaB/p65 in U1242 glioblastoma cells. *Turk Neurosurg*, 20, 277–285.

[156] do Carmo A, Patricio I, Cruz MT. et al. (2010). CXCL12 / CXCR4 promotes motility and proliferation of glioma cells. *Cancer Biol Ther*, 9, 56–65.

[157] Leirdal M, and Sioud M. (2000). Protein kinase Calpha isoform regulates the activation of the MAP kinase ERK1/2 in human glioma cells: involvement in cell survival and gene expression. *Mol Cell Biol Res Commun*, 4, 106–110.

[158] Lin CW, Shen SC, Chien CC, et al. (2010). 12-O-tetradecanoylphorbol-13-acetate-induced invasion/migration of glioblastoma cells through activating PKCalpha/ERK/NF-kappaB-dependent MMP-9 expression. *J Cell Physiol.*, 225, 472–481.

[159] Mishima K, Ohno S, Shitara N, et al. (1994). Opposite effects of the overexpression of protein kinase C gamma and delta on the growth properties of human glioma cell line U251 MG. *Biochem Biophys Res Commun*, 201, 363-372.

[160] Estève PO, Chicoine E, Robledo O, et al. (2002). Protein kinase C-zeta regulates transcription of the matrix metalloproteinase-9 gene induced by IL-1 and TNF-alpha in glioma cells via NF-kappa B. *J Biol Chem*, 277, 35150–35155.

[161] Uht RM, Amos S, Martin PM, et al. (2007). The protein kinase C-eta isoform induces proliferation in glioblastoma cell lines through an ERK/Elk-1 pathway. *Oncogene*, 26, 2885–2893.

[162] Okhrimenko H, Lu W, Xiang C, et al. (2006). Protein kinase C-epsilon regulates the apoptosis and survival of glioma cells. *Cancer Res*, 65, 7301–7309.

[163] Besson A, Wilson TL, and Yong VW. (2002). The anchoring protein RACK1 links protein kinase Cepsilon to integrin beta chains. Requirements for adhesion and motility. *J Biol Chem*, 277, 22073–22084.

[164] Baldwin RM, Barrett GM, Parolin DAE, et al. (2010). Coordination of glioblastoma cell motility by PKCι. *Mol Cancer*, 9, 1–13.

[165] Desai SR, Pillai PP, Patel RS, et al. (2012). Regulation of Cdk7 activity through a phosphatidylinositol (3)-kinase/PKC-ι-mediated signaling cascade in glioblastoma. *Carcinogenesis*, 33, 10–9.

[166] Silvani A, Gaviani P, Lamperti EA, et al. (2009). Cisplatinum and BCNU chemotherapy in primary glioblastoma patients. *J Neurooncol*, 94, 57–62.

[167] Stupp R, Mason WP, Van den Bent MJ, et al. (2005). Radiotherapy plus concomitant and adjuvant temozolomide for glioblastoma. *N Engl J Med*, 352, 987–96.

[168] Hegi ME, Diserens AC, Gorlia T, et al. (2005). MGMT gene silencing and benefit from temozolomide in glioblastoma. *N Engl J Med*, 352, 997–1003

[169] Vredenburgh JJ, Desjardins A, Reardon DA, et al. (2009). Experience with irinotecan for the treatment of malignant glioma. *Neuro-oncol*, 11, 80–91.

[170] Johnson LA and Sampson JH.(2010). Immunotherapy approaches for malignant glioma from 2007 to 2009. *Curr Neurol Neurosci Rep*, 10, 259–266.

[171] Weiner LM, Surana R and Wang S. (2010). Monoclonal antibodies: versatile platforms for cancer immunotherapy. *Nat Rev Immunol,* 10, 317–327.

[172] Ehrlich P. Collected Studies on Immunity. J. Wiley & Sons; New York: 1906.

[173] Peng D, Fan Z, Lu Y, et al. (1996). Anti-epidermal growth factor receptor monoclonal antibody 225 upregulates p27KIP1 and induces G1 arrest in prostatic cancer cell line DU145. *Cancer Res*, 56, 3666–3669.

[174] Wu X, Rubin M, Fan Z, et al. (1996). Involvement of p27KIP1in G1 arrest mediated by an anti-epidermal growth factor receptor monoclonal antibody. *Oncogene*, 12, 1397–1403

[175] Perrotte P, Matsumoto T, Inoue K, et al. (1999). Anti-epidermal growth factor receptor antibody C225 inhibits angiogenesis in human transitional cell carcinoma growing orthotopically in nude mice. *Clin Cancer Res,* 5, 257–265.

[176] Mandal M, Adam L, Mendelsohn J, et al. (1998). Nuclear targeting of Bax during apoptosis in human colorectal cancer cells. *Oncogene,* 17, 999–1007.

[177] Wu X, Fan Z, Masui H, et al. (1995). Apoptosis induced by an anti-epidermal growth factor receptor monoclonal antibody in a human colorectal carcinoma cell line and its delay by insulin. *J Clin Invest*, 95, 1897–1905.

[178] Rivera F, Vega-Villegas ME, and Lopez-Brea MF. (2008). Cetuximab, its clinical use and future perspectives. *Anticancer Drugs*, 19, 99–113.

[179] Eller JL, Longo SL, Kyle MM, et al. (2005). Anti-epidermal growth factor receptor monoclonal antibody cetuximab augments radiation effects in glioblastoma multiforme in vitro and in vivo. *Neurosurgery*, 56, 155–162.

[180] Combs SE, Heeger S, Haselmann R, et al. (2006). Treatment of primary glioblastoma multiforme with cetuximab, radiotherapy and temozolomide (GERT)--phase I/II trial: study protocol. *BMC Cancer*, 6, 133.

[181] Emrich JG, Brady LW, Quang TS, et al. (2002) Radioiodinated (I-125) monoclonal antibody 425 in the treatment of high grade glioma patients: ten-year synopsis of a novel treatment. *Am J Clin Oncol,* 25, 541–546.

[182] Quang TS and Brady LW. (2004). Radioimmunotherapy as a novel treatment regimen: 125I-labeled monoclonal antibody 425 in the treatment of high-grade brain gliomas. *Int J Radiat Oncol Biol Phys*, 58, 972–975.

[183] Luwor RB, Johns TG, Murone C, et al. (2001). Monoclonal antibody 806 inhibits the growth of tumor xenografts expressing either the de2-7 or amplified epidermal growth factor receptor (EGFR) but not wild-type EGFR. *Cancer Res*, 61, 5355–5361.

[184] Mishima K, Johns TG, Luwor RB, et al. (2001). Growth suppression of intracranial xenografted glioblastomas overexpressing mutant epidermal growth factor receptors by systemic administration of monoclonal antibody (mAb) 806, a novel monoclonal antibody directed to the receptor. *Cancer Res,* 61, 5349–5354.

[185] Scott AM, Lee FT, Tebbutt N, et al. (2007). A phase I clinical trial with monoclonal antibody ch806 targeting transitional state and mutant epidermal growth factor receptors. *Proc Natl Acad Sci U S A*, 104, 4071–4076.

[186] Shen J, Vil MD, Prewett M, et al. (2009). Development of a fully human *Neoplasia*, 11, 594-604.

[187] Shen J, Vil MD, Zhang H, et al. (2007). An antibody directed against PDGF receptor beta enhances the antitumor and the anti-angiogenic activities of an anti-VEGF receptor 2 antibody. *Biochem Biophys Res Commun,* 357, 1142–1147.

[188] Kim KJ, Li B, Winer J, et al. (1993). Inhibition of vascular endothelial growth factor-induced angiogenesis suppresses tumour growth in vivo. *Nature*, 362, 841–844.

[189] Rubenstein JL, Kim J, Ozawa T, et al. (2000). Anti-VEGF antibody treatment of glioblastoma prolongs survival but results in increased vascular cooption. *Neoplasia*, 2, 306–314

[190] Hoang T, Huang S, Armstrong E, et al. (2012). Enhancement of radiation response with bevacizumab. *J Exp Clin Cancer Res*, 31, 37.

[191] Lee CG, Heijn M, di Tomaso E, et al. (2000). Anti-vascular endothelial growth factor treatment augments tumor radiation response under normoxic or hypoxic conditions. *Cancer Res*, 60, 5565–5570.

[192] Dings RP, Loren M, Heun H, et al. (2007). Scheduling of radiation with angiogenesis inhibitors anginex and Avastin improves therapeutic outcome via vessel normalization. *Clin Cancer Res*, 13, 3395–3402.

[193] McGee MC, Hamner JB, Williams RF, et al. (2010). Improved intratumoral oxygenation through vascular normalization increases glioma sensitivity to ionizing radiation. *Int J Radiat Oncol Biol Phys*, 76, 1537–1545.

[194] Vredenburgh JJ, Desjardins A, Herndon JE, et al. (2007). Bevacizumab plus irinotecan in recurrent glioblastoma multiforme. *Clin Cancer Res*, 25, 4722–4729.

[195] Cloughsey TF, Prados MD, Wen PY, et al. (2008). A phase II, randomized, non-comparative clinical trial of the effect of bevacizumab (BV) alone or in combination with irinotecan (CPT) on 6-month progression free survival (PFS6) in recurrent, treatment-refractory glioblastoma (GBM). *J Clin Oncol*, 26, 2010b.

[196] Lu KV, and Bergers G. (2013). Mechanisms of evasive resistance *CNS Oncol,* 2, 49-65.

[197] Lucio-Eterovic AK, Piao Y, and de Groot JF. (2009). Mediators of glioblastoma resistance and invasion during antivascular endothelial growth factor therapy. *Clin Cancer Res*, 15, 4589-4599.

[198] Holash J, Davis S, Papadopoulos N, et al. (2002). VEGF-Trap: a VEGF blocker with potent antitumor effects. *Proc Natl Acad Sci U S A*, 99, 11393–11398.

[199] Scott BJ, Quant EC, McNamara MB, et al. (2010). Bevacizumab salvage therapy following progression in high-grade glioma patients treated with VEGF receptor tyrosine kinase inhibitors. *Neuro Oncol,* 12, 603–607.

[200] Kim ES, Serur A, Huang J, et al. (2002). Potent VEGF blockade causes regression of coopted vessels in a model of neuroblastoma. *Proc NatlAcad Sci USA*, 99, 11399–11404.

[201] Prewett M, Huber J, Li Y, et al. (1999). Antivascular endothelial growth factor receptor (fetal liver kinase 1) monoclonal antibody inhibits tumor angiogenesis and growth of several mouse and human tumors. *Cancer Res,* 59, 5209-5218.

[202] Spratlin JL, Cohen RB, Eadens M, et al. (2010). Phase I pharmacologic and biologic study of ramucirumab (IMC-1121B), a fully human *J Clin Oncol*, 28,780-787.

[203] Moscatello DK, Ramirez G and Wong AJ. (1997). A naturally occurring mutant human epidermal growth factor receptor as a target for peptide vaccine immunotherapy of tumors. *Cancer Res*, 57, 1419–1424.

[204] Kanaly CW, Ding D, Heimberger AB, et al. (2010). Clinical applications of a peptide-based vaccine for glioblastoma. *Neurosurg Clin N Am,* 21, 95–109.

[205] Yamanaka R. (2009). Dendritic-cell- and peptide-based vaccination strategies for glioma. *Neurosurg Rev*, 32, 265–273.

[206] Heimberger AB and Sampson JH. (2009). The PEPvIII-KLH (CDX-110) vaccine in glioblastoma multiforme patients. *Expert Opin Biol Ther*, 9, 1087–1098.

[207] Sampson JH, Archer GE, Mitchell DA, et al. (2009). An epidermal growth factor receptor variant III-targeted vaccine is safe and immunogenic in patients with glioblastoma multiforme. *Mol Cancer Ther,* 8, 2773–2779.
[208] Kohno M, Horibe T, Haramoto M, et al. (2011). A novel hybrid peptide targeting EGFR-expressing cancers. *Eur J Cancer,* 47, 773–783.
[209] Tada N, Horibe T, Haramoto M, et al. (2011). A single replacement of histidine to arginine in EGFR-lytic hybrid peptide demonstrates the improved anticancer activity. *Biochem Biophys Res Commun,* 407, 383–388.
[210] Kaplan CD, Krüger JA, Zhou H, et al. (2006). A novel DNA *Vaccine*, 24, 6994-7002.
[211] Zhou H, Luo, Mizutani M, et al. (2005). T cell-mediated suppression of angiogenesis results in tumor protective immunity. *Blood*, 106, 2026-2032.
[212] Feng K, Zhao H, Chen J, et al. (2004). Anti-angiogenesis *J Huazhong Univ Sci Technolog Med Sci*, 24, 389-391.
[213] Feng KK, Zhao HY, Qiu H, et al. (2005). Specific anti-glioma angiogenesis immune response induced by attenuated Salmonella typhimurium vaccine expressing vascular endothelial growth factor receptor-2. *Ai Zheng,* 24, 548-553.
[214] Feng KK, Zhao HY, Qiu H, et al. (2005). Combined therapy *Cancer Lett,* 221, 41-47.
[215] Karpel-Massler G, Schmidt U, Unterberg A, et al. (2009). Therapeutic inhibition of the epidermal growth factor receptor in high-grade gliomas: where do we stand? *Mol Cancer Res,* 7, 1000–1012.
[216] Mischel PS and Cloughesy TF. (2003). Targeted molecular therapy of GBM. *Brain Pathol,* 13, 52–61
[217] Moyer JD, Barbacci EG, Iwata KK, et al. (1997). Induction of apoptosis and cell cycle arrest by CP-358,774, an inhibitor of epidermal growth factor receptor tyrosine kinase. *Cancer Res,* 57, 4838–4848.
[218] Halatsch ME, Gehrke EE, Vougioukas VI, et al. (2004). Inverse correlation of epidermal growth factor receptor messenger RNA induction and suppression of anchorage-independent growth by OSI-774, an epidermal growth factor receptor tyrosine kinase inhibitor, in glioblastoma multiforme cell lines. *J Neurosurg,* 100, 523–533.
[219] Quatrale AE, Porcelli L, Silvestris N, et al. (2011). EGFR tyrosine kinases inhibitors in cancer treatment: in vitro and in vivo evidence. *Front. Biosci*, 16, 1962–1972.
[220] Van den Bent MJ, Brandes AA, Rampling R, et al. (2009). Randomized phase II trial *J Clin Oncol*, 27, 1268-1274.
[221] Brown PD, Krishnan S, Sarkaria JN, et al. (2008). Phase I/II trial *J Clin Oncol*, 26, 5603-5609.
[222] Mellinghoff IK, Wang MY, Vivanco I, et al.(2005). Molecular determinants of the response *N Engl J Med*, 353, 2012-2024.
[223] Knight LA, Di Nicolantonio F, Whitehouse P, et al. (2004). The in vitro effect of gefitinib ('Iressa') alone and in combination with cytotoxic chemotherapy on human solid tumours. *BMC Cancer*, 4, 83.
[224] Carrasco-García E, Saceda M, Grasso S, et al. (2011). Small tyrosine *Exp Cell Res*, 317, 1476-1489.
[225] Kang KB, Zhu C, Wong YL, et al. (2012). Gefitinib radiosensitizes stem-like glioma *Int J Radiat Oncol Biol Phys,* 83, e43-52

[226] Rich JN, Reardon DA, Peery T, et al. (2004). Phase II trial of gefitinib in recurrent glioblastoma. *J Clin Oncol,* 22, 133-142.

[227] Peereboom DM, Shepard DR, Ahluwalia MS, et al. (2010). Phase II trial *J Neurooncol*, 98, 93-99.

[228] O'Brien SG, Guilhot F, Larson RA, et al. (2003). Imatinib compared with interferon and low-dose cytarabine for newly diagnosed chronic-phase chronic myeloid leukemia. *N Engl J Med,* 348, 994–1004.

[229] Kilic T, Alberta JA, Zdunek PR, et al. (2000). Intracranial inhibition of platelet-derived growth factor-mediated glioblastoma cell growth by an orally active kinase inhibitor of the 2-phenylaminopyrimidine class. *Cancer Res*, 60, 5143–5150.

[230] Yang L, Xu ZY, Chen XH, et al. (2010). Effect of imatinib at different concentrations on rat C6 glioma *Nan Fang Yi Ke Da Xue Xue Bao*, 30, 1089-1091.

[231] Ranza E, Bertolotti A, Facoetti A, et al. (2009) Influence of imatinib mesylate on radiosensitivity of astrocytoma *Anticancer Res*, 29, 4575-4578.

[232] Kinsella P, Clynes M and Amberger-Murphy VJ. (2011). Imatinib and docetaxel *Neurooncol*, 101, 189-198.

[233] Majsterek I, Sliwinski T, Poplawski T, et al. (2006). Imatinib mesylate (STI571) abrogates the resistance *Mutat Res*, 603, 74-82.

[234] Kinsella P, Howley R, Doolan P, et al. (2012). Characterization and response *Exp Cell Res*, 318, 641-652.

[235] Wen PY, Yung WKA, Lamborn KR, et al. (2006). Phase I/II study of imatinib mesylate for recurrent malignant gliomas: North American Brain Tumor Consortium Study 99-08. *Clin Cancer Res*, 12, 4899–4907.

[236] Reardon DA, Egorin MJ, Quinn JA, et al. (2005). Phase II study of imatinib mesylate plus hydroxyurea in adults with recurrent glioblastoma multiforme. *J Clin Oncol,* 23, 9359-9368.

[237] De Boüard S, Herlin P, Christensen JG, et al. (2007). Antiangiogenic and anti-invasive effects of sunitinib on experimental human glioblastoma. *Neuro Oncol*, 9, 412-423.

[238] Chahal M, Xu Y, Lesniak D, et al. (2010) MGMT modulates glioblastoma angiogenesis and response to the tyrosine kinase inhibitor sunitinib. *Neuro-oncology,* 12, 822–833.

[239] Strawn LM, Kabbinavar F, Schwartz DP, et al. (2000) Effects of SU101 in combination with cytotoxic agents on the growth of subcutaneous tumor xenografts. *Clin Cancer Res*, 6, 2931–2940.

[240] Zhou Q, Guo P, Gallo JM, et al. (2008). Impact of angiogenesis inhibition by sunitinib on tumor distribution of temozolomide. *Clin Cancer Res*, 14, 1540–1549.

[241] Neyns B, Sadones J,Chaskis C, et al. (2011). Phase II study of sunitinib malate in patients with recurrent high-grade glioma. *J Neurooncol,* 103, 491–501.

[242] Reardon DA, Vredenburgh JJ, Coan A, et al. (2011). Phase I study of sunitinib and irinotecan for patients with recurrent malignant glioma *J Neurooncol*, 105, 621-627.

[243] Drappatz J, Norden AD, Wong ET, et al. (2010). Phase I study of vandetanib with radiotherapy *Int J Radiat Oncol Biol Phys*, 78, 85-90.

[244] Jane EP, Premkumar DR, Addo-Yobo SO, et al. (2009). Abrogation of mitogen *J Pharmacol Exp Ther*, 331, 327-337.

[245] Jo MY, Kim YG, Kim Y, et al. (2012). Combined therapy *Mol Med Rep*, 6, 88-92.

[246] Kreisl TN, McNeill KA, Sul J, et al. (2012). A phase I/II trial *Neuro Oncol*, 14, 1519-1526.

[247] Carra E, Barbieri F, Marubbi D, et al. (2013). Sorafenib selectively depletes human *Cell Cycle*, 12, 491-500.

[248] Siegelin MD, Raskett CM, Gilbert CA, et al. (2010). Sorafenib exerts anti-glioma *Neurosci Lett*, 478, 165-170.

[249] Yu C, Friday BB, Lai JP, et al. (2006). Cytotoxic synergy between the multikinase inhibitor *Mol Cancer Ther*, 5, 2378-2387

[250] Hainsworth JD, Ervin T, Friedman E, et al. (2010). Concurrent radiotherapy *Cancer*, 116, 3663-3669.

[251] Batchelor TT, Duda DG, di Tomaso E, et al. (2010). Phase II study of cediranib, an oral pan-vascular endothelial growth *J Clin Oncol*, 28, 2817-2823.

[252] Sorensen AG, Batchelor TT, Zhang WT, et al. (2008) Response criteria for glioma. *Nat Clin Pract Oncol,* 5, 634–635.

[253] Gerstner ER, Chen PJ, Wen PY, et al. (2010). Infiltrative patterns of glioblastoma spread detected via diffusion MRI after treatment with cediranib. *Neuro Oncol,* 12, 466–472.

[254] Batchelor TT, Sorensen AG, di Tomaso E, et al. (2007). AZD2171, a pan-VEGF receptor tyrosine kinase inhibitor, normalizes tumor vasculature and alleviates edema in glioblastoma patients. *Cancer Cell*, 11, 83–95.

[255] Kamoun WS, Ley CD, Farrar CT, et al. (2009). Edema control by cediranib, a VEGF targeted kinase inhibitor, prolongs survival despite persistent brain tumor growth in mice. *J Clin Oncol,* 27, 2542–2552.

[256] Sorensen AG, Batchelor TT, Zhang WT, et al. (2009). A vascular normalization index as potential mechanistic biomarker to predict survival after a single dose of cediranib in recurrent glioblastoma patients. *Cancer Res*, 69, 5296–5300.

[257] Winkler F, Kozin SV, Tong R, et al. (2004). Kinetics of vascular normalization by VEGFR2 blockade governs brain tumor response to radiation: Role of oxygenation, angiopoietin-1 and matrix metalloproteinases. *Cancer Cell*, 6, 553–563.

[258] di Tomaso E, Snuderl M, Kamoun WS, et al. (2011). Glioblastoma *Cancer Res*, 71, 19-28.

[259] Goldbrunner RH, Bendszus M, Wood J, et al. (2004). PTK787/ZK222584, an inhibitor *Neurosurgery*, 55, 426-432.

[260] Zhang YH, Yue ZJ, Zhang H, et al. (2010). Temozolomide/PLGA microparticles *Eur J Pharm Biopharm,* 76, 371-375.

[261] Conrad C, Friedman H, Reardon D, et al. (2004). A Phase I/II trial of single-agent PTK 787/ZK 222584 (PTK/ZK), a novel, oral angiogenesis inhibitor, in patients with recurrent glioblastoma multiforme (GBM). *J. Clin. Oncol*, 22, 1512.

[262] Conrad C, Friedman H, Reardon D, et al. (2004). A Phase I/II trial of PTK787/ZK222584 (PTK/ZK), a novel, oral angiogenesis inhibitor, in combination with either temozolomide or lomustine for patients with recurrent glioblastoma multiforme (GBM). *J. Clin. Oncol*, 22, 1512.

[263] Kefas B, Godlewski J, Comeau L, et al. (2008). microRNA *Cancer Res,* 68, 3566-3572.

[264] Yang H. (2010). Nanoparticle-mediated brain-specific drug delivery, imaging, and diagnosis. *Pharm Res*, 27, 1759–1771.

[265] Lee KM, Choi EJ, and Kim IA (2011). MicroRNA-7 increases radiosensitivity of human *Radiother Oncol*, 101, 171-176.

[266] Wu DG, Wang YY, Fan LG, et al. (2011). MicroRNA-7 regulates glioblastoma *Chin Med J (Engl)*, 124, 2616-2621.
[267] Wang W, Dai LX, Zhang S, et al. (2013). Regulation of epidermal growth *Neoplasma*, 60, 274-283.
[268] Sasaki A, Udaka Y, Tsunoda Y, et al. (2012). Analysis of p53 *Anticancer Res*, 32, 4709-4713
[269] Gao H, Zhao H, Xiang W, et al. (2013). Expression level of human *J Neurooncol,* 113, 221-228.
[270] Yu X, Zhang W, Ning Q, et al. (2012). MicroRNA-34a inhibits human *J Huazhong Univ Sci Technolog Med Sci*, 32, 370-374.
[271] Li WB, Ma MW, Dong LJ, et al. (2011). MicroRNA-34a targets notch1 and inhibits cell proliferation *Cancer Biol Ther*, 12, 477-483.
[272] Guessous F, Zhang Y, Kofman A, et al. (2010). MicroRNA-34a is tumor *Cell Cycle,* 9, 1031-1036.
[273] Sun L, Wu Z, Shao Y, et al. (2012). MicroRNA-34a suppresses cell proliferation *Technol Cancer Res Treat*, 11, 483-490.
[274] Silber J, Jacobsen A, Ozawa T, et al. (2012). miR-34a repression *PLoS One,* 7, e33844.
[275] Li Y, Guessous F, Zhang Y, et al. (2009). MicroRNA-34a inhibits glioblastoma *Cancer Res,* 69, 7569-7576.
[276] Hou SX, Ding BJ, Li HZ, et al. (2013). Identification of microRNA-205 as a potential prognostic indicator for human glioma. *J Clin Neurosci,* 20, 933-937.
[277] Adjei AA, Davis JN, Bruzek LM, et al. (2001). Synergy of the protein farnesyltransferase inhibitor SCH66336 and cisplatin in human cancer cell lines. *Clin Cancer Res*, 7, 1438-1445.
[278] Karp JE, Kaufmann SH, Adjei AA, et al. (2001). Current status of clinical trials of farnesyltransferase inhibitors. *Curr Opin Oncol*, 13, 470-476.
[279] Jiang K, Coppola D, Crespo NC, et al. (2000). The phosphoinositide 3-OH kinase/AKT2 pathway as a critical target for farnesyltransferase inhibitor-induced apoptosis. *Mol Cell Biol*, 20, 139-148.
[280] Wang CC, Liao YP, Mischel PS, et al. (2006). HDJ-2 as a Target for Radiosensitization of Glioblastoma Multiforme Cells by the Farnesyltransferase Inhibitor R115777 and the Role of the p53/p21 Pathway. *Cancer Res,* 66, 6756-6762.
[281] Delmas C, End D, Rochaix R, et al. (2003). The Farnesyltransferase Inhibitor R115777 Reduces Hypoxia and Matrix Metalloproteinase 2 Expression in Human. Glioma Xenograft. *Clin Cancer Res,* 9, 6062-6068.
[282] Cloughesy TF, Wen PY, Robins HI, et al. (2006). Phase II trial *J Clin Oncol,* 24, 3651-3656.
[283] Moyal EC, Laprie A, Delannes M, et al. (2007). Phase I trial *Int J Radiat Oncol Biol Phys,* 68, 1396-1401.
[284] Glass TL, Liu TJ and Yung WK. (2000). Inhibition of cell growth *Neuro Oncol.* 2, 151-158.
[285] Chaponis D, Barnes JW, Dellagatta JL, et al. (2011). Lonafarnib (SCH66336) improves the activity of temozolomide and radiation *J Neurooncol,* 104, 179-189.
[286] Yust-Katz S, Liu D, Yuan Y, et al. (2013). Phase 1/1b study of lonafarnib and temozolomide in patients with recurrent or temozolomide refractory glioblastoma *Cancer*, 119, 2747-2753.

[287] Nakamura JL, Karlsson A, Arvold ND et al. (2005). PKB/Akt mediates radiosensitization by the signaling inhibitor LY294002 in human malignant gliomas. *J Neurooncol*, 71, 215–222.

[288] Schmelzle T and Hall MN. (2000). TOR, a central controller of cell growth *Cell.* 103, 253-262.

[289] Newhart MS, Mellinghoff IK, Tran C, et al. (2001). Enhanced sensitivity of PTEN-deficient tumors to inhibition of FRAP/mTOR. *Proc Natl Acad Sci U S A*, 98, 10314-10319.

[290] Geoerger B, Kerr K, Tang CB, et al. (2001). Antitumor activity of the rapamycin analog CCI-779 in human *Cancer Res,* 61, 1527-1532.

[291] GalanisE, BucknerJC, Maurer MJ, et al. (2005). Phase II trial *J Clin Oncol*, 23, 5294-5304.

[292] Chang SM, Wen P, Cloughesy T, et al. (2005). Phase II study of CCI-779 in patients with recurrent glioblastoma *Invest New Drugs*, 23, 357-361.

[293] Mounier N, Vignot S and Spano JP, (2006). Update on clinical activity of CCI779 (temsirolimus), mTOR inhibitor *Bull Cancer*, 93, 1139-1143.

[294] Pitter KL, Galbán CJ, Galbán S, et al. (2011). Perifosine and CCI 779 co-operate to induce cell death *PLoS One*, 6, e14545.

[295] Hu X, Pandolfi PP, Li Y, et al. (2005). mTOR promotes survival *Neoplasia,* 7, 356-368.

[296] Reardon DA, Quinn JA, Vredenburgh JJ, et al. (2006). Phase 1 trial of gefitinib plus sirolimus in adults with recurrent malignant glioma. *Clin Cancer Res,* 12, 860-868.

[297] Kreisl TN, Lassman AB, Mischel PS, et al. (2009). A pilot study *J Neurooncol,* 92, 99-105.

[298] Hui AM, Zhang W, Chen W, et al. (2004). Agents with selective estrogen receptor (ER) modulator activity induce apoptosis in vitro and in vivo in ER-negative glioma cells. *Cancer Res*, 64, 9115-9123.

[299] Brandes AA, Ermani M, Turazzi S, et al. (1999). Procarbazine and high-dose tamoxifen as a second-line regimen in recurrent high-grade gliomas: a phase II study. *J Clin Oncol.* 17, 645-650.

[300] Spence AM, Peterson RA, Scharnhorst JD, et al. (2004). Phase II study of concurrent continuous Temozolomide (TMZ) and Tamoxifen (TMX) for recurrent malignant astrocytic gliomas. *J Neurooncol,* 70, 91-95.

[301] Galanis E and Buckner JC. (2010). Enzastaurin in the treatment *J Clin Oncol*, 28, 1097-1098.

[302] Graff JR, McNulty AM, Hanna KR, et al. (2005). The protein kinase C *Cancer Res*, 65, 7462-7469.

[303] Tabatabai G, Frank B, Wick A, et al. (2007). Synergistic antiglioma activity of radiotherapy *Ann Neurol,* 61, 153-161.

[304] Kreisl TN, Kim L, Moore K, et al. (2009). A phase I trial *Clin Cancer Res*, 15, 3617-3623.

[305] Wick W, Puduvalli VK, Chamberlain MC, et al. (2010). Phase III study of enzastaurin compared with lomustine in the treatment *J Clin Oncol*, 28, 1168-1174.

[306] Butowski N, Chang SM, Lamborn KR, et al. (2010). Enzastaurin plus temozolomide with radiation therapy in glioblastoma multiforme: a phase I study. *Neuro Oncol,* 12, 608-613.

In: Gliomas: Classification, Symptoms, Treatment and Prognosis ISBN: 978-1-63117-868-9
Editor: David Cory Adamson

Chapter 9

Identification of a Potent Antiglioma Agent from Pre-Clinical Screening*

***Shivaputra A. Patil*†1, *Lawrence M. Pfeffer*2 *and Duane D. Miller*‡1**

[1]Department of Pharmaceutical Sciences, College of Pharmacy,
[2]Department of Pathology and Laboratory Medicine,
College of Medicine, and the Center for Cancer Research,
University of Tennessee Health Science Center, Memphis, TN, US

Abstract

Chemotherapy has played a very important role in the treatment of glioblastoma multiforme (GBM). Although temozolomide is the current standard of care chemotherapeutic agent to treat GBM, the prognosis for most temozolomide-treated patients remains very poor. Therefore, new anticancer drugs are urgently needed to advance GBM treatment. The process of discovering new anticancer agents often begins with screening campaigns to identify pre-clinical lead compounds. Using this approach, we have identified **SP-6-27** as a potent lead antiglioma agent from GRI screening. The lead agent showed potent growth inhibition against 60 cell lines in the NCI panel. We describe the screening results of our lead **SP-6-27** (**NSC: D-771606/1**) in this short communication.

* Part of the paper is presented at 246th American Chemical Society National Meeting & Exposition, Indianapolis, IN, United States, 2013, September 8-12, MEDI 131.

† Author for correspondence: Department of Pharmaceutical Sciences, College of Pharmacy, The University of Tennessee Health Science Center, 847 Monroe Avenue, Room 327, Memphis, TN 38163, US, Tel.:+1 901 448 7837, Fax: +1 901 448 6828, E-mail addresses: spatil3@uthsc.edu (S. A. Patil)

‡ Author for correspondence: Department of Pharmaceutical Sciences, College of Pharmacy, The University of Tennessee Health Science Center, 881 Madison, Room 435, Memphis, TN 38163, US, Tel.:+1 901 448 76026, Fax: +1 901 448 3446, E-mail addresses: dmiller@uthsc.edu (D.D. Miller).

Introduction

Glioblastoma Multiforme (GBM, WHO grade IV) is the most aggressive form of glioma and accounts for nearly 53.8 % of malignant gliomas [1]. GBM remains difficult to treat because of the infiltrative growth of the tumor cells, and their resistance to standard therapy. The present treatment regimen for GBM involves surgery, radiation therapy and chemotherapy. Despite advances in GBM therapy, the prognosis remains poor [2-4]. Identification of biological peculiarities of GBM and study of genetic alterations and development of innovative therapies may provide new opportunities to develop effective treatment. Chemotherapy has an important adjuvant role in the treatment of GBM [5-6]. Various classes of chemotherapeutic agents including temozolomide are being studied in different brain tumor populations but have provided little improvement in patient survival [7-8]. Therefore, highly potent chemotherapeutic drugs are urgently needed to treat malignant gliomas. Development of antiglioma drugs is fraught with great challenges. To develop novel antiglioma agents, new families of compounds may need to be designed, synthesized and tested *in vitro* initially in various GBM cell lines [9-10]. Novel chemotherapeutic agents must be able to selectively inhibit the growth of GBM cells leaving normal cells unharmed. This selectivity is critical in identifying new chemotherapeutic agents for glioma. Scientists are testing a number of new drugs for GBM, but only a limited number of drugs have entered the clinical setting.

The process of design and development of new drugs to treat cancer mostly begins with screening processes to identify potential lead drug candidates. This process of pre-selection of drugs to treat GBM is very important. Drug screening can be performed using various *in vitro* assays. *In vitro* drug screening provides a quick, cost-effective method for selection of potent antiglioma compounds. Planning the course of effective screening mainly involves selection of a proper set of compounds built in-house or obtained from commercially available libraries. The main goal of the screening process is to identify the lead selective anticancer agent. Once the selective lead drug candidate is identified it can be further optimized using medicinal chemistry approached to optimize pharmaceutical issues such as absorption, distribution, metabolism, excretion, and toxicity (ADMET) of the drug.

The University of Cincinnati-Drug Discovery Center (UC-DDC) Library Screen

Various approaches are available to identify chemical starting points for drug discovery projects. Medicinal chemists are using mostly commercially available libraries as primary drivers for discovering initial hits for their particular interests. We recently used arginine-glycine-aspartate (RGD) and related analogs to perform the similarity searches against the University of Cincinnati-Drug Discovery Center (UC-DDC) Library consisting of 362,000 compounds [11]. Initially, we identified two compounds, 7-(4-bromocarbonyl-piperazin-1-yl)-1-cyclopropyl-6-fluoro-4-oxo-1,2,3,4-tetrahydro-quinoline-3-carboxylic acid (**GRI-102696**, a Ciprofloxacin analog) and 2-amino-4-(5-bromo-2-methoxy-phenyl)-7-hydroxy-4H-chromene-3-carbonitrile (**GRI-394837**) as initial hits (GRI stands for Genome Research Institute). Since **GRI-102696** is an alkylating agent, we turned our interest towards **GRI-**

394837, a chromene analog for further development (**Figure 1**). Development of potent lead agents using hits identified from the initial or primary screening process (hit-to-lead approach) presents considerable challenges. We used a synthetically feasible scaffold as a starting point in our program to identify the potent new antiglioma agent by designing and synthesizing a small set of chromenes and evaluating them against a panel of human GBM cell lines (T98, U87, LN18, A172). Thus, we developed a focused set of chromenes in our laboratory and screened for activity on established human glioma cell lines to identify a possible lead from the initial hit [12-13]. Fortunately, we identified **SP-6-27**, a novel chromene as our new lead antiglioma agent. **SP-6-27** has demonstrated selective cytotoxic activity against all four established human GBM cell lines (IC_{50} range = 7.4 to 640 nM) and it is particularly active against the A172 human glioma cell line (IC_{50} = 7.4 nM) as compared to normal primary astrocytes (IC_{50} = 2033 nM) *in vitro*. This compound was nearly ~8800-fold more potent than the standard care chemotherapy agent temozolomide (IC_{50} = 65000 nM) in our assay.

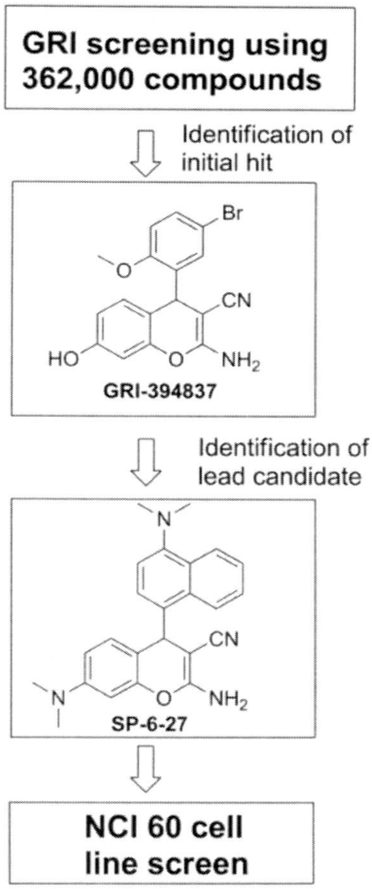

Figure 1. The general procedure followed to identify the lead candidate SP-6-27 from the initial screening process using compounds provided by University of Cincinnati, Drug Discovery Center's Genome Research Institute (GRI) library.

The National Cancer Institute-Development Therapeutics Program (NCI -DTP) 60 Cell Line Screen

The Development Therapeutics Program (DTP) of the National Cancer Institute's 60 human tumor cell line screen was developed as an *in vitro* drug discovery tool and it is a publicly available source worldwide for identifying compounds with high growth inhibitory or cytotoxic effects for cancer. The main mission of this program is to discover and develop novel anticancer agents. Details of the NCI 60 cell line drug development program are given elsewhere [14-15]. In brief, DTP's general drug screening procedure is shown in **Figure 2**.

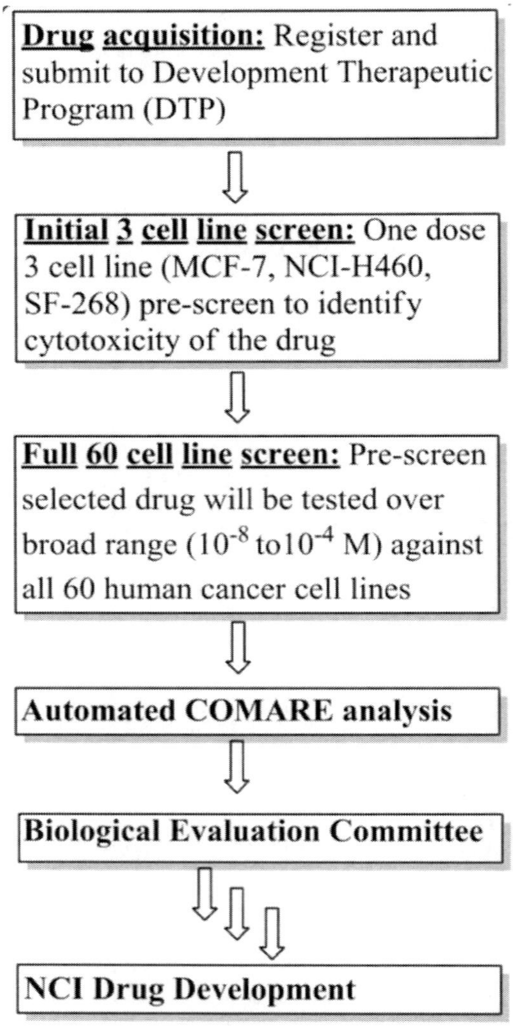

Figure 2. The NCI development therapeutics program's general pathway for the selection of compounds for the 60 cell line screen and further development.

The DTP utilizes 60 different human tumor cell lines representing nine major cancers (leukemia, non-small cell lung, central nervous system, colon, melanoma, ovarian, renal, prostate, and breast). Researchers from all over the world can register and submit the natural or synthetic compounds to the DTP. They provide information about the testing rationale and chemical structures of the submitted compounds. First, three cell lines (MCF-7 breast cancer; NCI-H460 large-cell lung cancer; SF-268 glioma) are used in a pre-screen to identify compounds with anti-proliferative activity. This procedure eliminates the inactive compounds but preserve active agents for 60 cell line screening. Pre-screen selected compounds are tested over a broad concentration range against every cell line from the 60 cell line panel (**Figure 2**). The screening procedure has been given in detail elsewhere and presently DTP uses the sulforhodamine B (SRB) assay [16-20].

We submitted our lead candidate **SP-6-27** along with its close analog **SP-6-19** to the DTP for the 60 cell lines screen. Both compounds were tested over a broad range of concentration against every cell line in the panel (five 10-fold dilutions starting from 10^{-4} M concentration). **Figure 3** shows the dose response curves for our lead compound **SP-6-27**. From these dose response curves three end points are calculated (GI_{50}: 50% of growth inhibition; TGI: total growth inhibition; LC_{50}: 50% of lethal concentration).

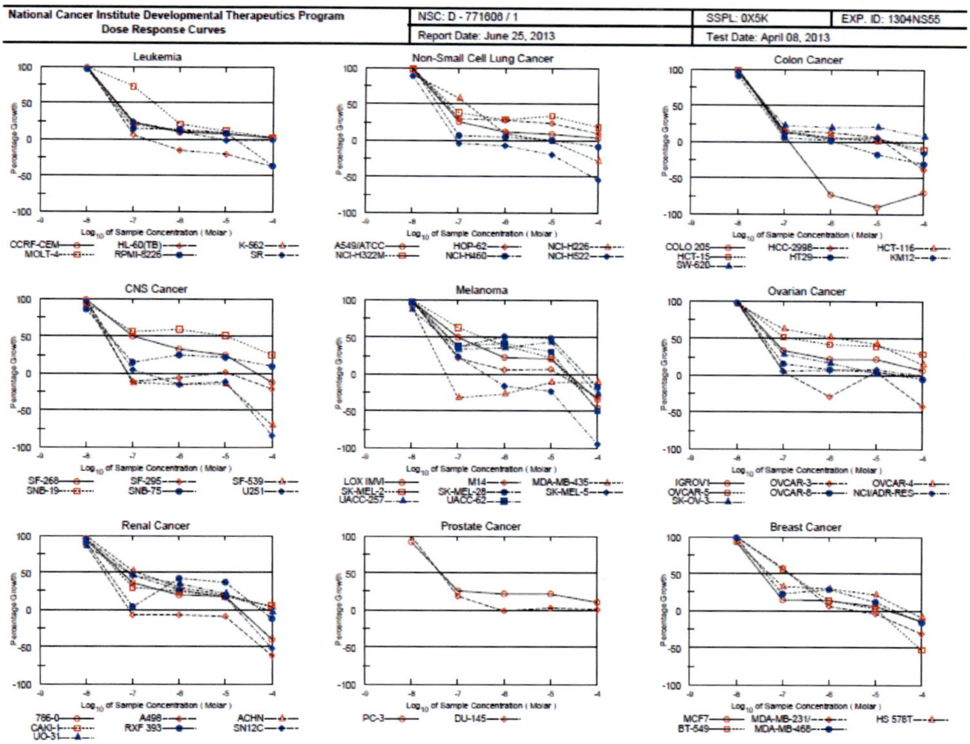

Figure 3. Dose response curves derived from screening of SP-6-27 (NSC: D-771606/1) in 60 cell line screen using nine major human cancer cell lines (leukemia, non-small cell lung cancer, colon cancer, CNS cancer, melanoma, ovarian cancer, renal cancer, prostate cancer and breast cancer).

Our lead molecules, **SP-6-27** (**NSC: D-771606/1**) and its close analog **SP-6-19 (NSC: D–761347/1)** demonstrated a cytostatic effect towards most of the cancer cell lines tested. Compounds **SP-6-27** (**NSC: D-771606/1**) and **SP-6-19** (**NSC: D–761347/1**) showed significant cytotoxic effect (LC_{50}: 0.52 μM and 2.9 μM) towards COLO205 (colon cancer), respectively. In general, both compounds showed a broad spectrum of antiproliferative activity towards all nine major cancers (**Table 1A & Table 1B**).

Table-1A. NCI *in vitro* testing results of SP-6-27 (μM)

Panel/Cell line	GI_{50} (μM)	TGI (μM)	LC_{50} (μM)	Panel/Cell line	GI_{50} (μM)	TGI (μM)	LC_{50} (μM)
Leukemia				MDA-MB-435	0.021	0.055	>100
CCRF-CEM	0.044	>100	>100	SK-MEL-2	0.351	21.2	>100
HL-60(TB)	0.034	0.189	>100	SK-MEL-28	-	55.1	>100
K-562	0.044	>100	>100	SK-MEL-5	0.046	0.404	24.2
MOLT-4	0.279	>100	>100	UACC-257	0.050	42.8	>100
RPMI-8226	0.037	15.7	>100	UACC-62	0.063	24.3	>100
SR	0.044	8.72	>100	**Ovarian Cancer**			
Non-small cell Lung				IGROV1	0.058	>100	>100
A549/ATCC	0.046	>100	>100	OVCAR-3	0.035	-	>100
HOP-62	0.052	>100	>100	OVCAR-4	1.59	>100	>100
NCI-H226	0.147	>100	>100	OVCAR-5	0.160	>100	>100
NCI-H322M	0.063	>100	>100	OVCAR-8	0.038	31.3	>010
NCI-H460	0.035	12.1	>100	NCI/ADR-RES	0.035	92.8	>100
NCI-H522	0.026	0.091	77.4	SK-OV-3	0.052	>100	>100
Colon Cancer				**Renal Cancer**			
COLO 205	0.037	0.12	0.52	786-0	0.058	20.3	>100
HCC-2998	0.039	14.0	>100	A498	0.024	0.084	59.9
HCT-116	0.038	>100	>100	ACHN	0.120	>100	>100
HCT-15	0.037	22.4	>100	CAKI-1	0.049	>100	>100
HT29	0.030	1.31	>100	RXF 393	0.029	57.2	>100
KM12	0.036	19.2	>100	SN12C	0.084	17.8	93.7
SW-620	0.041	>100	>100	UO-31	0.081	75.7	>100
CNS Cancer				**Prostate Cancer**			
SF-268	0.104	48.2	>100	PC-3	0.043	>100	>100
SF-295	0.026	-	>100	DU-145	0.044	-	>100
SF-539	0.030	0.078	44.2	**Breast Cancer**			
SNB-19	11.1	>100	>100	MCF7	0.036	19.7	>100
SNB-75	0.032	>100	>100	MDA-MB-231/ATCC	0.142	3.72	>100
U251	0.032	0.176	34.0	HS 578T	0.052	51.7	>100
Melanoma				BT-549	0.141	11.2	88.1
LOX IMVI	0.103	24.0	>100	MDA-MB-468	0.044	27.0	>100
M14	0.044	15.1	>100				

In this study, we mainly present the results of our lead agent **SP-6-27** (**NSC: D-771606/1**) in the glioma cell line panel (SF-268, SF-295, SF-539, SNB-19, SNB-75, U251) of the NCI. Interestingly, it showed notable LC_{50} (44.2 μM) towards the SF-539 cell line. Total growth inhibition (TGI) was observed for the SF-539 and U251 cell lines at 0.078 μM and 0.176 μM, respectively. More importantly, it showed nanomolar range GI_{50}'s towards several glioma cell lines (GI_{50}: SF-268- 0.104 μM; SF-295- 0.026 μM; SF-539-0.030 μM; SNB-75-0.032 μM; U251-0.032 μM) except SNB-19 cell line for which a GI_{50}: 11.1 μM was observed.

Table 1B. ***In vitro*** **testing results of SP-6-27 (NSC: D - 771606/1)**

National Cancer Institute Developmental Therapeutics Program
In-Vitro Testing Results

NSC : D - 771606 / 1	Experiment ID : 1304NS55	Test Type : 08	Units : Molar
Report Date : June 25, 2013	Test Date : April 08, 2013	QNS :	MC :
COMI : SP-6-27 (124977)	Stain Reagent : SRB Dual-Pass Related	SSPL : 0X5K	

			Log10 Concentration												
	Time		Mean Optical Densities					Percent Growth							
Panel/Cell Line	Zero	Ctrl	-8.0	-7.0	-6.0	-5.0	-4.0	-8.0	-7.0	-6.0	-5.0	-4.0	GI50	TGI	LC50
Leukemia															
CCRF-CEM	0.520	2.930	2.904	1.078	0.757	0.707	0.559	99	23	10	8	2	4.42E-8	> 1.00E-4	> 1.00E-4
HL-60(TB)	1.055	3.133	3.146	1.174	0.897	0.846	0.669	101	6	-15	-20	-37	3.41E-8	1.89E-7	> 1.00E-4
K-562	0.205	2.043	2.111	0.584	0.430	0.343	0.268	104	21	12	8	3	4.43E-8	> 1.00E-4	> 1.00E-4
MOLT-4	0.758	2.815	2.859	2.259	1.198	0.996	0.821	102	73	21	12	3	2.79E-7	> 1.00E-4	> 1.00E-4
RPMI-8226	0.779	2.758	2.700	1.072	1.052	0.954	0.499	97	15	14	9	-36	3.73E-8	1.57E-5	> 1.00E-4
SR	0.524	2.740	2.671	1.060	0.759	0.521	0.517	97	24	11	-1	-1	4.41E-8	8.72E-6	> 1.00E-4
Non-Small Cell Lung Cancer															
A549/ATCC	0.519	2.193	2.152	0.959	0.728	0.676	0.579	98	26	12	9	4	4.65E-8	> 1.00E-4	> 1.00E-4
HOP-62	0.689	2.055	2.067	1.097	1.075	1.022	0.829	101	30	28	24	10	5.21E-8	> 1.00E-4	> 1.00E-4
NCI-H226	1.253	2.554	2.437	2.007	1.385	1.236	0.896	91	58	10	-1	-28	1.47E-7	7.56E-6	> 1.00E-4
NCI-H322M	0.599	1.639	1.634	0.994	0.901	0.948	0.792	99	38	29	34	19	6.38E-8	> 1.00E-4	> 1.00E-4
NCI-H460	0.340	3.111	3.144	0.535	0.469	0.361	0.312	101	7	5	1	-8	3.50E-8	1.21E-5	> 1.00E-4
NCI-H522	1.247	2.506	2.371	1.201	1.159	1.010	0.575	89	-4	-7	-19	-54	2.65E-8	9.13E-8	7.74E-5
Colon Cancer															
COLO 205	0.470	1.775	1.839	0.585	0.126	0.046	0.139	105	9	-73	-90	-70	3.73E-8	1.28E-7	5.21E-7
HCC-2998	0.528	1.639	1.632	0.708	0.675	0.601	0.325	99	16	13	7	-38	3.93E-8	1.40E-5	> 1.00E-4
HCT-116	0.264	2.247	2.279	0.543	0.384	0.274	0.267	102	14	6	1		3.89E-8	> 1.00E-4	> 1.00E-4
HCT-15	0.331	2.024	2.004	0.563	0.432	0.422	0.298	99	14	6	5	-10	3.74E-8	2.24E-5	> 1.00E-4
HT29	0.260	1.390	1.294	0.333	0.285	0.217	0.183	91	6	2	-17	-30	3.07E-8	1.31E-6	> 1.00E-4
KM12	0.665	2.964	2.911	0.960	0.754	0.802	0.566	98	13	4	6	-15	3.65E-8	1.92E-5	> 1.00E-4
SW-620	0.408	2.727	2.582	0.951	0.866	0.886	0.603	94	23	20	21	8	4.19E-8	> 1.00E-4	> 1.00E-4
CNS Cancer															
SF-268	0.612	2.199	2.186	1.411	1.129	1.006	0.542	99	50	33	25	-12	1.04E-7	4.82E-5	> 1.00E-4
SF-295	0.899	2.904	2.788	0.802	0.848	0.948	0.713	94	-11	-6	2	-21	2.64E-8		> 1.00E-4
SF-539	0.979	2.315	2.425	0.851	0.832	0.845	0.295	108	-13	-15	-14	-70	3.02E-8	7.80E-8	4.42E-5
SNB-19	0.755	2.308	2.222	1.625	1.672	1.549	1.150	94	56	59	51	25	1.11E-5	> 1.00E-4	> 1.00E-4
SNB-75	0.959	1.788	1.672	1.081	1.170	1.140	1.046	86	15	25	22	10	3.20E-8	> 1.00E-4	> 1.00E-4
U251	0.585	2.126	2.083	0.661	0.497	0.520	0.093	97	5	-15	-11	-84	3.25E-8	1.76E-7	3.40E-5
Melanoma															
LOX IMVI	0.658	3.136	3.097	1.907	1.227	1.172	0.435	98	50	23	21	-34	1.03E-7	2.40E-5	> 1.00E-4
M14	0.546	2.070	2.068	0.887	0.633	0.648	0.379	100	22	6	7	-31	4.40E-8	1.51E-5	> 1.00E-4
MDA-MB-435	0.544	2.434	2.290	0.370	0.398	0.484	0.486	92	-32	-27	-11	-11	2.19E-8	5.53E-8	> 1.00E-4
SK-MEL-2	0.753	1.257	1.288	1.070	0.952	0.869	0.399	106	63	39	23	-47	3.51E-7	2.12E-5	> 1.00E-4
SK-MEL-28	0.592	1.502	1.546	0.929	1.059	1.037	0.491	105	37	51	49	-17		5.51E-5	> 1.00E-4
SK-MEL-5	0.929	2.954	2.973	1.419	0.783	0.717	0.060	101	24	-16	-23	-94	4.61E-8	4.04E-7	2.42E-5
UACC-257	0.905	1.859	1.735	1.231	1.245	1.327	0.672	87	34	36	44	-26	5.02E-8	4.28E-5	> 1.00E-4
UACC-62	0.902	2.805	2.755	1.635	1.710	1.492	0.458	97	38	42	31	-49	6.38E-8	2.43E-5	> 1.00E-4
Ovarian Cancer															
IGROV1	0.486	1.717	1.767	0.903	0.753	0.760	0.576	104	34	22	22	7	5.89E-8	> 1.00E-4	> 1.00E-4
OVCAR-3	0.705	1.962	2.024	0.766	0.503	0.763	0.410	105	5	-29	5	-42	3.54E-8		> 1.00E-4
OVCAR-4	0.559	1.071	1.050	0.881	0.824	0.780	0.635	96	63	52	43	15	1.59E-6	> 1.00E-4	> 1.00E-4
OVCAR-5	0.593	1.295	1.312	0.959	0.886	0.872	0.799	102	52	42	40	29	1.60E-7	> 1.00E-4	> 1.00E-4
OVCAR-8	0.588	2.367	2.323	0.873	0.739	0.683	0.556	98	16	8	5	-5	3.83E-8	3.13E-5	> 1.00E-4
NCI/ADR-RES	0.543	2.117	2.200	0.632	0.646	0.672	0.542	105	6	7	8		3.59E-8	9.28E-5	> 1.00E-4
SK-OV-3	0.584	1.322	1.351	0.795	0.707	0.604	0.588	104	29	17	3		5.20E-8	> 1.00E-4	> 1.00E-4
Renal Cancer															
786-0	0.584	2.480	2.387	1.275	0.965	0.926	0.348	95	36	20	18	-40	5.87E-8	2.03E-5	> 1.00E-4
A498	1.700	2.568	2.452	1.583	1.583	1.542	0.652	87	-7	-7	-9	-62	2.46E-8	8.44E-8	5.99E-5
ACHN	0.411	1.720	1.768	1.089	0.801	0.669	0.460	104	52	30	20	4	1.20E-7	> 1.00E-4	> 1.00E-4
CAKI-1	0.648	2.617	2.528	1.236	1.141	1.000	0.752	95	30	25	18	5	4.93E-8	> 1.00E-4	> 1.00E-4
RXF 393	0.948	1.878	1.795	0.986	1.343	1.297	0.834	91	4	42	37	-12	2.97E-8	5.72E-5	> 1.00E-4
SN12C	0.643	2.735	2.644	1.613	1.211	1.006	0.309	96	46	27	17	-52	8.43E-8	1.78E-5	9.37E-5
UO-31	0.655	1.834	1.675	1.203	1.062	0.917	0.635	86	46	35	22	-3	8.16E-8	7.57E-5	> 1.00E-4
Prostate Cancer															
PC-3	0.698	2.247	2.129	1.106	1.037	1.035	0.869	92	26	22	22	11	4.38E-8	> 1.00E-4	> 1.00E-4
DU-145	0.460	1.873	1.968	0.734	0.457	0.496	0.477	107	19	-1	3	1	4.46E-8		> 1.00E-4
Breast Cancer															
MCF7	0.419	2.348	2.220	0.717	0.695	0.535	0.359	93	15	14	6	-14	3.60E-8	1.97E-5	> 1.00E-4
MDA-MB-231/ATCC	0.681	1.624	1.638	1.228	0.734	0.653	0.473	101	58	6	-4	-31	1.42E-7	3.72E-6	> 1.00E-4
HS 578T	1.268	2.301	2.232	1.611	1.574	1.491	1.159	93	33	30	22	-9	5.25E-8	5.17E-5	> 1.00E-4
BT-549	1.240	2.112	2.127	1.732	1.360	1.263	0.582	102	56	14	3	-53	1.41E-7	1.12E-5	8.81E-5
MDA-MB-468	0.767	1.676	1.670	0.979	1.032	0.879	0.643	99	23	29	12	-16	4.45E-8	2.70E-5	> 1.00E-4

Figure 4 demonstrates a mean graph pattern for the lead agent **SP-6-27** (**NSC: D-771606/1**). Mean graphs are created for GI_{50}, TGI, and LC_{50} by plotting positive and negative values termed as deltas generated from dose response curves. More sensitive cell lines are displayed as bars that project to the right of the mean, whereas the less sensitive cell lines are displayed with bars projected to the left. The length of each bar is proportional to the relative sensitivity of the agent with the mean determination. In GI_{50} mean graphs, the lead agent **SP-6-27** (**NSC: D-771606/1**) is active towards the SF-295, SF-539, SNB-75 and U251 cell lines.

In the case of TGI and LC_{50} mean graphs SF-539 and U251 are active cell lines. In summary, NCI screening results confirmed that the lead agent **SP-6-27 (NSC: D-771606/1)** has cytostatic activity towards most of the cancer cell lines except the COLO-205 cell line for which it is cytotoxic. The **SP-6-27 (NSC: D-771606/1)** has been selected for further *in vivo* screening at the NCI and outcomes of the NCI screening along with our *in vivo* findings will be published in near future.

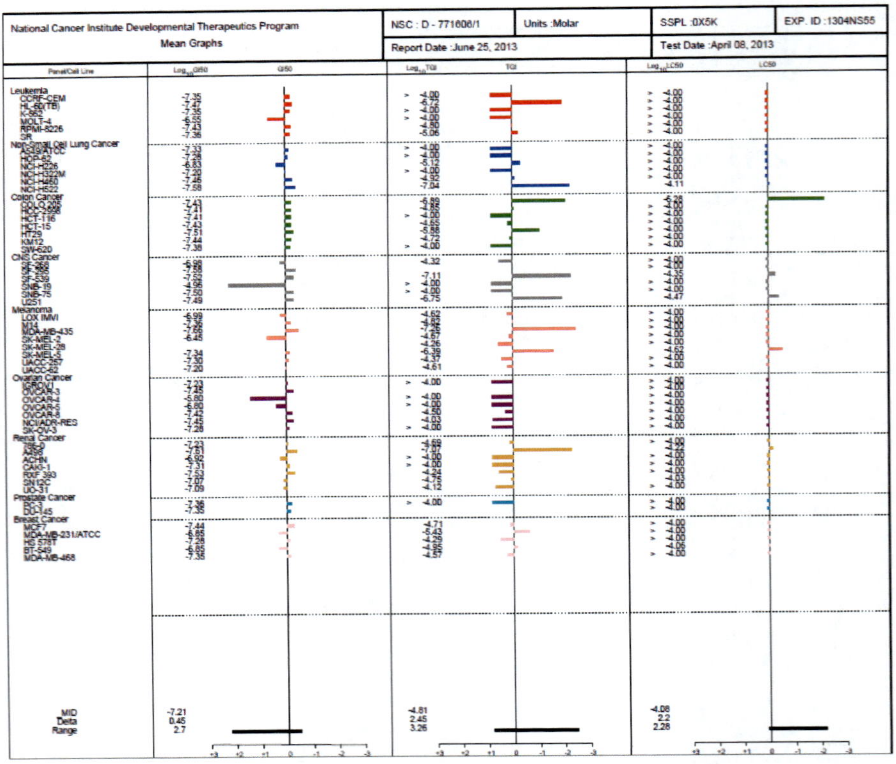

Figure 4. The mean graph representation of antitumor effects of SP-6-27 (NSC: D-771606/1). The GI50 (50% of growth inhibition), TGI (total growth inhibition) and LC50 (50% of lethal concentration) mean graphs derived from the dose response curves using figure 3 from the initial screening.

Conclusion

Preclinical *in vitro* screening is a very important initial process in drug discovery and development. It helps to identify and prioritize lead drug candidates from initial hits for the further development. A main criterion behind screening is that the lead candidate should have selective growth inhibitory effect towards the cancer cell lines and not affect the growth of normal cells. The identified potent cytotoxic candidate (lead) is further modified through medicinal chemistry techniques to enhance its drug like properties. In the present study we identified **SP-6-27 (NSC: D-771606/1)** as an initial lead agent through our screening processes and its growth inhibitory effect was confirmed by the NCI 60 cell line screening. This promising lead will be further optimized to advance it towards *in vivo* pre-clinical studies.

Acknowledgment

The screening of **SP-6-27** against 60 human cancer cell lines of NCI's developmental therapeutic programs (DTP) is gratefully acknowledged. This work was supported by the Van Vleet Professorship (DDM), the Pilot Data Program Research Fund, UTHSC Research Office (SAP) and Dean's Enhancement Program for Seed Research Grant (SAP)

References

[1] *http://www.cbtrus.org/*

[2] Arko, L; Katsyv, I; Park, GE; Luan, WP; Park JK. (2010) Experimental approaches for the treatment of malignant gliomas. *Pharmacol Ther*, 128(1), 1-36.

[3] Van Meir, EG; Hadjipanayis, CG; Norden, AD; Shu, HK; Wen, PY; Olson, JJ. (2010) Exciting new advances in neuro-oncology: the avenue to a cure for malignant glioma. *CA Cancer J Clin*, 60(3), 166-193.

[4] Reardon, DA; Wen, PY. (2006) Therapeutic advances in the treatment of glioblastoma: Rationale and potential role of targeted agents. *The Oncologist,* 11, 152–164.

[5] Kreisl TN. (2009) Chemotherapy for Malignant Gliomas. *Semin Radiat Oncol*, 19, 150-154.

[6] Minniti, G; Muni, R; Lanzetta, G; Marchetti, P; Enrici RM. (2009) Chemotherapy for glioblastoma: current treatment and future perspectives for cytotoxic and targeted agents. *Anticancer Res*, 29(12), 5171-84.

[7] Villano, JL; Seery, TE; Bressler, LR. (2009) Temozolomide in malignant gliomas: current use and future targets. *Cancer Chemother Pharmacol*, 64(4), 647-55.

[8] Reardon, DA; Wen, PY. (2006) Therapeutic advances in the treatment of glioblastoma: Rationale and potential role of targeted agents. *The Oncologist*, 11, 152–164.

[9] Patil, SA; Hosni-Ahmed, A; Jones, TS; Patil, R; Pfeffer, LM; Miller, DD. (2013) Novel approaches to glioma drug design and drug screening. *Expert Opin Drug Discov*. [Epub ahead of print].

[10] Sathornsumetee, S; Rich, JN. (2008) Designer Therapies for Glioblastoma Multiforme. *Ann NY Acad Sci*, 1142, 108–132

[11] *http://www.drugdiscovery.uc.edu*

[12] Patil, SA; Wang, J; Li, XS; Chen, J; Jones, TS; Hosni-Ahmed, A; Patil, R; Seibel, WL; Li, W; Miller DD. (2012) New substituted 4H-chromenes as anticancer agents. *Bioorg Med Chem Lett*, 22(13), 4458-61.

[13] Patil, SA; Jones, TS; Hosni-Ahmed, A; Wang, J; Patil, R; Li, W; Miller, DD. (2012), *New substituted 4H-chromenes as antiglioma agents*. 244th ACS National Meeting & Exposition, Philadelphia, PA, United States, August 19-23, MEDI-53.

[14] *http://dtp.nci.nih.gov/*

[15] Shoemaker, RH. (2006) The NCI60 human tumour cell line anticancer drug screen. *Nat Rev Cancer*, 6(10):813-23.

[16] Boyd, MR; Paull, KD. (1995) Some practical considerations and applications of the National Cancer Institute in vitro anticancer drug discovery screen. *Drug Dev Res*, 34, 91–109.

[17] Holbeck, SL; Collins, JM; Doroshow, JH. (2010) Analysis of Food and Drug Administration-approved anticancer agents in the NCI60 panel of human tumor cell lines. *Mol Cancer Ther*, 9(5), 1451-60.

[18] Covell, DG; Huang, R; Wallqvist, A. (2007) Anticancer medicines in development: assessment of bioactivity profiles within the National Cancer Institute anticancer screening data. *Mol Cancer Ther*, 6(8), 2261-70.

[19] Skehan, P; Streng, R; Scudiero, D; Monks, A; McMahon, J; Vistica, D; Warren, JT; Bokesch, H; Kenney, S; Boyd, M. (1990) New colorimetric cytotoxicity assay for anticancer-drug screening. *J. Natl. Cancer Inst*, 82: 1107–1112.

[20] Monks, A; Scudiero, D; Skehan, P; Shoemaker, R; Paull, K; Vistica, D; Hose, C; Langley, J; Cronise, P; Vaigro-Wolff, A; Gray-Goodrich, M; Campbell, H; Mayo, J; Boyd, M. (1991) Feasibility of a high-flux anticancer drug screen using a diverse panel of cultured human tumor cell Lines. *J. Natl. Cancer Inst,* 11: 757–766.

In: Gliomas: Classification, Symptoms, Treatment and Prognosis ISBN: 978-1-63117-868-9
Editor: David Cory Adamson

Chapter 10

The Relationship between P53-ROS Pathway and Programmed Cell Death in C6 Glioma Cells

***Gang Wang*[*1,3], JunJie Wang,[1] ShiMing Du[1] and DongSheng Li[2]**
[1] Department of Hospital Pharmacy, Binzhou Medical University Hospital, Binzhou City, Shandong Province, China
[2] University of Hubei Medicine, Shiyan City, Hubei Province Hubei Province, China
[3] Department of Pharmacy, Chendu Traditional Chinese Medical University, Chendu City, Sichuan Province, China

Abstract

Background and purpose: As one of the major types of programmed cell death (PCD), necrosis has been observed and demonstrated to be responsible for cell death and the mechanisms responsible for necrosis are still not very clear. This study reviews that programmed cell death (PCD), including apoptosis and necrosis for C6 glioma cells is related to p53-reactive oxygen species (ROS).

Experimental approach: The C6 glioma cells were treated with N-acetylcysteine (NAC) and assayed for cell survival, cellular ROS levels by flow cytometry assays, and western blot assay for P53 expression. C6 glioma cells were compared to downregulation of ROS levels and p53 expression, respectively pretreated with p-fifty three inhibitor-alpha (PFT-α) and N-acetylcysteine (NAC).

Key results: C6 glioma cells showed a significant decrease (~2-fold) in DHE-fluorescence after NAC treatment. Interestingly, the accumulation of ROS was elevated with P53 expression in C6 glioma cells. The increase in ROS levels was followed by a decrease in cell growth and viability, and increase in the percentage of cells with necrosis.

[*] Corresponding Author: Gang Wang, PhD, Department of hospital pharmacy, Binzhou Medical University Hospital, Yellow River two Road, No. 661, Binzhou City, Shandong Province 256603,China, Phone: +86 13972481839, Email: 13972481839@163.com.

Conclusions and implications: p53 overexpression enhanced p53-induced ROS-accumulation, which was accompanied by an increase in cell death with necrosis. These results support the hypothesis that there is a close relationship between regulating p53-induced ROS–accumulation and apoptosis and necrosis in C6 glioma cells.

Keywords: C6 Glioma, ROS, p53, programmed cell death (PCD), Cell Necrosis

Abbreviations

PCD	programmed cell death;
ROS	reactive oxygen species;
PFT-α,	p-fifty three inhibitor-alpha;
NAC	N-acetylcysteine;
LDH	lactate dehydrogenase

Introduction

As the major types of programmed cell death (PCD), a wide variety of modes of glioma cell death have been reported, including apoptotic, necrotic, and autophagic cell death (Hotchkiss et al., 2009). On occasion, necrosis and apoptosis occur simultaneously after stress; at other times, only necrosis or apoptosis is observed (Okada and Mak, 2004). The mechanisms responsible for necrosis are still not very clear.

In recent years, it has become apparent that reactive oxygen species (ROS) play an important role during apoptosis induction (Fleury et al., 2002). Accumulation of ROS could result in oxidative damage to critical cellular biomolecules (nucleic acids, protein, and lipids) resulting in cytotoxicity (Biaglow et al., 1992). Many stimuli such as anticancer drugs, and chemotherapeutic agents stimulate cells to produce intracellular ROS as well as endogenous sources (mitochondrial electron transport chain and oxygen metabolizing enzymes) (Simizu et al., 1998; Park et al., 2005; Kuwabara et al., 2008).Increased production of ROS may derive from the NADPH oxidase and from the mitochondria (Haendeler et al.,2004). Intracellular production of ROS can directly lead to activation of the mitochondrial permeability transition and to loss of mitochondrial membrane potential (Chan et al., 2003).

Gliomas are the most frequent primary tumors in the central nervous system, and patients with malignant glioma have a very poor prognosis (Castro et al., 2011). Unfortunately, during tumor progression towards drug resistance, the tumor's apoptotic machinery, consisting of anti-apoptotic and pro-apoptotic proteins, becomes unbalanced and favors cell survival following cytotoxic insults. In such a scenario, agents that initiate non-apoptotic cell death may easily overcome the inherent deficiencies of the apoptotic machinery in cancer cells. As a result, targeting alternative cell death pathways may represent an attractive approach to increasing overall tumor cell kills. In this review, we demonstrate that N-acetylcysteine (NAC) can induce cell death distinct from apoptosis and autophagy, and is associated with the loss of mitochondrial membrane potential and the induction of ROS.

A previous study reported (Macip et al., 2003) a correlation between ROS levels to human glioma's response to chemotherapy. Necrosis is often defined as the default cell death pathway. To date, however, the exact mechanism by which ROS regulate necrosis in glioma cells is still poorly understood. Thus, the purpose of this review is to elucidate the relationship between necrosis and apoptosis in C6 glioma cells and to uncover the molecular mechanism that might be involved.

NAC Induces Apoptosis and Necrosis in C6 Glioma Cells

To examine whether N-acetylcysteine (NAC) induced cell death in C6 glioma cells, C6 glioma cells were treated with NAC, and cell death was measured by flow-cytometric analysis with Propidium Iodide staining. Treatment effectively induced cell death in C6 glioma cells after 12-24 h of incubation with NAC.

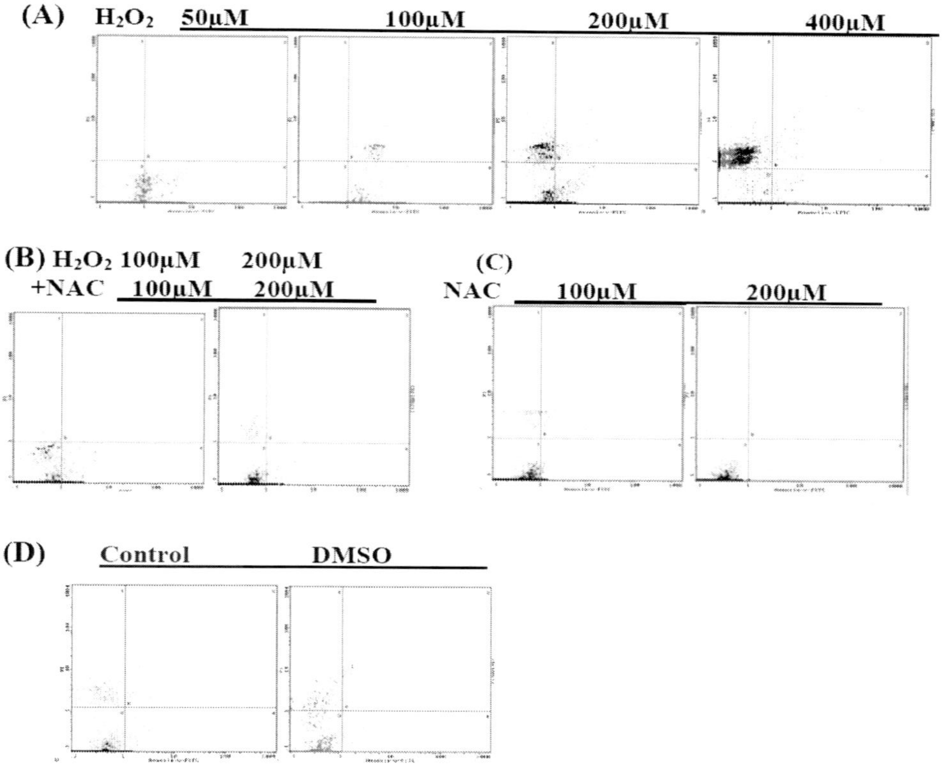

Figure 1. Apoptosis and necrosis in C6 glioma cells induced by H_2O_2. C6 glioma cells were treated with the indicated concentration of nano-liposome of quercetin (H2O2) in the absence or presence of NAC or PFT-α for 24 h. (A) H_2O_2 induces dose-dependent apoptosis and necrosis in C6 glioma cells. Cells were stained with annexin V-FITC and analyzed by flow cytometry. (B) H_2O_2-induced apoptosis and necrosis of C6 glioma cells were treated with NAC or for 24 h. Cells stained with annexin V-FITC and analyzed by flow cytometry. (C) C6 glioma cells were respectivly treated with NAC for 24 h and stained with annexin V-FITC and analyzed by flow cytometry. (D) Control cells, including blank, DMSO. The values of cell death (apoptosis and necrosis) reported represent the mean ± SD of three separate experiments. *$P < 0.05$, **$P < 0.01$ compared with control cells.

Next, the C6 glioma cells were treated with H_2O_2 and pretreated with N-acetylcysteine (NAC). Assays for necrosis and apoptosis showed protection for C6 glioma cells from NAC. As control cells exhibited normal nuclei with uniform and finely dispersed chromatin, surrounded by cytoplasm with normal appearing mitochondria. In this study, necrotic cells were decreased in C6 glioma cells after pretreatment with NAC treatment. Moreover, there is a time- and dose-dependent decrease of cell death in C6 glioma cells (Figure 1). These results provided further evidence that NAC induced necrosis in C6 glioma cells.

P53 Participates in the Regulation of Necrosis in C6 Glioma Cells

To evaluate the function of the antioncogene p53 in necrosis, C6 glioma cells were treated with H_2O_2 and pretreated with 60, 120μmol/L p-fifty three inhibitor-alpha(PFT-α). Treatment efficiency was estimated by Western blot analysis. Results show that p53 protein expression significantly decreased in PFT-α- treated C6 glioma cells (Figure 2).

Compared with C6 cells treated with H_2O_2, expression of p53 was promoted. In contrast, PFT-α decreased the level of p53 in C6 glioma cells. All these results corroborate the observation that necrosis was partially promoted by expression of p53 and decreased by p53 inhibitor.

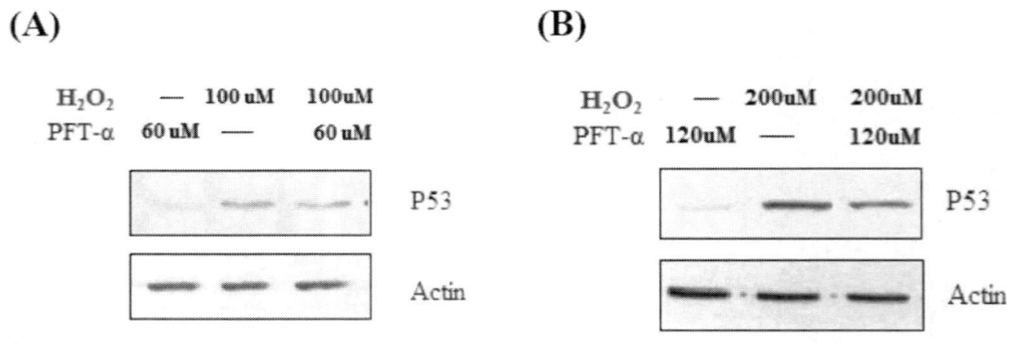

Figure 2. P53 participated in the regulation of necrosis induced by H_2O_2. C6 glioma cells ($5x10^6$/ml) were treated with H_2O_2 in the absence or presence of PFT-α for 24 h then harvested for associated protein expressions estimated using Western blotting as described in Materials and Methods. (A) C6 glioma cells were respectivly treated with the indicated concentrations of 100μmol/L H_2O_2 in the absence or present of 60μmol/L PFT-α for 24 h. The alteration of p53 and actin was analyzed by western blotting. (B) 200μmol/L H_2O_2-induced increase of p53 proteins is inhibited with 120μmol/L PFT-α. The alteration of p53 and actin was analyzed by western blotting.

ROS Participate in the Regulation of Necrosis in C6 Glioma Cells

To evaluate the function of reactive oxygen species (ROS)-related necrosis induced by H_2O_2, C6 glioma cells were treated with N-acetylcysteine (NAC). Treatment efficiency was estimated by flow cytometer analysis. ROS activity significantly increased in C6 glioma cells while NAC decreased the level of ROS.

To further address the function of ROS in the regulation of necrosis, we compared the levels of ROS after cells treated with H_2O_2 and pretreated with NAC. Results show that NAC significantly inhibited the effect of necrosis in C6 glioma cells. In contrast, H_2O_2 led to obviously increased ROS accumulation compared to C6 glioma cells treated without NAC (Figure 3). Compared with C6 glioma cells where high levels of ROS enhanced the necrosis induced by H_2O_2, the levels of ROS decreased and were associated with bright green fluorescence more after H_2O_2 treatment in C6 glioma cells and cells pretreated with NAC.

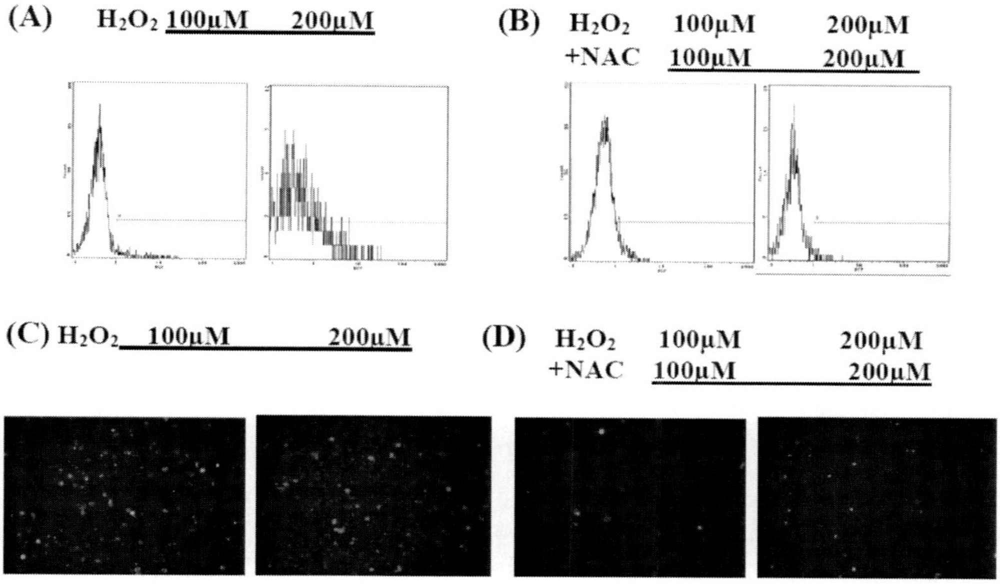

Figure 3. Apoptosis and necrosis of C6 glioma cells is involved in mediating ROS accumulation induced by H_2O_2. C6 glioma cells were treated with the indicated concentration of nano-liposome of quercetin (H_2O_2) for 24 h in the presence or absence of NAC. Cells were loaded with DCFH-DA for 30 min. **(A)** ROS in C6 glioma cells treated with H_2O_2 alone was estimated by flow cytometer analysis. **(B)** ROS in C6 glioma cells treated with NAC in combination with H_2O_2 was estimated by flow cytometer analysis. **(C, D)** The DCF fluorescence was visualized using fluorescence microscope.

Necrosis in C6 Glioma Cells Is Facilitated by P53-Mediated ROS Signaling

To look for the possible pathways that ROS signaling might be involved in p53-regulated necrosis in C6 glioma cells, we measured p53 expression and levels of ROS in C6 glioma cells after H_2O_2 treatment (Figure 4). These results show that the increased level of ROS expression induced by H_2O_2 was enhanced by overexpression of p53. Inhibition of p53 resulted in decreased ROS activation. These results suggest that p53 has a direct interaction with endogenous ROS. In H_2O_2 treated cells, more p53 combined with ROS, thereby inhibiting necrosis through the classic p53- mediated ROS pathway. In contrast, ROS inhibitor- NAC decreased necrosis, likely related to ROS activation.

We also investigated whether p53-mediated ROS, important in regulating cell apoptosis and necrosis, was involved in H_2O_2 induced ROS-regulated necrosis. H_2O_2 treatment causes a significant increase in the level of ROS and downregulated expression of the phosphorylation of p53. Thus, we speculated that p53-mediated ROS induced necrosis might act through the p53-mediated ROS signaling pathway. To test our hypothesis, we measured the phosphorylation of p53 after treatment of cells with H_2O_2. Compared with the untreated cells, H_2O_2 induced down-regulation of phosphorylation of p53 was remarkably enhanced by overexpression of ROS. In contrast, ROS inhibitor NAC increased expression of phosphorylation of p53. Collectively, these results indicated that necrosis in C6 glioma cells is mediated by p53-mediated ROS signaling pathways.

(A) H2O2 200μM **(B) H2O2 +NAC 200μM 200μM** **(C) NAC 200μM**

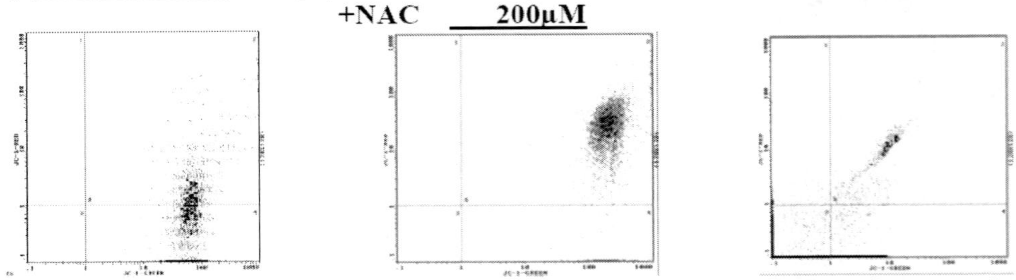

(Area of D2 means the normal mitochondrial membrane potential of C6 glioma cells, Area of D4 means the decreased mitochondrial membrane potential normal of C6 glioma cells)

(D)

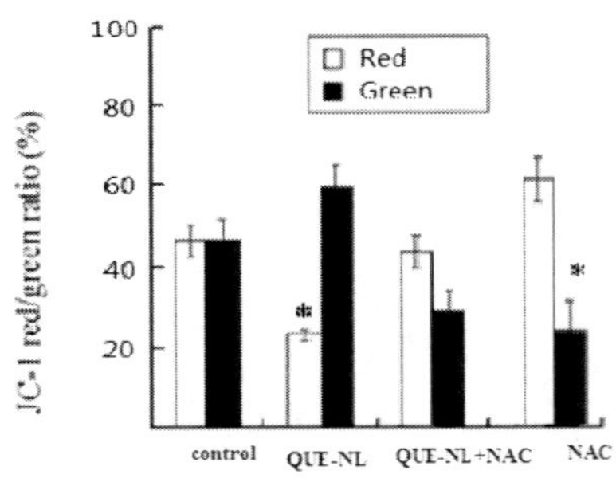

Figure 4. H_2O_2 induced necrosis is associated with loss of mitochondrial membrane potential and the changes of ROS. (A)H_2O_2-Induced Mitochondrial Membrane Potential and mitochondrial dynamics and regulated by H_2O_2. Mitochondrial membrane potential of cells was determined by retention of DiOC6(3) (40μM) added during the last 30 min of the treatment. The amount of retained DiOC6(3) was measured by flow cytometry. (B) C6 glioma cells were respectivly treated with the indicated concentrations of 200μmol/L H_2O_2 in the absence or presence of 200μmol/L N-acetylcysteine(NAC) for 24 h. (C) C6 glioma cells were respectivly treated with 200μmol/L N-acetylcysteine(NAC) alone for 24 h. (D)H_2O_2-induced loss of mitochondrial membrane potential is inhibited with NAC. The alteration of mitochondrial membrane potential was analyzed by flow cytometer. The values reported represent the mean ±SD of three separate experiments. *$P < 0.05$, compared with control cells.

Conclusion

Gliomas are the most common primary brain tumors in adults (Preusser M, et al., 2011). Malignant gliomas are resistant to various pro-apoptotic therapies, such as radiotherapy and conventional chemotherapy (Stewart, 2002); glioma cells are also resistant to conventional pro-apoptotic cancer therapeutics (Lefranc et al., 2005). Therefore, effective treatment of malignant gliomas may rely on the development of novel strategies for inducing nonapoptotic cell death, such as necrotic cell death, which has been recently described as an important alternative cell death pathway (Okada and Mak, 2004).

In this study, we demonstrated that necrosis or apoptosis in C6 glioma cells is through a p53-mediated ROS/ mitochondrial signaling pathway (Figure 5). Our results indicate that necrosis occurred with an increase in the protein level of p53. p53 is a antioncogene, and results in accumulation of ROS.

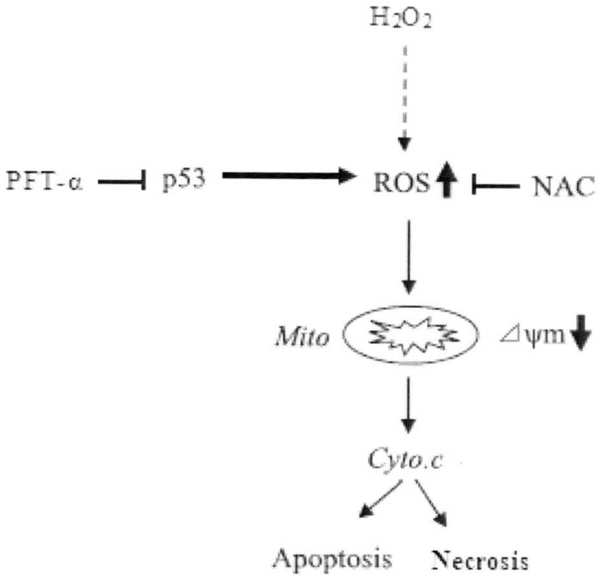

Figure 5. Diagram of mechanisms underlying the synergy between H_2O_2 induced necrosis and apoptosis.

Accumulation of intracellular ROS in response to diverse stimuli has been shown to lead to mitochondrial membrane permeability and subsequent activation of cell death machinery (Fleury et al., 2002). Moreover, recent studies provide evidence for the role of p53 as the potential inducer of ROS activation during necrotic cell death in response to a variety of different stimuli (Fleury et al., 2002; Park et al., 2006; Kuwabara et al., 2008). In this study, we provide further evidence that activation of ROS is involved in cell death. It is possible that ROS activation is caused by ROS-dependent DNA damage because recent reports show ROS-mediated DNA damage after hydrogen peroxide injury or in neurodegenerative disease triggers P53 activation and subsequent cell death (de Vries et al., 2008).

ROS involved in the cellular response to DNA damage plays a role in DNA damage mitochondrial signaling and repair (Ditsworth et al., 2007). Recent evidence indicates that excessive activation of ROS via intracellular NAD^+ and ATP generation can lead to necrotic or apoptotic cell death (Ditsworth et al., 2007; Mathews and Berk, 2008). Our results show p53 overexpression promotes accumulation of ROS, which is associated with ROS-induced necrosis. This is prevented with N-acetylcysteine (NAC) by blocking ROS induced loss in C6 glioma cells.

Thus, the p53-mediated ROS/mitochondrial signaling pathway can contribute to glioma cell death. We speculate that the ROS/p53-mediated cell death and the extrinsic pathway of apoptosis predominates in the present system. These findings might help guide new anti-cancer strategies.

In summary, this study provides rational evidence for further preclinical development of preferentially targeting alternative cell death pathways. Regulating the p53-mediated ROS/ mitochondrial signaling pathway in glioma treatment may result in improved preclinical outcomes.

Conflict of Interest

The authors state no conflict of interest.

Supplementary Material

Refer to Web version on PubMed Central for supplementary material.

Acknowledgments

We thank Dr. Li R M for the cell lines, Hubei Provincial Key Laboratory of embryo stem cells provided the facility for assisting with the experiments, Mr. Liu Z Q and Feng J B for assisting with the flow cytometry facility for assisting with flow cytometry, and Dr. Li D S for chemistry discussion. Funding from the project of Hubei Provincial Education Department and Pharmacy of Department in Taihe hospital supported this work.

References

Biaglow JE, Mitchell JB, Held K.(1992). The importance of peroxide and superoxide in the X-ray response. *Int J Radiat Oncol Biol Phys.* 22:665–669.

Castro MG, Cowen R, Williamson IK, David A, Jimenez-Dalmaroni MJ, Yuan X, Bigliari A, Williams JC, Hu J, Lowenstein PR. (2003).Current and future strategies for the treatment of malignant brain tumors. *Pharmacol Ther.*98:71–108.

Chan WH, Wu CC, Yu JS. (2003). Curcumin inhibits UV irradiation-induced oxidative stress and apoptotic biochemical changes in human epidermoid carcinoma A431 cells. *J Cell Biochem* 90:327–338.

de Vries HE, Witte M, Hondius D, et al. (2008).Nrf2-induced antioxidant protection: a promising target to counteract ROS-mediated damage in neurodegenerative disease? *Free Radic Biol Med.* 45:1375-1383.

Ditsworth D, Zong WX, Thompson CB.(2007).Activation of poly(ADP)-ribose polymerase (PARP-1) induces release of the pro-inflammatory mediator HMGB1 from the nucleus. *J Biol Chem.* 282:17845-17854.

Fleury C, Mignotte B, and Vayssie`re JL. (2002). Mitochondrial reactive oxygen species in cell death signaling. *Biochimie.*84**:**131–141.

Fleury C, Pampin M, Tarze A, Mignotte B. (2002).Yeast as a model to study apoptosis? *Biosci Rep.* 22:59-79.

Haendeler J, Hoffmann J, Diehl JF, Vasa M, Spyridopoulos I, Zeiher AM, Dimmeler S. (2004) Antioxidants inhibit nuclear export of telomerase reverse transcriptase and delay replicative senescence of endothelial cells. *Circ Res.*94: 768–775

Hotchkiss RS, Strasser A, McDunn JE, Swanson PE. Cell death.(2009).*N Engl J Med.*361: 1570– 1583.

Kuwabara M, Asanuma T, Niwa K, Inanami O. (2008).Regulation of cell survival and death signals induced by oxidative stress. *J Clin Biochem Nutr.* 43:51-57.

Kuwabara M, Asanuma T, Niwa K, Inanami O.(2008). Regulation of cell survival and death signals induced by oxidative stress. *J Clin Biochem Nutr.* 43:51–57.

Lefranc, F., Brotchi, J., and Kiss, R. (2005). Possible future issues in the treatment of glioblastomas: Special emphasis on cell migration and the resistance of migrating glioblastoma cells to apoptosis. *J. Clin. Oncol.* 23:2411–2422.

Lockshin RA, Zakeri Z. (2004). Caspase-independent cell death? *Oncogene.* 23:2766-2773.

Macip S, Igarashi M, Berggren P, Yu J, Lee SW, Aaronson SA. (2003). Influence of induced reactive oxygen species in p53-mediated cell fate decisions. *Mol Cell Biol.*23: 8576–8585

Mathews MT, Berk BC.(2008).PARP-1 inhibition prevents oxidative and nitrosative stress-induced endothelial cell death via transactivation of the VEGF receptor 2. *Arterioscler Thromb Vasc Biol.* 28:711-717.

Okada H, Mak TW. (2004). Pathways of apoptotic and non-apoptotic death in tumour cells. *Nat Rev Cancer.* 4:592–603.

Park CM, Park MJ, Kwak HJ, et al. (2006). Induction of p53-mediated apoptosis and recovery of chemosensitivity through p53 transduction in human glioblastoma cells by cisplatin. *Int J Oncol.* 28:119-125.

Park MT, Kim MJ, Kang YH, et al. (2005). Phytosphingosine in combination with ionizing radiation enhances apoptotic cell death in radiation-resistant cancer cells through ROS dependent and -independent AIF release. *Blood.* 105:1724–1733.

Preusser M, de Ribaupierre S, Wöhrer A, et al. (2011).Current concepts and management of glioblastoma. *Ann Neurol.* 70:9-21.

Scherz-Shouval R, Elazar Z. (2007). ROS, mitochondria and the regulation of autophagy. *Trends Cell Biol.* 17:422-427.

Stewart, L. A. (2002). Chemotherapy in adult high-grade glioma: A systematic review and meta-analysis of individual patient data from 12 randomised trials. *Lancet.*359:1011–1018.

Wabnitz GH, Goursot C, Jahraus B, et al. (2010). Mitochondrial translocation of oxidized cofilin induces caspase-independent necrotic-like programmed cell death of T cells. Cell Death Dis. 22;1:e58.

In: Gliomas: Classification, Symptoms, Treatment and Prognosis ISBN: 978-1-63117-868-9
Editor: David Cory Adamson

Chapter 11

Nanoparticles and other Vectors for Delivering Targeted Therapeutics to Malignant Gliomas

Sai An, Xi He, Yuyang Kuang, Jianfeng Li, Yubo Guo, Haojun Ma and Chen Jiang*

Key Laboratory of Smart Drug Delivery, Ministry of Education,
Department of Pharmaceutics, School of Pharmacy, Fudan University, China

Abstract

Gliomas account for the vast majority of malignant brain tumors, making up about 80%. Due to the inherent nature of infiltration and the existence of the blood-brain-barrier (BBB), common therapies can rarely provide an ideal cure for malignant brain gliomas. Therefore, targeting nanoscaled delivery systems for chemical drugs and therapeutic genes are more and more extensively explored as novel strategies for brain glioma therapy. To achieve favourable targeting efficiency, functional molecules are designed more for BBB crossing then glioma targeting. Because of the high need for nutrients of gliomas, excess receptors and transporters are expressed on the surface of the BBB as well as the tumor cells, mediating various kinds of transcytosis and endocytosis passageways. Diversified substrates to these receptors and transporters are exploited as the brain-targeting functional molecules. In addition to targeting efficiency, the size of the delivery system is also critical for glioma therapy. Therefore, promising carriers are able to precisely control the size of the delivery system in nanoscale amounts. In this paper, recent advances on various kinds of vectors as well as the diversified targeting functional molecules are reviewed to provide insight into the burgeoning targeting therapies for malignant gliomas (MGs).

Keywords: Malignant gliomas; targeting; gene therapy; chemotherapy; vector.

* Corresponding author: Prof. Chen Jiang, Department of Pharmaceutics, School of Pharmacy, Fudan University, 826 Zhangheng Road, Shanghai 201203, China, Tel.: +86-21-5198-0079, Fax: +86-21-5198-0079, E-mail: jiangchen@shmu.edu.cn.

1. Introduction

Gliomas originally arise from glial cells, and commonly located in the brain [1]. Gliomas account for the vast majority of malignant brain tumors, making up about 80% of all [2]. Low-grade gliomas include WHO grade I astrocytomas, grade Ⅱ well-differentiated astrocytomas, and grade II oligodendroglioma. High-grade gliomas include WHO grade Ⅲ anaplastic astrocytomas, grade III anaplastic oligodendrogliomas, grade III anaplastic oligoastrocytomas, and grade Ⅳglioblastoma multiforme (malignant gliomas [MGs]) [3]. According to clinical experience, the prognosis of the MGs is generally very poor.

MGs are some of the most devastating human diseases, the treatment of which is considered one of the greatest challenges in cancer therapy. MGs are highly-vascular tumors with a strong tendency to infiltrate [4]. These natural features cause great difficulties for permanent cure. Although a large number of advanced treatments have had impacts on medical management for other tumors, the development of effective therapeutic methods for MGs still remains a great challenge.

To seek an efficacious therapy for MGs, multiple treatments have been under attempt for decades. Tumor excision is the most direct therapeutic method by removing tumor tissue through surgical resection. However, because of the inherent nature of angiogenesis as well as the intrinsic tendency to infiltrate, recurrence always occurs even after complete surgical excision of all visible tumor [5]. Radiotherapy is commonly applied to MGs because of its ability to control cell growth, whereas a range of side effects have limited the utility of this treatment [6]. For example, nausea, vomiting, fatigue, and skin irritation may expose patients to more additional challenges during their treatment.

Chemotherapy in the form of gene therapy has become a more popular area of research for MGs over the past few decades, since it has great potential to cause tumor cell apoptosis in a specific fashion. Nonspecific chemotherapies kill tumor cells that divide rapidly or degrade the abnormally expressed proteins that are essential for uncontrolled cell growth [7]. But for gene therapy, tumor cell death is caused by changing the genetic material that is expressed or not expressed and critical to the process of cell survival [8]. Either one is able to effectively induce tumor cell death, but a combination of chemotherapy and targeted gene therapy may cause an additive and potentially curative effect.

However, for either chemical or genetic therapeutic agents, the existence of the blood-brain-barrier (BBB) proves to be a major obstacle to get agents into the brain parenchyma freely [9]. High renal clearance and nonspecific organ distribution also limit the therapeutic effect and cause many unexpected side effects for patients [8]. Moreover, poor drug penetration from vessels into tumors influences the treatment effects of many therapeutic agents [10]. In particular for gene therapy, the enzymatic stability is also a very important factor to be taken into consideration. Therefore, using nanoscale delivery systems for chemical drugs and therapeutic genes are more and more in need to be explored as novel strategies for MGs therapy.

Nanotechnology has been extensively researched for decades. According to reports, drug delivery systems of nanoscale size are prone to be taken up efficiently by tumor cells through mechanisms like endocytosis [12]. As a result, they have a better chance of crossing biological barriers in vivo, such as the complex BBB. With specific surface characteristics, nanoparticles can have good targeting ability for certain organs, such as the brain, and sometimes even specifically targeting tumor tissue. Moreover, nanoscale drug delivery systems are able to effectively raise the drug loading capacity and drug stability during circulation. Meanwhile, the release of drug can also be strictly controlled by changing the design of the drug delivery system.

To achieve favorable targeting efficiency, various kinds of functional molecules have been engineered in the delivery systems for BBB crossing and glioma targeting. Because of the high need for nutrients during development and progression of MGs, numerous receptors and transporters are expressed on the surface of tumor cells, mediating various kinds of transcytosis and endocytosis passageways [11]. As a result, numerous varied substrates to these receptors and transporters have been exploited as targeting functional molecules in recent work.

In addition to targeting efficiency, the size of the delivery system is also critical for MG therapy. Therefore, multiple kinds of promising carriers have been explored in order to precisely control the size of the delivery system in nanoscale proportions. Many organic polymers as well as inorganic materials have been applied for drug delivery systems. Carriers, which have both the capacity to combine the therapeutics tightly during the circulation and release them freely in tumor cells are the most promising ones [13].

In this chapter, recent advances on various kinds of vectors as well as the various targeting functional molecules are reviewed to provide an overall review on the burgeoning targeting strategies for MGs.

2. Targeting Functional Molecules

To achieve an efficient targeting therapy for MGs, strategies with different drug delivery pathways have been under investigation for decades (Fig. 1). Correspondingly, various kinds of targeting functional molecules have been exploited.

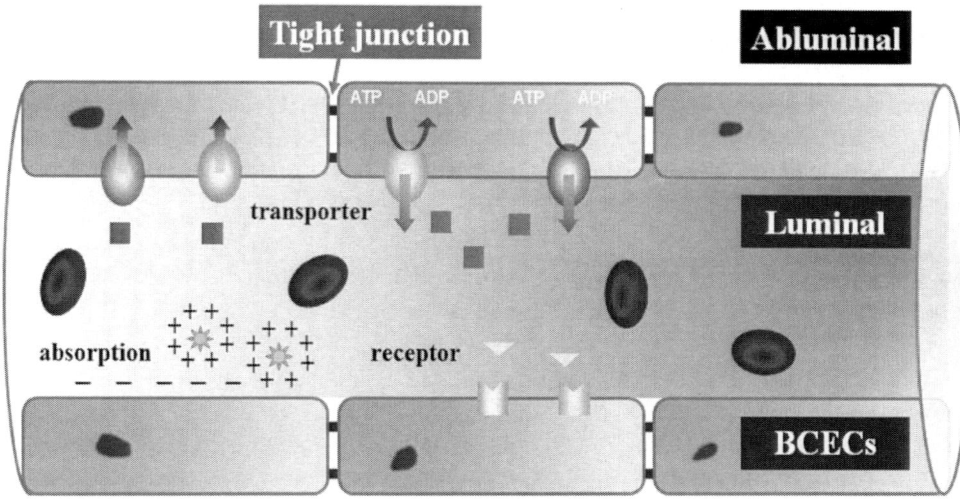

Figure 1. Different strategies for therapeutic drug delivery.

2.1. Receptor-Mediated Transcytosis

Targeted delivery of therapeutic agents for MGs can be achieved by conjugating ligands to drug delivery systems which bind to specific receptors. Some receptors demonstrate high expression both on the BBB and MGs cells, while some are only expressed on the membrane of tumor cells. According to the physiological characteristics during the growth of gliomas, different receptors could be selected as the target for therapeutic drug delivery.

2.1.1. Low Density Lipoprotein Receptor

Low density lipoprotein receptor (LDL-R) is one of the receptors that are over-expressed both on the membranes of brain capillary endothelial cells (BCECs) and many tumor cells, including MGs. Peptide-22 (Ac–[cMPRLRGC]c–NH2), which shows special affinity for LDL-R without competition with endogenous LDL, has been expressed on poly(lactic acid) (PLA) nanoparticles for dual-targeting therapy, firstly by crossing the BBB and then targeting MGs cells, and reveals great potential [14]. Angiopep-2 (TFFYGGSRGKRNNFKTEEY) has proven to possess high affinity to low-density lipoprotein receptor-related protein (LRP) [15]. Several investigators have taken advantage of this peptide to modify nanoparticles made of dendrimers, such as polyamidoamine dendrime (PAMAM) and dendrigraft poly-L-lysine (DGL), making them target to MGs for efficient gene therapy [16, 17]. In addition to these two kinds of peptides, more than 40 different ligands of LRP ranging from lipoproteins, protease/protease inhibitor complexes, extracellular matrix proteins and viruses to growth factors and cytokines have been reported, which are all potential targeting molecules for MGs.

2.1.2. Transferrin Receptor

Transferrin receptor (TfR) is a type II transmembrane glycoprotein involved in iron uptake and cell growth regulation [18]. It is expressed on brain capillary vascular endothelium at much higher levels than in most human tissues. It has up to 100-fold higher expression on glioma cells than normal astrocytes and is correlated with cancer progression and tumor stage [19], making TfR a highly promising target for the delivery of therapeutics to the MGs. As the most common ligand to TfR, transferrin (Tf) has been widely used for targeting therapy. For example, it was coupled via biotin–avidin to the surface of micelles of PEG-PLA biotin (Tf–PEG-PLA) with the aim of targeting MGs [20]. T7 (HAIYPRH) is reported to be another peptide targeting to TfR through a cavity on the surface of TfR and then transport into cells via endocytosis with the help of Tf. It has been successfully conjugated to PEG-PAMAM polymer and further loaded with doxorubicin (DOX), formulating PAMAM-PEG-T7/DOX nanoparticles (NPs), which has been studied as potential glioma-targeting drug delivery system [21]. In addition to these, OX26, a mouse monoclonal antibody against the rat TfR1, has also been explored for brain tumor targeting behind the BBB. In one study, it was conjugated to the hydrophilic anticancer drug methotrexate by a hydrazone bond for glioma therapy [22]. And in another one, OX26, coupled with streptavidin (SA), was conjugated to [111In] DTPA-EGF-PEG3400-biotin, achieving distinct in vivo imaging of gliomas [23].

2.1.3. Lactoferrin Receptor

Lactoferrin receptor (LfR) is another receptor that is highly expressed on the surface of glioma cells as well as the BBB. As the ligand to LfR, lactoferrin (Lf) has been reported as one of the most widely used targeting ligands for MGs. Lf is a bilobed cationic iron-binding glycoprotein (80 kDa), consisting of approximately 690 amino acids. Upon binding with its receptor, Lf can cross the BBB unidirectionally and enter glioma cells through receptor-mediated transcytosis, with no apparent intraendothelial degradation [24]. To achieve brain tumor targeting chemotherapeutical delivery, Lf has been modified on the surface of doxorubicin-loaded procationic liposomes (DOX-Lf-PCLs). An effective therapeutic potential for MGs with DOX-Lf-PCLs has been demonstrated [25]. Lf has also been exploited to develop a novel antitumor agent loaded drug delivery system, Lf-conjugated biodegradable polymersome holding doxorubicin and tetrandrine (Lf-PO-Dox/Tet). This system integrates both a BBB and glioma-targeting moiety and multidrug resistance (MDR) inhibitor, with great therapeutic potential for gliomas [26].

2.1.4. Epidermal Growth Factor Receptor

The Epidermal Growth Factor Receptor (EGFR) is transmembrane receptor responsible for binding epidermal growth factor (EGF) and mediating transcytosis. Amplification of the EGFR gene and overexpression of EGFR is common in MGs, making it a prime target for therapy. Ligands of EGFR, which include EGF, transforming growth factor-α (TGF-α), and amphiregulin (AREG), are reported to be transmembrane precursors that are cleavage by matrix metalloproteinases (MMPs) to become mature ligand peptides [27]. A boronated monoclonal antibody (cetuximab [IMC-C225]) developed against the wild type and mutant isoforms of EGFRs as boron-delivering agents for intracerebral gliomas in boron neutron capture therapy has been widely studied [28].

2.1.5. Folate Receptor

The Folate Receptor (FR) is a 38 kDA glycosyl-phosphatidylinositol-anchored glycoprotein overexpressed in most kinds of tumors compared with the expression in normal tissues, which is an important characteristic for targeting. Folic acid (also known as folate) is a form of the water-soluble vitamin B9, which is indispensable for gene replication during cell proliferation [29]. Due to the high specificity to FR, folic acid (FA) has become one of the most investigated targeting ligands in cancer therapeutic targeting. FA-PAMAM conjugates have been synthesized for delivering therapeutic antisense oligonucleotides (ASODN) to inhibit the growth of glioma cells. FA demonstrates efficient glioma-targeting efficiency [30]. In another studies, FA has been used to label PEGylated grafted-hyperbranched-PEI for tumor-targeted gene delivery. FA-PEG-PEI/pDNA complexes show significantly higher transgene activity in reporter assays than other groups [31].

2.2. Transporter-Mediated Transcytosis

Transporters are another kind of protein expressed on the surface of BCECs almost at the same level as receptors. MG cells are reported to have accelerated metabolism, high nutrition requirements, and increased nutrition uptake. Enhanced tumor uptake of nutrient is facilitated by the overexpression of different transporter proteins on tumor cells. Because of the high affinity to substrates, transporters have been developed as a novel transcytosis pathway for brain tumor targeted delivery. The common researched transporters include the glucose transporter, choline transporter and amino acid transporters.

Mammalian cells depend on glucose as a major substrate for energy production, which acts as the primary source for the generation of ATP with high affinity to transporters. Glucose enters cells via two different types of membrane associated carrier proteins, the Na+ coupled glucose transporter (SGLT) as well as glucose transporter facilitator (GLUT) [32]. Molecules with similar structures to glucose, such as 2-deoxyglucose, galactose, mannose, and glucose analogs, demonstrate high affinity to GLUT [33]. Based on the overexpression of GLUT both on BCECs and glioma cells, 2-deoxy-d-glucose was modified on poly(ethylene glycol)-co-poly(trimethylene carbonate) nanoparticles (dGlu-NP) for potential dual-targeted drug delivery, achieving efficient BBB penetration via GLUT-mediated transcytosis and glioma drug accumulation via GLUT-mediated endocytosis [34]. Considering the specific affinity to GLUT1, p-aminophenyl-α-D-manno-pyranoside (MAN), a mannose analog, was incorporated onto the surface of Tf-modified liposomes, achieving dual-targeting of daunorubicin delivery to treat MGs [33].

Choline transporter (ChT) is another kind of transporter that has proven to be highly expressed on the BBB as well as glioma cells. The most common native substrate to the ChT is reported to be choline [35]. A quaternary ammonium group and a free hydroxyl group are suggested as the key requirements for BBB ChT substrates [36]. Based on these findings, some choline derivatives have been synthesized and developed as ChT targeting molecules. These molecules have been modified on DGL nanoparticles for targeted delivery. Enhanced brain and glioma targeting have been observed both in vivo and in vitro [37, 38].

Until now, transporter-mediated transcytosis has not been as extensively explored as receptor-mediated transcytosis. However, different substrates to all kinds of transporters have been researched and assessed for affinity as well as permeability [39]. Substrates with ideal affinity to transporters may hold the promise as MGs targeting molecules.

2.3. Adsorptive-Mediated Transcytosis

Adsorptive-mediated transcytosis (AMT) transcytosis that is triggered by electrostatic interactions between the positively charged moieties of proteins and negatively charged microdomains on the membrane surface of cells. Drug delivery, which is based on AMT, can be achieved by exploiting cationic proteins and basic oligopeptides such as cell-penetrating peptides (CPPs) for good BBB crossing efficiency. In this way large therapeutic agents as well as drug-encapsulated vectors such as liposomes and nanoparticles are able to get access to brain parenchyma easily by conjugating with these cationic molecules [40]. Protamine is one of the most common cationic proteins that has been used for AMT-based drug delivery. In a recent study, protamine-stabilized mRNA was used to induce tumor regression and long-term anti-tumor immunity for gliomas in mice [41]. And in another one, activatable low molecular weight protamine was conjugated to PEG-PCL nanoparticles for paclitaxel delivery as a smart drug delivery system for enhanced targeted glioblastoma therapy [42]. Both results showed efficient AMT mediated by cationic protamine. CPPs are small peptides derived from protein-transduction domains with an ability to open the cellular membrane and enter the cell interior. For CPPs, two main families belonging to the TAT-derived peptides and Syn-B vectors have been extensively used in drug delivery systems. TAT protein is an 86 amino acid peptide [43]. It is covalently conjugated with cholesterol for preparing doxorubicin-loaded liposomes for glioma therapy and demonstrates a rapid uptake by cells and concentration in the nucleus [44]. Other CPPs like poly-arginine and poly-lysine are also used. For example, poly-arginine has been exploited to deliver the ubiquitination-resistant p53 protein into cancer cells and inhibit the proliferation of malignant glioma cells [45].

3. Drug Delivery Vectors

For decades, nanotechnology has played a pivotal role in significant breakthroughs in drug delivery. Drug delivery systems in nanoscale dimensions are reported to have great potential in effectively raising drug loading capacity and drug stability during circulation. Viral-based vectors have an extensive history, but are often limited by shortcomings such as immunogenicity and high costs [46]. As a result, only non-viral vectors are reviewed here, including liposomes, micelles, solid lipid nanoparticles, dendrimer nanoparticles and inorganic nanoparticles (Fig. 2).

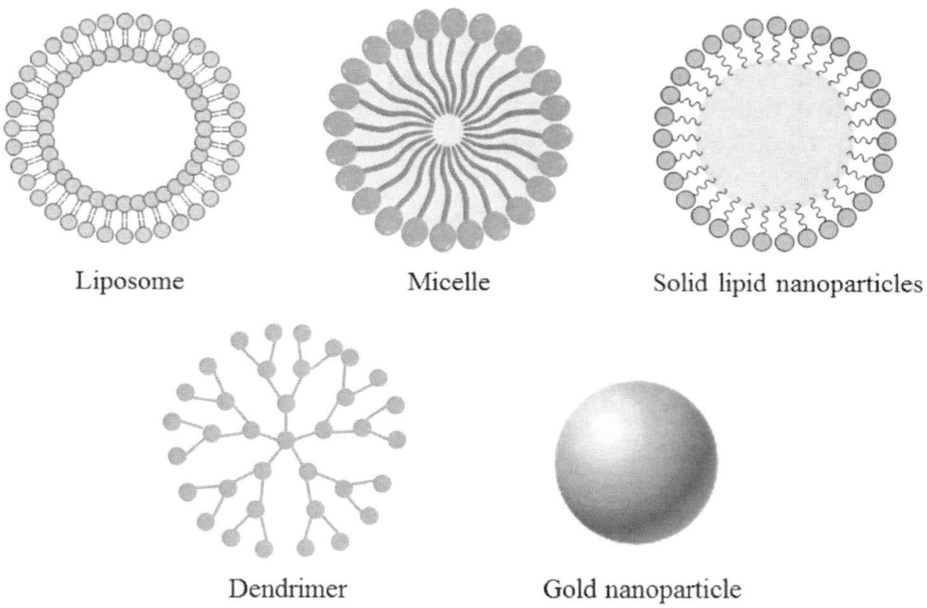

Figure 2. Various vectors used in therapeutic drug delivery.

3.1. Liposomes

A liposome is an artificially-prepared vesicle composed of a lipid bilayer, which can be used as a vehicle for administration of pharmaceutical drugs. A large number of studies have found that liposomes are expected to be one of the most promising delivery systems for therapeutic agents to treat brain tumors, especially MGs. The transfer of anticancer agents using liposomes has been studied by numerous investigators and found to effectively induce regression of experimental gliomas [47]. Recently, Tf-modified cisplatin liposomes were prepared to achieve effective glioma therapy through sequential targeting ability [48]. DOX liposomes labeled with FA and Tf simultaneously were developed for duel-targeting of gliomas [49]. Therapeutic genes can also be co-delivered with chemical antitumor drugs. For example, O6-methylguanine-DNA methyltransferase (MGMT) siRNA has been delivered together with temozolomide in one liposome to improve cytotoxity for gliomas [50]. pEGFP-hTRAIL (a therapeutic gene encoding human tumor necrosis factor-related apoptosis-inducing ligand) and paclitaxel have been co-delivered by an angiopep-conjugated liposome for a promising dual targeting therapeutic strategy against glioma [51].

3.2. Micelles

A micelle is an aggregate of surfactant molecules dispersed in a liquid colloid. A typical micelle in aqueous solution forms an aggregate with the hydrophilic "head" regions in contact with surrounding solvent, sequestering the hydrophobic single-tail regions in the micelle center [52]. Block copolymer micelles have been extensively explored for decades, and shown great potential in drug delivery. Compared with traditional nanoparticle formulations, micelles have overcome many drawbacks including in vivo instability and fast clearance from the blood [53]. Tf modified c[RGDfK]-paclitaxel conjugate loaded hybrid micelles have been developed for sequential BBB penetration and glioma targeting [54]. SN-38, an anticancer plant alkaloid 7-ethyl-10-hydroxy-camptothecine, has been incorporated into micelles to form the NK012 micelles, which act as a prodrug of SN-38 and passively target cells [55].

3.3. Solid Lipid Nanoparticles

Solid lipid nanoparticles (SLNs) are typically spherical nanoparticles with a solid lipid core matrix that can solubilize lipophilic molecules. According to studies, the lipid core exhibits high affinity to hydrophobic drugs and is usually stabilized by surfactants. The outer layer lipid of SLNs includes triglycerides, diglycerides, monoglycerides, fatty acids and so on [56]. SLNs are efficacious in carrying anticancer compounds, overcoming the drawbacks like tissue toxicity, poor specificity and stability, and the high incidence of drug resistance in tumor cells [57]. Catanionic solid lipid nanoparticles (CASLNs) (composed of cationic and anionic surfactants), loaded with DOX and grafted with anti-EGFR, have been applied to suppress propagation of MGs cells [58]. Another kind of innovated CASLNs carrying carmustine grafted with anti-EGFR has been developed by the same group and inhibits the propagation of human MGs cells [59]. Therapeutic genes can also be delivered by SLNs. SLNs, reconstituted from natural components of protein-free low-density lipoprotein, have been conjugated to PEGylated c-Met siRNA. The corresponding complex efficiently down-regulates c-Met expression, as well as decreases cell proliferation of MGs cells [60].

3.4. Dendrimer Nanoparticles

Dendrimers are repetitively branched molecules. Dendrimer nanoparticles represent unique symmetric and spherical structures [61]. The outershell of dendrimers have rich peripheral reactive sites easily modified with small functional molecules. Therefore, higher generation dendrimers possess more exposed functional groups on the surface and are easily customized for more applications [62]. As a result, dendrimers have been extensively developed to provide promising delivery of molecular cargos ranging in size from small molecules and peptides to proteins and DNA for MGs therapy [63]. A combination glioma therapy has been investigated by our group via co-delivery of a therapeutic gene encoding pORF-hTRAIL and DOX using tumor-targeting peptide T7 modified PEGylated PAMAM [64]. Another combination of gene therapy and chemotherapy conducted by our group is a co-delivery system of pORF-hTRAIL and DOX with a choline-derivate modified PEGylated DGL, which has also proven to be a promising approach for MGs therapy [38].

3.5. Inorganic Nanoparticles

Compared to organic nanoparticles, inorganic ones possess better stability in blood circulation against biodegradation and more precise control of particle size with additional functions for tumor imaging or photothermal effect [65]. Common inorganic nanoparticles, which have been extensively studied, include iron oxide nanoparticles, gold nanoparticles (Au NPs), and mesoporous silica nanoparticles. For decades, inorganic nanoparticles have been explored as novel vectors for therapeutic agents against gliomas. Iron oxide nanoparticles conjugated with TRAIL induce apoptosis in cancer cells but not in normal cells, and exhibit increased anti-tumor activities in glioma cells [66]. The novel nanovector, composed of an iron oxide magnetic nanoparticle core coated with three different functional molecules: PEI, siRNA, and chlorotoxin, has been designed with dual targeting specificity and dual therapeutic effect for targeted MGs imaging and therapy [67]. Including a photothermal treatment effect of gliomas, Au NPs can also be used for anticancer drug delivery. Hydrophobic photodynamic therapy (PDT) drugs can induce DNA and cell membrane damage to cancer cells and can be conjugated non-covalently to Au NPs. The resulting therapeutic system performs a rapid drug release and deep penetration of the drug into tumors through passive accumulation [68]. Glioma tumor targeting peptide EGF has been modified on the surface of this PDT-Au conjugant, resulting in a glioma targeting therapeutic system, which shows high efficiency in glioma therapy. This delivery system has demonstrated to hold promise for future delivery of a wide range of hydrophobic therapeutic drugs for the treatment of hard-to-reach cancers [69].

3.6. Peptide-Drug Conjugate

Recently, a peptide-drug conjugate named ANG-1005 has been developed as a new drug for glioma therapy. ANG-1005 stands for a paclitaxel–Angiopep-2 conjugate, which has demonstrated great potential to treat MGs [70]. Paclitaxel is highly efficacious in the treatment of many kinds of tumors. Because of the influence by P-glycoprotein 1 (P-gp) as well as the BBB, limited amounts of paclitaxel could reach the therapeutic target. To solve this problem, three paclitaxel molecules have been conjugated to one Angiopep-2 molecule, which specifically binds to the LDL-R expressed on the BBB and glioma cells [71]. The antitumor potential of ANG1005 has proven to be ideal for inhibiting the growth of glioma and significantly increase the survival of mice with intracerebral implantation of U87 MG glioblastoma cells [72].

Conclusion and Future Perspective

The development of promising drug delivery systems and strategies has improved the outlook for better management of MGs. Different targeting moieties utilized on these delivery systems induce selective targeting behavior. Nowadays, dual modification of targeting molecules is common and provides a sequential targeting method for delivering agents across the BBB first and then into tumor tissues, resulting in enhanced tumor accumulation. Novel nanovectors that increase drug loading efficiency, prolong the blood circulation time, and rapidly release drug in tumor, are under extensive development. Vectors with additional antitumor effects or tumor imaging functions are getting more popular. Antitumor agents able to self-assemble into nanoparticles and act as vectors and carry cargo simultaneously is burgeoning research area. The co-delivery of genes with chemotherapeutics which can provide a rapid tumor-killing effect and alter gene expression at the same time is being widely studied. Although abundant research on MGs therapy has been done, few delivery systems have reached the clinical stage. Thus, future research is most likely to address translational issues for the development of safe and effective therapy for MGs.

References

[1] Targeted delivery of antitumoral therapy to glioma and other malignancies with synthetic chlorotoxin (TM-601). Mamelak AN, Jacoby DB. *Expert Opin Drug Deliv.* 2007; 4(2): 175-86.

[2] Genetics of adult glioma. Goodenberger ML, Jenkins RB. *Cancer Genet.* 2012; 205(12): 613-21.

[3] Understanding high grade glioma: Molecular mechanism, therapy and comprehensive management. Wang Y, Jiang T. *Cancer Lett.* 2013; 331(2):139-46.

[4] Primary brain tumours in adults. Behin A, Hoang-Xuan K, Carpentier AF, Delattre JY. *Lancet.* 2003; 361(9354), 323–331.

[5] Glioma extent of resection and its impact on patient outcome. Sanai N, Berger MS. *Neurosurgery.* 2008; 62(4), 753–764.

[6] Glioblastoma multiforme: a review of where we have been and where we are going. Adamson C, Kanu OO, Mehta AI et al. *Expert Opin. Inv. Drug.* 2009; 18(8), 1061–1083.

[7] Chemotherapy for high-grade glioma. Glioma Meta-Analysis Trialists (GMT) Group. *Cochrane Database Syst Rev.* 2002; (4).

[8] Impact of genetic targets on primary brain tumor therapy: what's ready for prime time? Zalatimo O, Zoccoli CM, Patel A, Weston CL, Glantz M. *Adv Exp Med Biol.* 2013; 779:267-89.

[9] Blood–brain barrier disruption in the treatment of brain tumors. Blanchette M, Fortin D. *Methods Mol. Biol.* 2011; 686, 447–463.

[10] Temozolomide for high grade glioma. Hart MG, Grant R, Garside R, Rogers G, et al. *Cochrane Database Syst Rev*. 2008; (4).

[11] Gateways for the intracellular access of nanocarriers: a review of receptor-mediated endocytosis mechanisms and of strategies in receptor targeting. Zaki NM, Tirelli N. *Expert Opin Drug Deliv*. 2010; 7(8):895-913.

[12] The role of drug transporters at the blood–brain barrier. De Boer AG, Van Der Sandt ICJ, Gaillard PJ. Annu. Rev. Pharmacol. Toxicol. 2003; 43, 629–656.

[13] Is there a clinical future for polymeric nanoparticles as brain-targeting drug delivery agents? Costantino L, Boraschi D. *Drug Discov. Today*. 2012; 17(7–8), 367–378.

[14] LDLR-mediated peptide-22-conjugated nanoparticles for dual-targeting therapy of brain glioma. Zhang B, Sun X, Mei H, Wang Y, et al. *Biomaterials*. 2013; 34(36):9171-82.

[15] Identification and design of peptides as a new drug delivery system for the brain. Demeule M, Régina A, Ché C, Poirier J, et al. *J Pharmacol Exp Ther*. 2008; 324(3):1064-72.

[16] Gene delivery targeted to the brain using an Angiopep-conjugated polyethyleneglycol-modified polyamidoamine dendrimer. Ke W, Shao K, Huang R, Han L, et al. *Biomaterials*. 2009; 30(36):6976-85.

[17] Dual targeting effect of Angiopep-2-modified, DNA-loaded nanoparticles for glioma. Huang S, Li J, Han L, Liu S, et al. *Biomaterials*. 2011; 32(28):6832-8.

[18] Transferrin receptor expression and the control of cell growth. Neckers LM, Trepel JB. *Cancer Invest*. 1986; 4(5):461–470.

[19] Expression of transferrin receptor and ferritin H-chain mRNA are associated with clinical and histopathological prognostic indicators in breast cancer. Yang DC, Wang F, Elliott RL, Head JF. *Anticancer Res*. 2001; 21(1B):541-9.

[20] Development of transferrin functionalized poly (ethylene glycol)/poly (lactic acid) amphiphilic block copolymeric micelles as a potential delivery system targeting brain glioma. W.H. Ren, J. Chang, C.H. Yan, X.M. Qian, et al. *J Mater Sci Mater Med*. 2010; 21(9):2673-81.

[21] Peptide-conjugated PAMAM for targeted doxorubicin delivery to transferrin receptor overexpressed tumors. Han L, Huang R, Liu S, Huang S, et al. *Mol Pharm*. 2010; 7(6):2156-65.

[22] Anti-transferrin receptor antibody and antibody-drug conjugates cross the blood-brain barrier. Friden PM, Walus LR, Musso GF, Taylor MA, et al. *Proc Natl Acad Sci U S A*. 1991; 88(11):4771-5.

[23] Epidermal growth factor radiopharmaceuticals: 111In chelation, conjugation to a blood-brain barrier delivery vector via a biotin-polyethylene linker, pharmacokinetics, and in vivo imaging of experimental brain tumors. Kurihara A, Deguchi Y, Pardridge WM. *Bioconjug Chem*. 1999; 10(3):502-11.

[24] Lactoferrin-conjugated poly (ethylene glycol)-coated Fe3O4 nanoparticles. *Shan L. Molecular Imaging and Contrast Agent Database* (MICAD) [Internet]. Bethesda (MD): National Center for Biotechnology Information (US); 2004-2013.

[25] Lactoferrin modified doxorubicin-loaded procationic liposomes for the treatment of gliomas. Chen H, Qin Y, Zhang Q, Jiang W, et al. *Eur J Pharm Sci*. 2011; 44(1-2):164-73.

[26] Lactoferrin-conjugated biodegradable polymersome holding doxorubicin and tetrandrine for chemotherapy of glioma rats. Pang Z, Feng L, Hua R, Chen J, et al. *Mol Pharm.* 2010; 7(6):1995-2005.
[27] The epidermal growth factor receptor and its ligands in cardiovascular disease. Makki N, Thiel KW, Miller FJ. *Int J Mol Sci.* 2013; 14(10):20597-613.
[28] Neutron capture therapy of epidermal growth factor (+) gliomas using boronated cetuximab (IMC-C225) as a delivery agent. Barth RF, Wu G, Yang W, Binns PJ, Riley KJ, et al. *Appl Radiat Isot.* 2004; 61(5):899-903.
[29] Describes the ligand-based dendritic system for tumor targeting and discusses basic information of lectin, folate, epidermal and transferrin receptors. Agarwal A, Saraf S, Asthana A, Gupta U, et al. *Int. J. Pharm.* 2008; 350,3–13.
[30] Evaluation of folate-PAMAM for the delivery of antisense oligonucleotides to rat C6 glioma cells in vitro and in vivo. Kang C, Yuan X, Li F, Pu P, et al. *J Biomed Mater Res A.* 2010; 93(2):585-94.
[31] Synthesis and characterization of folate-PEG-grafted-hyperbranched-PEI for tumor-targeted gene delivery. Liang B, He ML, Xiao ZP, Li Y, et al. *Biochem Biophys Res Commun.* 2008; 367(4):874-80.
[32] The glucose transporter families SGLT and GLUT: molecular basis of normal and aberrant function. Scheepers A, Joost HG, Schürmann A. *JPEN J Parenter Enteral Nutr.* 2004; 28(5):364-71.
[33] Dual-targeting daunorubicin liposomes improve the therapeutic efficacy of brain glioma in animals. Ying X, Wen H, Lu WL, Du J, et al. *J Control Release.* 2010; 141(2):183-92.
[34] Nanoparticles of 2-deoxy-d-glucose functionalized poly(ethylene glycol)-co-poly(trimethylene carbonate) for dual-targeted drug delivery in glioma treatment. Jiang X, Xin H, Ren Q, Gu J, et al. *Biomaterials.* 2013. pii: S0142-9612(13)01194-0.
[35] The blood-brain barrier choline transporter. Geldenhuys WJ, Allen DD. *Cent Nerv Syst Agents Med Chem.* 2012; 12(2):95-9.
[36] The blood-brain barrier choline transporter as a brain drug delivery vector. Allen DD, Lockman PR. *Life Sci.* 2003; 73(13):1609-15.
[37] Choline-derivate-modified nanoparticles for brain-targeting gene delivery. Li J, Zhou L, Ye D, Huang S, et al. *Adv Mater.* 2011; 23(39):4516-20.
[38] Choline transporter-targeting and co-delivery system for glioma therapy. Li J, Guo Y, Kuang Y, An S, et al. *Biomaterials.* 2013; 34(36):9142-8.
[39] Structure-based ligand discovery for the Large-neutral Amino Acid Transporter 1, LAT-1. Geier EG, Schlessinger A, Fan H, Gable JE, et al. *Proc Natl Acad Sci U S A.* 2013; 110(14):5480-5.
[40] CNS delivery via adsorptive transcytosis. Hervé F, Ghinea N, Scherrmann JM. *AAPS J.* 2008; 10(3):455-72.
[41] Therapeutic anti-tumor immunity triggered by injections of immunostimulating single-stranded RNA. Scheel B, Aulwurm S, Probst J, Stitz L, et al. *Eur J Immunol.* 2006; 36(10):2807-16.
[42] PEG-co-PCL nanoparticles modified with MMP-2/9 activatable low molecular weight protamine for enhanced targeted glioblastoma therapy. Gu G, Xia H, Hu Q, Liu Z, et al. *Biomaterials.* 2013; 34(1):196-208.

[43] TAT-based drug delivery system--new directions in protein delivery for new hopes? Rapoport M, Lorberboum-Galski H. *Expert Opin Drug Deliv*. 2009; 6(5):453-63.
[44] Liposome formulated with TAT-modified cholesterol for improving brain delivery and therapeutic efficacy on brain glioma in animals. Qin Y, Chen H, Zhang Q, Wang X, et al. *Int J Pharm. 2011*; 420(2):304-12.
[45] Ubiquitination-resistant p53 protein transduction therapy facilitates anti-cancer effect on the growth of human malignant glioma cells. Michiue H, Tomizawa K, Matsushita M, Tamiya T, et al. *FEBS Lett*. 2005; 579(18):3965-9.
[46] *Current status of non-viral vectors for siRNA delivery*. Yang FF, Huang W, Li YF, Gao ZG. Yao Xue Xue Bao. 2011; 46(12):1436-43.
[47] Clinical gene therapy for brain tumors. Liposomal delivery of anticancer molecule to glioma. Yoshida J, Mizuno M. *J Neurooncol*. 2003; 65(3):261-7.
[48] Characteristics of sequential targeting of brain glioma for transferrin-modified cisplatin liposome. Lv Q, Li LM, Han M, Tang XJ, et al. *Int J Pharm*. 2013; 444(1-2):1-9.
[49] Glioma targeting and blood-brain barrier penetration by dual-targeting doxorubincin liposomes. Gao JQ, Lv Q, Li LM, Tang XJ, et al. *Biomaterials*. 2013; 34(22):5628-39.
[50] Efficient delivery of liposome-mediated MGMT-siRNA reinforces the cytotoxity of temozolomide in GBM-initiating cells. Kato T, Natsume A, Toda H, Iwamizu H, et al. *Gene Ther*. 2010; 17(11):1363-71.
[51] Co-delivery of pEGFP-hTRAIL and paclitaxel to brain glioma mediated by an angiopep-conjugated liposome. Sun X, Pang Z, Ye H, Qiu B, et al. *Biomaterials*. 2012; 33(3):916-24.
[52] Peptide delivery using phospholipid micelles. Banerjee A, Onyuksel H. Wiley *Interdiscip Rev Nanomed Nanobiotechnol*. 2012; 4(5):562-74.
[53] Tailoring polymeric micelles to optimize delivery to solid tumors. Li W, Feng S, Guo Y. *Nanomedicine* (Lond). 2012; 7(8):1235-52.
[54] Transferrin-modified c[RGDfK]-paclitaxel loaded hybrid micelle for sequential blood-brain barrier penetration and glioma targeting therapy. Zhang P, Hu L, Yin Q, Feng L, et al. *Mol Pharm*. 2012; 9(6):1590-8.
[55] Potent antitumor effect of SN-38-incorporating polymeric micelle, NK012, against malignant glioma. Kuroda J, Kuratsu J, Yasunaga M, Koga Y, et al. *Int J Cancer*. 2009; 124(11):2505-11.
[56] High melting lipid based approach for drug delivery: solid lipid nanoparticles. Kumar S, Randhawa JK. *Mater Sci Eng C Mater Biol Appl*. 2013; 33(4):1842-52.
[57] Poly (ethylene)-glycol conjugated solid lipid nanoparticles of noscapine improve biological half-life, brain delivery and efficacy in glioblastoma cells. Madan J, Pandey RS, Jain V, Katare OP, et al. *Nanomedicine*. 2013; 9(4):492-503.
[58] Catanionic solid lipid nanoparticles carrying doxorubicin for inhibiting the growth of U87MG cells. Kuo YC, Liang CT. *Colloids Surf B Biointerfaces*. 2011; 85(2):131-7.
[59] Inhibition of human brain malignant glioblastoma cells using carmustine-loaded catanionic solid lipid nanoparticles with surface anti-epithelial growth factor receptor. Kuo YC, Liang CT. *Biomaterials*. 2011; 32(12):3340-50.
[60] In vivo specific delivery of c-Met siRNA to glioblastoma using cationic solid lipid nanoparticles. Jin J, Bae KH, Yang H, Lee SJ, et al. *Bioconjug Chem*. 2011; 22(12):2568-72.

[61] Dendrimers and the development of new complex nanomaterials for biomedical applications. Gardikis K, Micha-Screttas M, Demetzos C, Steele BR. *Curr Med Chem.* 2012; 19(29):4913-28.

[62] Dendritic nanoparticles: the next generation of nanocarriers? Pearson RM, Sunoqrot S, Hsu HJ, Bae JW, et al. *Ther Deliv.* 2012; 3(8):941-59.

[63] Advances in applications of dendritic compounds. Ma N, Ma C, Deng Y, Wang T, He N. *J Nanosci Nanotechnol.* 2013;13(1):33-9.

[64] Plasmid pORF-hTRAIL and doxorubicin co-delivery targeting to tumor using peptide-conjugated polyamidoamine dendrimer. Han L, Huang R, Li J, Liu S, et al. *Biomaterials.* 2011; 32(4):1242-52.

[65] Liposomes and inorganic nanoparticles for drug delivery and cancer imaging. Heneweer C, Gendy SE, Peñate-Medina O. *Ther Deliv.* 2012; 3(5):645-56.

[66] TRAIL conjugated to nanoparticles exhibits increased anti-tumor activities in glioma cells and glioma stem cells in vitro and in vivo. Perlstein B, Finniss SA, Miller C, Okhrimenko H, et al. *Neuro Oncol.* 2013; 15(1):29-40.

[67] pH-Sensitive siRNA nanovector for targeted gene silencing and cytotoxic effect in cancer cells. Mok H, Veiseh O, Fang C, Kievit FM, et al. *Mol Pharm.* 2010; 7(6):1930-9.

[68] Deep penetration of a PDT drug into tumors by noncovalent drug-gold nanoparticle conjugates. Cheng Y, Meyers JD, Broome AM, Kenney ME, et al. *J Am Chem Soc.* 2011; 133(8):2583-91.

[69] Addressing brain tumors with targeted gold nanoparticles: a new gold standard for hydrophobic drug delivery? Cheng Y, Meyers JD, Agnes RS, Doane TL, et al. *Small.* 2011; 7(16):2301-6.

[70] Influence of glioma tumour microenvironment on the transport of ANG1005 via low-density lipoprotein receptor-related protein 1. Bertrand Y, Currie JC, Poirier J, Demeule M, et al. *Br J Cancer.* 2011; 105(11):1697-707.

[71] Uptake of ANG1005, a novel paclitaxel derivative, through the blood-brain barrier into brain and experimental brain metastases of breast cancer. Thomas FC, Taskar K, Rudraraju V, Goda S, et al. *Pharm Res.* 2009 Nov;26(11):2486-94.

[72] Antitumour activity of ANG1005, a conjugate between paclitaxel and the new brain delivery vector Angiopep-2. Régina A, Demeule M, Ché C, Lavallée I, et al. *Br J Pharmacol.* 2008; 155(2):185-97.

Index

B

C

D

E

H

I

J

K

L

N

O

P

Q

R

S

U

V

W

X

Y

Z